Soft Tissue Rheumatic Pain

Recognition, Management, Prevention

Soft Tissue Rheumatic Pain
Recognition, Management, Prevention

ROBERT P. SHEON, M.D.
*Clinical Professor of Medicine
Medical College of Ohio at Toledo
Consultant in Rheumatology, Toledo Hospital
Senior Rheumatologist, Toledo Clinic, Inc.,
and Flower Memorial Hospital, Sylvania, Ohio*

ROLAND W. MOSKOWITZ, M.D.
*Professor of Medicine
Case Western Reserve University School of Medicine
Director, Division of Rheumatic Diseases
University Hospitals
Cleveland, Ohio*

VICTOR M. GOLDBERG, M.D.
*Professor of Orthopaedics
Case Western Reserve University School of Medicine
Attending Orthopaedist
University Hospitals and Veterans' Administration Hospital
Cleveland, Ohio*

Illustrations by

Claire B. Kirsner
Roy C. Schneider
Alan Weintraub

Second Edition

Lea & Febiger   Philadelphia   1987

Lea & Febiger
600 Washington Square
Philadelphia, PA   19106-4198
U.S.A.
(215) 922-1330

First Edition, 1982
Second Edition, 1987

Library of Congress Cataloging-in-Publication Data

Sheon, Robert P.
  Soft tissue rheumatic pain.

  Includes bibliographies and index.
  1. Nonarticular rheumatism. 2. Pain.
I. Moskowitz, Roland W.   II. Goldberg, Victor M.,
1939–   .   III. Title. [DNLM: 1. Connective
Tissue Diseases. 2. Rheumatism.   WE 544 S546s]
RC927.5.N65S48   1986   616.7'7   86-7342
ISBN 0-8121-1048-X

PRINTED IN THE UNITED STATES OF AMERICA

Print number: 5 4 3 2 1

To Irma, Peta, and Harriet

for their love and support

Preface

In the present revolution in health care, government and industry seek more efficient and economic health care delivery. This has resulted in greater scrutiny of the processes that physicians use in providing health care. In the area of musculoskeletal problems, the use of ambulatory care is increasingly stressed. Therefore, the methods outlined by this book are ever more timely. Because of our aging population, these disabilities continue to be our number one national health problem. The first edition of this book and a German edition have received wide readership throughout the world. Many readers have provided feedback to us. Most were enthusiastic. The Network for Continuing Medical Education produced a 55-minute videotape based on the first edition. A book relative to this area of interest for the general public is currently under contract to McGraw-Hill and will be published soon. This is most gratifying.

The second edition has been modified in an effort to increase its practicality and to provide additional emphasis on soft tissue injuries that arise in the worker or the individual engaged in sport and calisthenic activities. We have added over 1,000 references including those that describe new diagnostic and treatment techniques and that document efficacy of treatment measures. Also, we have added seventeen new topics, including a new chapter on etiology and pathogenesis; descriptions of over 40 additional disorders; 51 new tables; 14 anatomic plates; and 26 new illustrations. Several illustrations have been redone for further clarity.

To each body region we have added tables detailing a Danger List, Joint Protection Measures, Exercises, and a Decision Chart. These tables may be photocopied for handouts to your patients. Tables of differential diagnosis have been added where appropriate.

Since the first edition, we have seen scintigraphy gain importance in documenting axial joint arthropathy (in patients with spondyloarthropathy who lack peripheral arthritis or other features of spondylitis). Similarly, computed tomography has helped define spinal stenosis. Arthroscopic examination has become a widely available technique. We will soon evaluate magnetic resonance imaging in soft tissue problems. The use of scales (clinometrics) has recently been introduced in order to provide a measurement of subjective phenomena. Physical medicine techniques have expanded as well. Friction massage and ice massage are helpful techniques that are described in this edition.

Appreciation is gratefully acknowledged to Ken Bussy and the editorial staff of Lea & Febiger; to the library staff of Toledo Hospital and Flower Memorial Hospital; to the media services department of Toledo Hospital; to our colleagues in practice at Toledo Clinic and Case Western Reserve University School of Medicine; to research secretaries, Cathy LaCourse and Sandra Needler; and to our families who never complain about the many hours we have spent preparing this text.

Toledo, Ohio   Robert P. Sheon, M.D.
Cleveland, Ohio   Roland W. Moskowitz, M.D.
Cleveland, Ohio   Victor M. Goldberg, M.D.

Contents

Introduction   **An Overview of Diagnosis and Management** **1**

Anatomic Plates and Trigger Point Map

Impact of Musculoskeletal Pain on Society   2

An Overview of the Diagnosis of Soft Tissue Rheumatic Pain   3

New Diagnostic Techniques Useful for Soft Tissue Rheumatic Pain
     Disorders   6

Six Points for Managing Myofascial Soft Tissue Pain   7

An Overview of the Injured Worker   10

The Psychology of Injury   11

Outcome Appraisal Techniques   12

Chapter 1   **Etiology and Pathogenesis** **16**

Regional Myofascial Pain and Fibrositis   16

Tendinitis   19

Bursitis   20

Nerve Entrapment Disorders   21

Chapter 2   **The Head and Neck** **26**

Temporomandibular Joint Dysfunction Syndrome   26

Anterior Neck and Face Pain   30

The Cervical Syndrome: Sprain (Whiplash); Myofascial Neck Pain . . .   34

Torticollis   40

Impingement of the Fifth Cervical Nerve Root   41

Cervicothoracic Interspinous Bursitis   42

Muscle Contraction Headache   43

Occipital Neuralgia   44

Chapter 3   **The Thoracic Outlet Region** **48**

The Thoracic Outlet and Related Syndromes   48

Reflex Sympathetic Dystrophy (RSD)   56

Pancoast's Syndrome   59

Chapter 4   **The Shoulder Girdle Region** **62**

Musculotendinous Rotator Cuff Disorders   65

Frozen Shoulder (Adhesive Capsulitis)   83

Scapular Region Disorders   88

Other Shoulder Region Disorders   92

Chapter 5   **The Elbow** **98**

Tennis Elbow   99

Olecranon Bursitis   104

Other Bursal and Cystic Swellings at the Elbow   107

Tendinitis   107

Nerve Entrapment Syndromes   108

Chapter 6   **The Wrist and Hand** **112**

Disorders of the Lower Arm and Wrist   112

Systemic Diseases Affecting the Wrist and Hand   113

Joint Laxity and the Hypermobility Syndrome.................... 115
Psychophysiologic Disorders of the Hand 119
Disorders of the Thumb.. 121
Disorders of the Palm and Fingers............................ 124
Dorsal Edema of Secretan 128
Nerve Entrapment Disorders of the Wrist and Hand 128
Neurovascular Disorders of the Wrist and Hand 131
Nodules.. 134

Chapter 7   **The Thoracic Cage and Dorsal Spine Region** **141**
Myofascial Chest Wall Syndromes 143
Tietze's Syndrome.. 149
Juvenile Kyphosis (Scheuermann's Disease) 150
Osteoporosis and Osteomalacia (Osteopenia) 152
Herniated Dorsal Intervertebral Disc 156

Chapter 8   **The Low Back** **159**
Pathophysiology of Low Back Pain 162
The Pain Syndromes... 164
    Mechanical Low Back Pain 164
    Sciatica and Other Nerve Entrapment Syndromes 165
    Myofascial Back Pain 169
    Psychogenic Back Pain 171
    History and Physical Examination 173
    Laboratory and Roentgenographic Examination 183
    Differential Diagnosis 185
    Management 185
    Outcome and Additional Suggestions...................... 194
Pain Syndromes of the Pelvis 197
Entrapment Neuropathies 200

Chapter 9   **The Hip and Thigh Region** **207**
Myofascial Pain Syndromes 211
Bursitis 212
Entrapment Neuropathies 214

Chapter 10   **The Knee** **217**
Arthroscopic Examination 222
Quadriceps Mechanism Derangement 224
Disturbances of the Patella 225
Bursitis About the Knee...................................... 229
Popliteal Cyst (Baker's Cyst) 231
Miscellaneous Disorders of the Knee.......................... 233
Bowleg and Knock Knee 235

Chapter 11   **The Foreleg Region** **237**
Shin Splints 237
Other Leg Pain and Dysfunction 238
Nodules.. 241

Chapter 12   **The Ankle and Foot** **243**
Soft Tissue Injury of the Ankle 246
Heel Pain 249
Plantar Fasciitis 250
Midfoot and Metatarsal Pain 251

	Flexible Flatfeet	255
	Toe Disorders	258
	Hammertoe Deformity	259
	Entrapment Neuropathies	259
	Night Cramps	264
Chapter 13	**Generalized Soft Tissue Rheumatic Disorders**	**267**
	Fibrositis Syndrome	267
	Psychogenic Rheumatism	275
	Polymyalgia Rheumatica	276
	Eosinophilic Fasciitis	276
Chapter 14	**Chronic Persistent Pain**	**280**
	Psychogenic Pain Disorder	280
	Psychologic Factors in Patients with Chronic Persistent Pain	281
	Gate Control Theory Updated	282
	Differential Diagnosis	283
	The Examination	283
	Management	286
	Anti-Pain Modalities	287
	Exercise Therapy	288
Chapter 15	**Intralesional Soft Tissue Injection Technique**	**293**
	Indications	294
	Contraindications	294
	Hazards	295
	Technique	299
Chapter 16	**Physical and Occupational Therapy**	**301**
	Goals of Therapeutic Exercise	302
	Evaluation for an Exercise Plan	302
	The Type of Exercise	302
	Exercise for Conditioning and Fitness	303
	Adjuncts to an Exercise Plan	304
	Passive Exercises	306
	Occupational Therapy	307
	Appendix	**315**
	Index	**317**

INTRODUCTION

An Overview of Diagnosis and Management

Subjective complaints of pain, spasm, and "disability" often lack objective measurement. Therefore scientific advances in the soft tissue rheumatic disorders have not kept up with the advances made in other rheumatic disorders. Furthermore, prospective studies are hampered by the simultaneous occurrence of several disorders in one patient, with each having numerous causal attributes. For these reasons, much of what we report is anecdotal, and to some extent arbitrary, and at times controversial. But application of the principles of a careful and intelligent history and physical examination may lead to prompt diagnosis and probable causation *without* expensive invasive procedures. Treatment is often empiric, safe, and economical. This book is, then, to some extent, a "What it is" and "How to treat it" book.

The conditions discussed include localized disease problems that result from trauma, spasm, inflammation, degeneration, or congenital abnormalities. Included among the many entities discussed are tendinitis, bursitis, carpal tunnel and other nerve entrapment syndromes, disc and low back syndromes, other structural derangements of the musculoskeletal system, myofascial pain, other pain syndromes including reflex sympathetic dystrophies, psychogenic rheumatism, and the fibrositis syndrome. Fasciitis includes plantar fasciitis, gluteal and presacral fasciitis, and fascia lata fasciitis.

We have tried to detail each disorder or syndrome as the patients commonly present to the physician. Aggravating factors are stressed. Specific well-defined methods of management are given where available. In those entities where specific therapy is unavailable, empirical modes of treatment that appear to be effective and safe are described. In many cases treatment regimens may require extensive patient education and cooperation; therefore, we have tried to present an expected outcome. However, if further care is needed, guidelines are provided for additional diagnostic procedures and therapy. Most patients with these entities respond well to treatment if all the steps outlined are considered. A common mistake is to provide only one or two therapeutic modalities when a more comprehensive program is necessary. Furthermore, several causative mechanisms may coexist and must be discerned; therefore, the clinician must be thorough in his evaluation of the patient.

Prospective studies are hampered by the simultaneous occurrence of several disorders in one patient, with each contributing many variables to the problem.

Over 150 painful and disabling musculoskeletal disorders are described. No doubt, experienced physicians could add many more to those we have presented. For example:

*Back-pocket sciatica is caused by pressure on the sciatic nerve in the gluteal region [Gould]. We now record another related neuromuscular condition, ponderous-purse disease in shoulder-purseuses. Both

---

*W.K. Engel, Editorial. Reprinted by permission N. Engl. J. Med., 299:557, 1978.

disorders are highly sex-limited, back-pocket sciatica to men and ponderous-purse disease to women, although the latter can affect men of certain habit.

Ponderous-purse disease is manifest by pain, tenderness and spasm in upper shoulder and lateral neck muscles, especially trapezius, supraspinatus and rhomboideus, and is sometimes accompanied by radicular pains.

The pathogenic mechanism is neuromuscular. Constant contraction of the shoulder elevator and neck stabilizer muscles attempting to carry the load on the side of the shouldered purse results in pain, tenderness and focal spasms of those muscles. The muscle contractions can cause abnormal neck posture and provocation of cervical nerve radiculopathy. An informal assay of a series of feminine purse weights and contents revealed weights up to 5 kg. and internal milieus that can modestly and summarily, for the uninitiated, be pursimoniously likened to the contents of a goat's stomach. The profligate-credit-card factor and coins-for-eating-machines factor are links with back-pocket sciatica, but the instruments, bottles, boxes, tubes, jars, packets, and spray cans of material necessary for beauty are unique to ponderous purses.

Prevention of ponderous-purse disease is so logical that to point it out may be considered purscilious. The physician's advice has almost no patient pursuance. An unfavored but sometimes patient-tried remedy is contralateral shifting of the shoulder purse, usually followed by contralateralling of the pain and needless pursponement of the cure. Switching to a hand-held purse is subjectively objectionable and objectively often complicated by purse partings, with resulting hot pursuits, purspirations and panic from loss of beauty aids (and credit cards). Another approach, reduction of the shoulder purse contents, is apparently more of a pain in the neck than the pain in the neck.

And so, like hookworms in unsanitary societies who won't wear shoes, ponderous-purse disease appears destined to remain endemic in ours.

One of our colleagues has labeled these disorders "wastebasket rheumatism"!* In our ignorance of the pathogenesis of many of the persistent musculoskeletal pain syndromes, classification has been difficult. "Nonarticular (soft tissue) rheumatism is a term embracing a large group of miscellaneous conditions with a common denominator of musculoskeletal pain and stiffness."[1]

We have tried to stay with the concept that the nonarticular and soft tissue rheumatic disorders are noninflammatory; but because of their importance to differential diagnosis, the systemic inflammatory spondyloarthropathies with their tendinopathies, eosinophilic fasciitis, and polymyalgia rheumatica are included in appropriate chapters.

Although systemic diseases can produce similar syndromes, we hope the physician will gain confidence in the early recognition and treatment of a *primary* soft tissue rheumatic pain disorder, thus preventing the establishment of a chronic pain-spasm-pain cycle.

The reader is encouraged to review the regional anatomy related to the syndromes described. Knowledge of anatomy and muscle function will aid the clinician in diagnosis and therapy of soft tissue rheumatism. The functional anatomy of the locomotor system is well described in Rene Cailliet's monograph, *Soft Tissue Pain and Disability.*[2] (Plates I to XV.)

IMPACT OF MUSCULOSKELETAL PAIN ON SOCIETY

Musculoskeletal disorders, including soft tissue rheumatic pain disorders, are among the leading causes of time lost from work, and a major reason for disability payments in the United States. One third of these disabled persons are younger than 45 years of age. Chronic "medical absences from work" due

*Courtesy of Allan B. Kirsner, M.D.

ANATOMIC PLATES
and
TRIGGER POINT MAP

Plates I to XIII from *Gray's Anatomy*, 30th American Edition,
used with permission from Lea & Febiger, Philadelphia, 1985.

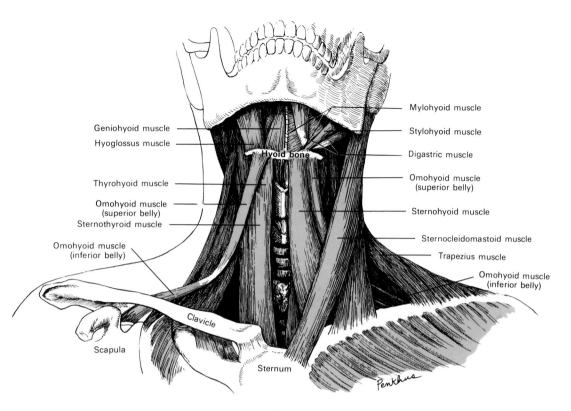

Geniohyoid muscle

Hyoglossus muscle

Thyrohyoid muscle

Omohyoid muscle
(superior belly)

Sternothyroid muscle

Omohyoid muscle
(inferior belly)

Hyoid bone

Clavicle

Scapula

Sternum

Mylohyoid muscle

Stylohyoid muscle

Digastric muscle

Omohyoid muscle
(superior belly)

Sternohyoid muscle

Sternocleidomastoid muscle

Trapezius muscle

Omohyoid muscle
(inferior belly)

Penthus

Plate I.   Muscles of the neck. Anterior view.

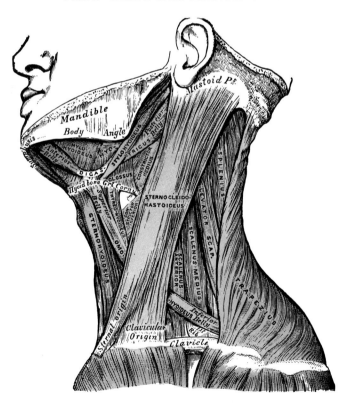

Plate II.   Muscles of the neck. Lateral view.

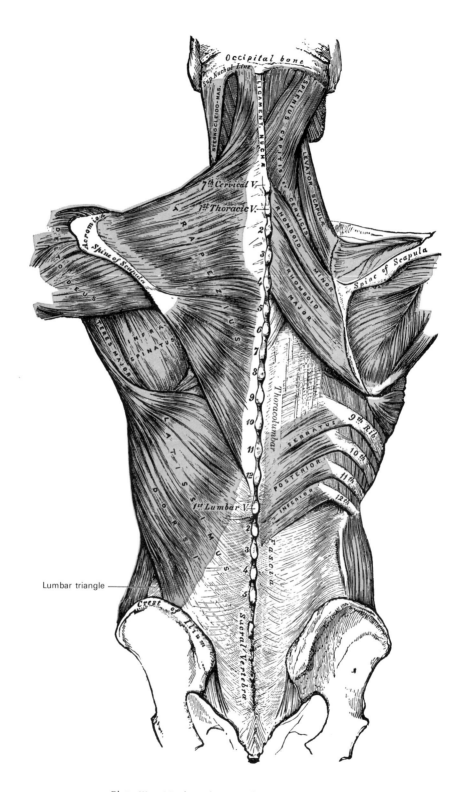

Lumbar triangle

Plate III.　Neck and upper thorax, posterior view.

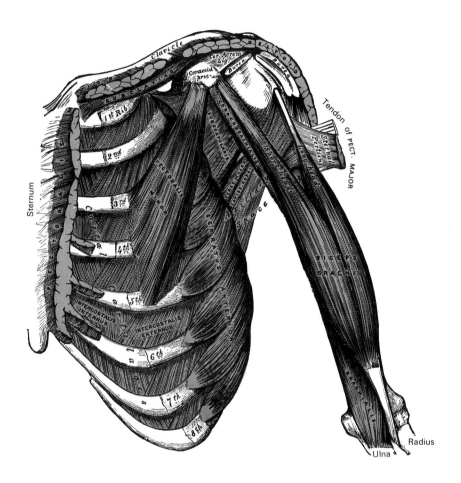

Plate IV.   Shoulder, anterior view.

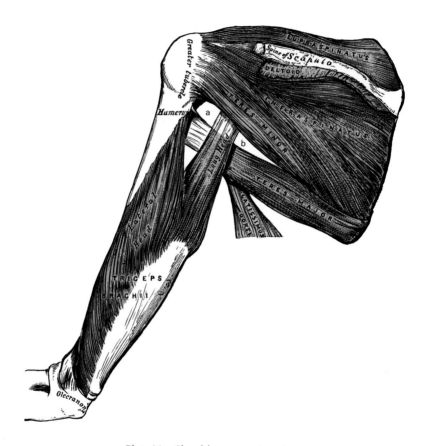

Plate V.   Shoulder, posterior view.

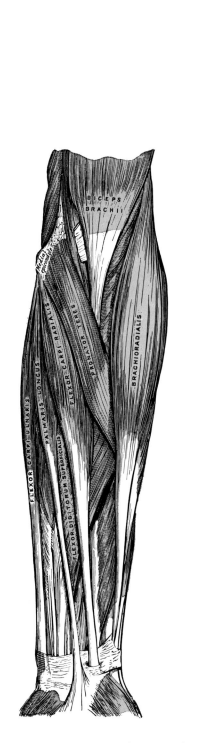

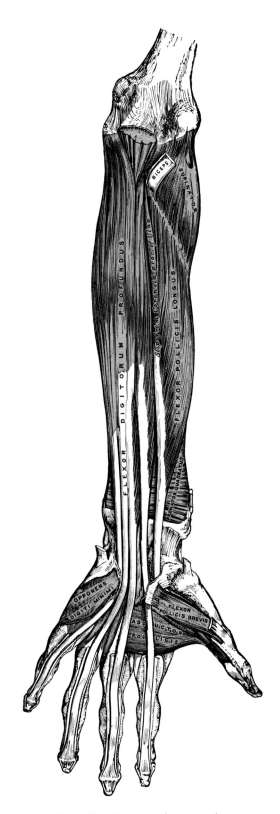

Plate VI.   Forearm, superficial muscles.   Plate VII.   Forearm, deep muscles.

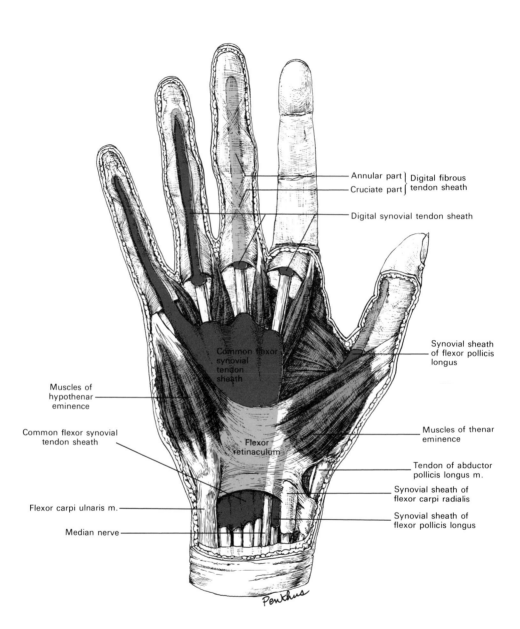

Annular part | Digital fibrous
Cruciate part ∫ tendon sheath

Digital synovial tendon sheath

Synovial sheath
of flexor pollicis
longus

Muscles of thenar
eminence

Tendon of abductor
pollicis longus m.

Synovial sheath of
flexor carpi radialis

Synovial sheath of
flexor pollicis longus

Common flexor
synovial
tendon
sheath

Muscles of
hypothenar
eminence

Common flexor synovial
tendon sheath

Flexor carpi ulnaris m.

Median nerve

Flexor
retinaculum

Penthus

Plate VIII.   Hand, palmar aspect.

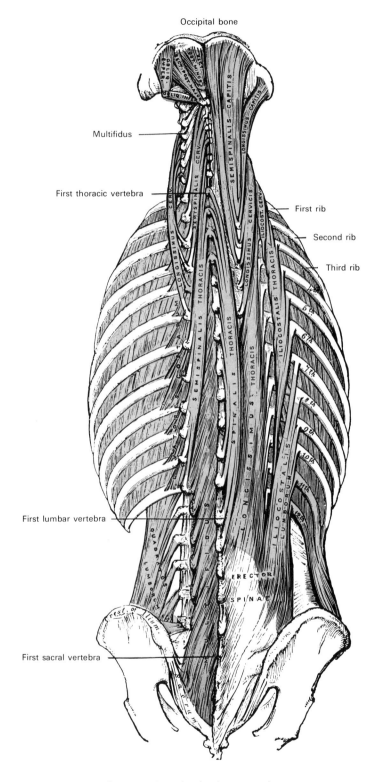

Occipital bone

Multifidus

First thoracic vertebra

First rib

Second rib

Third rib

First lumbar vertebra

First sacral vertebra

Plate IX.   Low back, deep muscles.

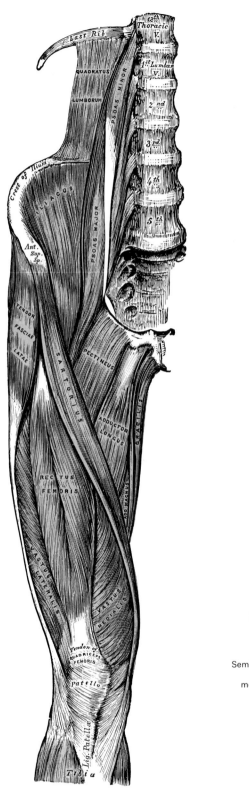

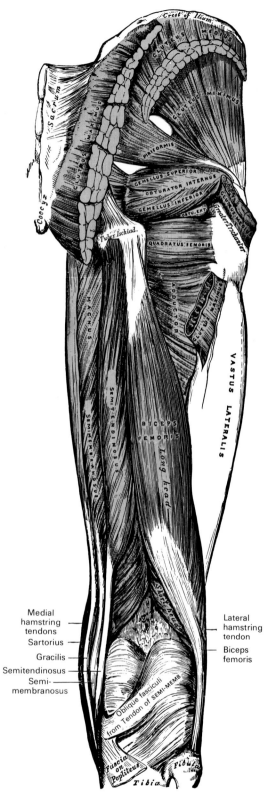

Plate X.   Anterior hip and thigh.

Plate XI.   Posterior hip and thigh.

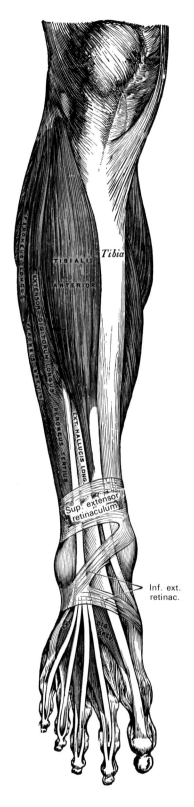

Plate XII.   Anterior foreleg and foot.

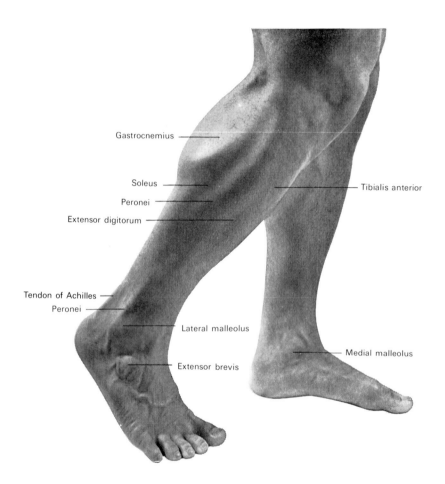

Gastrocnemius

Soleus

Peronei

Extensor digitorum

Tibialis anterior

Tendon of Achilles

Peronei

Lateral malleolus

Medial malleolus

Extensor brevis

Plate XIII.   Right side of leg to show surface contours of muscles and bones.

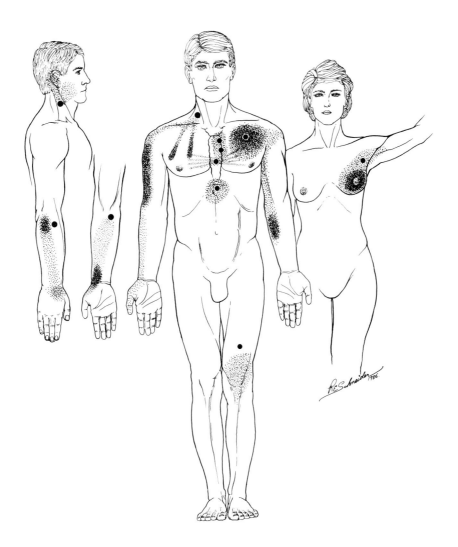

Plate XIV.   Myofascial trigger points and zones of pain referral. Front view.

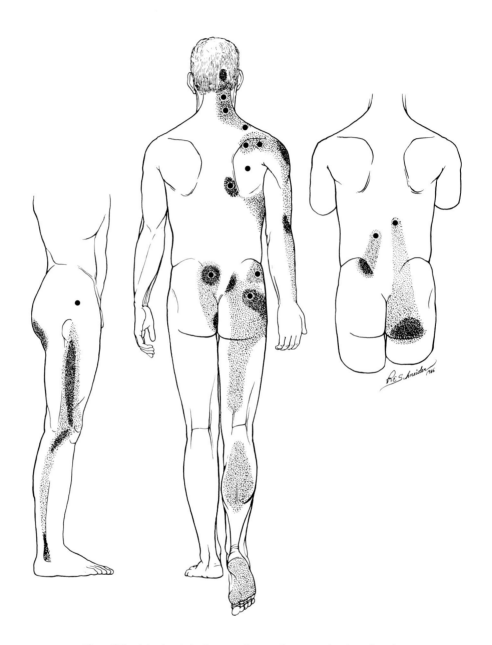

Plate XV.   Myofascial trigger points and zones of pain referral.
Posterior view.

to musculoskeletal disorders exceed medical absences due to circulatory, mental, and neoplastic disorders combined. Of the five leading diseases causing disability, four involve the musculoskeletal system.[3-5] The prevalence of musculoskeletal disorders has increased 24% in the past decade.[6] Of visits to practitioners of medicine, 15 to 25% are estimated to be due to complaints related to the musculoskeletal system.[7] The Mayo Clinic's Department of Physical Medicine reports that 30% of visits were the result of soft tissue musculoskeletal disorders.[8] Of workers who take early retirement, 16% do so as a result of musculoskeletal disorders.[9] Yet, in one study of the 1978 Social Security Survey of Disability and Work, those with rheumatic diseases had the same commitment to work as did those persons with other chronic conditions.[10]

Hopefully, early recognition of these disorders, recognition and avoidance of aggravating factors, and treatment will have a significant impact on the financial and emotional exhaustion that these patients experience. The lack of interest in nonarticular rheumatism in our major teaching centers may result from the fact that such tertiary centers do not see these problems often. Thus, in a 1977 survey, nonacademic rheumatologists saw two to three times more patients with nonarticular rheumatic disorders than their academic colleagues.[11]

AN OVERVIEW OF THE DIAGNOSIS OF SOFT TISSUE RHEUMATIC PAIN

These soft tissue rheumatic pain disorders can be diagnosed with reasonable certainty by taking a careful history and applying simple physical examination tests and maneuvers that accentuate or reproduce the symptoms. The numerous disorders described in this book fall into five major groups as presented in Table 1.

Myofascial Pain

Muscle injury usually involves only one body region, and is of brief duration. When

Table 1. Soft Tissue Rheumatic Pain Disorders

1. Regional Myofascial Pain: Regional pain with trigger point (See Plates XIV and XV)
2. Tendinitis and Bursitis
3. Structural disorders: Examples include short leg, scoliosis, lateral patellar subluxation, flat feet
4. Neurovascular entrapment: Examples include thoracic outlet syndrome, carpal tunnel syndrome and tarsal tunnel syndromes
5. Generalized pain disorders: Examples include the fibrositis syndrome, chronic benign pain syndrome, reflex sympathetic dystrophy, and psychogenic rheumatism.

local muscular pain is more prolonged and is accompanied by tender hard places in muscle, called "trigger points" or "tender points", the condition is termed "myofascial pain".[12-14]

Recognition and management of myofascial pain is an art as well as a science. The pain is of a deep aching quality, occasionally accompanied by a sensation of burning or stinging. The trigger points often feel indurated to palpation, and palpation reproduces the pain. The trigger points are reliably located within the center of a muscle belly or at other locations as specified throughout the chapters of this book. They cause pain in a "target zone" that is distant from the trigger point. The trigger point locations and their target zones of pain reference were popularized by Janet Travell and her colleagues based on the examinations of 1,000 patients.[14-16] Simons and Travell suggest that the trigger point is sometimes accompanied by satellite and secondary trigger points. The secondary trigger points may be activated by irritation of the primary trigger point. These secondary trigger points also result in pain at some distance away. "Tender points" may also occur, but the tenderness associated with tender points is located adjacent to the tender point. Tender points are not activated by other trigger points.[16]

Trigger and tender points may result from acute trauma or minor injury, repeated minor microtrauma of daily living, or from the chronic strain of sedentary living habits. Trigger point maps are provided in Plates XIV–XV.

Palpation of the trigger point may cause a muscle twitch, and electromyographic response.[17] Trigger points cause pain in muscles, fascial structures, ligamentous insertion sites, and in some fatty locations.[14] They also occur in systemic inflammatory disorders or infections. Visible swelling is rare.

Bonica suggested that chronicity often resulted from a pain-spasm-pain cycle.[14] The etiology and pathogenesis of trigger points are discussed more fully in the other chapters.

Tendinitis and Bursitis

Tendinitis is a clinical and pathologic disorder with common features of local pain and dysfunction. Sport and calisthenic activities, hobbies, and jobs that require repetitive motion may give rise to inflammation and degeneration. Triggering is a unique disturbance associated with tendinitis. Usually a digit will suddenly lock up and must be pulled passively for release. A snapping is perceived as the digit "unlocks". Triggering occurs in 20% of upper limb occurrences of tendinitis.

Tendinitis that results from inflammatory rheumatic diseases or from metabolic disturbances may have a single site of occurrence; a careful history will often suggest the systemic rheumatic disorder. Spondyloarthropathies, and other diseases that affect the tendinous attachments to bone, the entheses, are discussed in Chapter 1. The entheses are the site of attachment of a muscle or ligament to bone. These locations have predilection for many inflammatory diseases.

Bursitis is an inflammation of the sac-like structures that form in utero to protect the soft tissues from underlying bony prominences. Common sites for inflammation of these sacs are the olecranon, prepatellar, and trochanteric bursae. The origin of the term "bursitis" as recalled by Bywaters is of interest.[18] Monro provided the first atlas of some 40 bursae. At the time (1788), the society that had followed the second bourgeois revolution consisted of princes and their political power,

laborers and freeman who provided the basic work, and the new middlemen—the purse ('la bourse')—the businessmen and the banks, ensuring that lubrication made for a frictionless and easy running society. Hence the aptly applied term—the bursa!

Structural Disorders

Structural disorders must be kept in mind as important causes of soft tissue injury among athletes and those participating in conditioning activities. In a study of medical students, 69% had from one, to as many as seven, different musculoskeletal structural abnormalities. Joint laxity was the most common; next was restricted joint motion.[19] Other common findings are scoliosis, short leg, and lateral patellar subluxation. In another group of 90 medical students who were injured in sports events, (226 injuries in them) abnormal musculoskeletal findings included persistent loss of joint range of motion, temporomandibular joint dysfunction syndrome, synovitis, bursitis, tendinitis, and joint laxity. In runners, neither shoe type nor type of running surface correlated with any finding or symptom.[20] Physical findings of musculoskeletal structural disorders are common to those participating in athletic activities and should be documented before as well as afterward. Further studies are needed to determine any correlation of structural disorders to injury and morbidity in those who participate in sports and conditioning programs.

Neurovascular Entrapment Disorders

Neurovascular entrapment disorders may occur within the spinal canal (spinal stenosis) or along the course of a peripheral nerve. A sensation of swelling and pain and paresthesias distal to the site of entrapment should suggest the condition.

The *generalized pain disorders* will be discussed in Chapters 13 and 14.

Evaluation

A careful history requires that the clinician discern what pain the patient is experiencing throughout the day and night. The pain quality (aching, burning, numbness, throbbing) must be elicited; the physician should not prejudge the severity of the patient's pain.[21] Objective swelling must be distinguished from a *sensation* of swelling. Is "swelling" limited to a joint area, is it periarticular, or more diffuse? Is motion impaired, and if so, is the limited motion constant or intermittent?

What precipitating events preceded the pain? These may include injury from overstretching, a direct blow to the body, repetitive activity or prolonged inactivity from driving long distances or performing prolonged sedentary tasks. What therapeutic endeavors were tried by the patient and with what results?

The patient's general condition must be considered. Evaluation of the condition should proceed in an orderly, logical manner. Localized syndromes may reflect local limited areas of disease. Many local disorders result from "misuse injury."[22] Similar manifestations may result from a systemic disorder or may be drug-induced (e.g., drug lupus, serum sickness). If a systemic disease process is present, the physician must consider whether it is the cause of myofascial pain or coincidental. A comprehensive examination includes body development, posture, gait, movement, motivation, and emotional status in addition to the usual evaluations[23-24] (Fig. 1).

The physical examination of patients with nonarticular rheumatism includes special maneuvers unique to defining the syndromes described in this book. Each chapter describes the performance of these essential clinical tests; these tests often reproduce the symptoms.

The examining physician should observe the patient while sitting, when rising from a chair, or while bending and walking. In this manner, structural disorders can be recognized. Laying on of hands to palpate tender, indurated, trigger points of muscle, to determine joint passive range of movement, or to elicit joint hypermobility is particularly important. Careful joint palpation for synovial thickening or synovial effusion is essential to

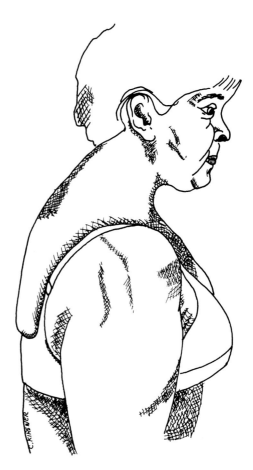

Fig. 1. The clinician observes the heavy breasts, improper brassiere with tight straps, heavy arms, forward sloping shoulder, and forward inclination of the neck. The patient is a good candidate for thoracic outlet syndrome, cervical myofascial pain or muscle contraction headaches.

detect these subtle manifestations of various connective tissue diseases.

The diagnosis of myofascial origin of pain can be compared to the diagnosis of migraine headaches. The physician must first learn the specific features of such headaches. A careful history of the quality, location, and duration of the headache must be elicited. Associated characteristic symptoms include visual scotomata, nausea and vomiting, transient neurologic deficits, and personality features that occur with sufficient frequency to be recognized as a syndrome called "migraine." The possible aggravating features of bright light and mental stress are sought.[25] Treatment is specific, and is associated with a good response in most patients. *Relief from pain becomes a corroborative part of the syndrome recognition.* A majority of patients with non-articular rheumatic disorders respond favorably to treatment, which often helps corroborate or establish the diagnosis.

Nonarticular rheumatic pain disorders have clinical features that are also helpful in diagnosis (Table 2). First, the usual physical findings and tests of inflammation, and roentgenographic features of arthritis are normal or expected for age. Second, symptoms often are worse after resting. Whereas intra-articular disease is worse with use and relieved by rest, these conditions often will awaken the patient from sleep or will be accentuated after sitting and relieved with movement. Of course, overuse may aggravate them as well. Third, most of these conditions have aggravating factors that lead to recurrences. These include improper resting positions, prolonged repetitive movements, lack of respect for pain, and a personality trait that leads to "I'm going to finish this even if it kills me!" attitude. Fourth, physical examination tests and maneuvers can reproduce or exacerbate symptoms. Lastly, simple office management can provide relief, and this response to treatment will corroborate the diagnosis.

NEW DIAGNOSTIC TECHNIQUES USEFUL FOR SOFT TISSUE RHEUMATIC PAIN DISORDERS

Diagnosis of many soft tissue rheumatic pain disorders has been hampered by the lack

---

Helpful Hints
1. Laying on of the examiner's hands often provides more useful information than do roentgenograms.
2. Osteoarthritis seen on roentgenograms is often unrelated to the pain syndrome.
3. Localized musculoskeletal pain disorders may be layered over another established disease process.
4. When morning stiffness does not *mainly* involve the hands and feet, rheumatoid arthritis is an unlikely diagnosis.
5. Pain so severe that the limbs cannot be touched (the touch-me-not syndrome), and with no discernible spasm, is usually of psychogenic origin.
6. Pain localized to a body quadrant seldom is due to a psychogenic cause.
7. Observing the patient while seated, while rising from a chair, while standing, and while bending forward can lead to recognition of basic *structural* alterations. "Misuse" of the musculoskeletal system may also be observed.
8. Drugs may be the least important part of treatment. Stretching exercises and avoiding aggravating factors often provide more sustained benefit than pills.

---

of reproducible measurements. When, after World War II, electrodiagnostic studies provided measurement of impaired nerve conduction, the nerve entrapment disorders gained validity and recognition. Presently, great interest lies in newer technologies for measurement and diagnosis of soft tissue rheumatic pain problems. These new methods include scintigraphy, computed tomography, thermography, and magnetic resonance imaging.

Radionuclide scanning has proved of value in a number of the soft tissue rheumatic disorders. In addition to its use in reflex sympathetic dystrophy,[26-27] scintigraphy (using methylene diphosphonate[28] has been reported of value in the diagnosis of frozen shoulder, for evaluation of inflammatory muscle disease using 99 pyrophosphate (TcPYP) nuclear scans,[29-30] for assessment of sacroiliac joint involvement in low back pain,[31] for os-

Table 2. Clinical Features of Non-Articular Rheumatism

1. No positive signs or tests of systemic inflammation
2. Pain is often worse with rest and improved with movement
3. Aggravating factors are common and cause recurrences
4. Physical examination tests and maneuvers reproduce symptoms
5. Treatment provides relief; this corroborates diagnosis

teonecrosis as a cause for knee pain,[32] and for detection of anarthritic rheumatoid arthritis.[33]

Computed tomography has been used for aiding the diagnosis of back and neck problems, particularly tumors, prolapsed discs, and spinal stenosis;[34–37] hip pain (lipoma, cysts, bursitis)[38] and may demonstrate the possible role of stenosis of the carpal canal as a cause for carpal tunnel syndrome.[39]

Thermography is becoming of greater interest as the technique gains refinement in quality. Infrared emission from the body can be recorded by telethermogrpahy, contact thermography, and microwave thermography. It may provide a noninvasive, simple, permanent record of sympathetic nervous system change in association with impingement of nerve roots, myofascial pain, and with pain referred from cardiac or visceral diseases.[40–44] Although trigger point identification has been described,[45] this has not been our experience. Thermography has been advocated for objective diagnosis of tennis elbow[46] and for identification of metatarsophalangeal inflammation as a cause for foot pain.[47] One study reports changes in thermogram images coincident with the pain relief that followed use of a transcutaneous electric stimulator in patients with lumbar disc disease.[48] Nevertheless, thermography remains a research tool; it is not yet accepted as a reliable test method.[49]

Magnetic resonance imaging (MRI) is another new and noninvasive technique.[50] In the first 1000 consecutive studies performed at the Mayo clinic, 115 were for musculoskeletal disorders. Of these, 29 were for trauma. The authors considered MRI a significantly useful technique for noninvasive visualization of tendon, ligamentous and muscular injuries.[51] This technique may be of diagnostic value in metabolic myopathies,[30] mass lesions of the spine or extremities (e.g., popliteal cysts)[52] or for spinal stenosis with lateral canal entrapment.[53] Compared to computed tomography for spinal disorders, one study suggests that MRI is superior to CT scan for disc degeneration, and disc space in-

fections.[54] Drawbacks to MRI are slowness of the procedure, cost, and the inability to image patients with implanted pacemakers or metallic clips.[50] Acoustic arthrography and tenography can provide an objective and reproducible record of pathology involving joints and tendons.[55] This noninvasive technique may allow objectivity in future studies of treatment modalities.

SIX POINTS FOR MANAGING MYOFASCIAL SOFT TISSUE PAIN

Six points of management can often be initiated during the patient's *first visit*, even before appropriate laboratory and radiographic findings are available.

1. Exclude systemic disease.
2. Recognize and eliminate aggravating factors.
3. Provide an explanation to the patient.
4. Provide instruction in self-help exercises.
5. Provide relief from pain.
6. Project an expected outcome (Fig. 2).

Exclude Systemic Disease. Satisfy yourself and the patient that serious systemic disease is not present. Systemic inflammatory connective tissue disorders must be excluded as well as such entities as diabetes mellitus, thyroid dysfunction, occult neoplasm, and drug reactions. *Treatment need not wait for results from such tests* in many patients. If roentgenographs are likely to add little information to the findings, they may be deferred until results of the treatment program are evaluated a few weeks later. Expensive, time-consuming, and possibly hazardous procedures (e.g., angiography for a thoracic outlet syndrome) should only be considered if they are clinically justified. More often, such procedures can and should be reserved for patients who fail to benefit from the conservative therapy initiated on the first visit. We would certainly order appropriate screening tests, including complete blood counts, urinalysis, sedimentation rate, and appropriate serum chemistries. If radiographs have been done

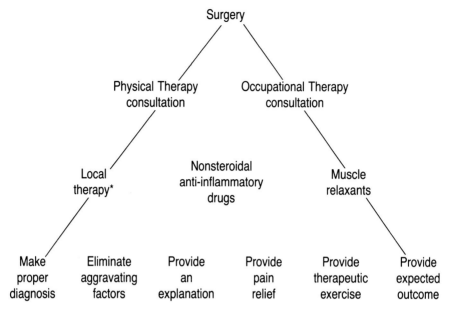

Fig. 2. A pyramid of management for nonarticular soft tissue rheumatic disorders. The pyramid builds from the six essential points of management at the base. *Local therapy may be injection(s) and/or vasocoolant spray. (From Sheon, RP[103])

elsewhere recently, the films may be requested for review.

Recognize and Eliminate Aggravating Factors. Events and activities preceding the pain state must be reviewed in an effort to recognize aggravating activities *that can cause recurrences.* Improper resting, sitting, or working positions are common precipitating factors (Fig. 3). Strain resulting from job performance, a new hobby, or repetitive tiring tasks should be recognized and altered. Strain resulting from structural disorders, such as flatfeet or heavy pendulous breasts, can also be altered with appropriate instructions. Joint protection advice is detailed for each body region and in Chapter 16. Chronic pain causes anxiety, depression, physical tension, and disturbed sleep. Let the patient know that emotional stress can be an aggravating factor, and may not only play a primary role in the pain syndrome, but may lower a patient's pain threshold and compound the pain-spasm-pain cycle. Similarly, secondary gain resulting in dependent interpersonal relationships can prolong treatment. Frank discussion usually leads to a satisfactory solution.

Somatic delusions that accompany certain psychoses may confound the clinician. The need for psychiatric care in such patients soon becomes obvious.

Provide an Explanation to the Patient. The physician should provide the patient with a suspected cause for her symptoms. For example, if after the examination, a benign hypermobility syndrome (see Chapt. 6) is considered to be the cause of the patient's symptoms, this may be explained to the patient and she may be reassured immediately. Hypermobility syndrome is a more welcome diagnosis than systemic lupus erythematosus, or rheumatoid arthritis. When a myofascial pain syndrome such as gluteal fasciitis, or trochanteric bursitis, is superimposed upon another disorder, such as osteoarthritis of the hip, the patient's comprehension of the findings is vital to future care. The myofascial or bursitis pain may cause more suffering than the coexisting arthritis. Alternatively, nonarticular rheumatic pain may disrupt a physical therapy program that is essential for treatment of the accompanying arthritis. Treatment of the bursitis or fasciitis provides

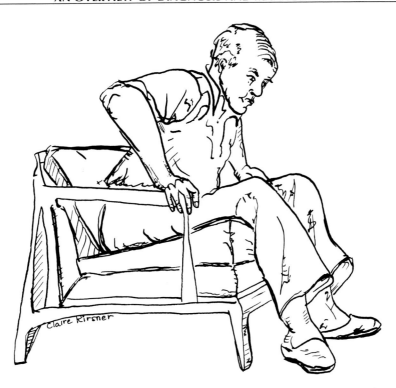

Fig. 3. Illustration of a patient arising from a chair demonstrating the following faults: (1) Hands and wrists used to push off from the side of the chair; this promotes quadriceps weakness and carpal tunnel syndrome. (2) The chair is too low; this impedes use of the quadriceps during the act of arising. (3) The neck is unsupported and the chair is overstuffed; this promotes muscular strain about the head and neck. (4) House slippers promote metatarsalgia.

relief from pain, and furthermore allows the patient to follow conservative care necessary for the arthritis. If a myofascial pain syndrome has been found and trigger points identified, the patient can be informed that the pain is real, and that a pain-spasm-pain cycle may be prolonging the condition.

Provide Instruction in Self-Help Exercises. A prescription program of home physical therapy and exercises should be outlined on the first visit. Myofascial pain syndromes appear to respond best to a twice daily regimen performed first thing in the morning and last thing at night. Even if pain has subsided, twice daily stretching exercises should be continued until the involved region no longer tightens up during sleep. The ease or flexibility of morning stretching should be compared to the ease of stretching the preceding evening. The exercises should be continued until the morning and evening exercise regimens appear equally flexible. Exercises are described throughout the text.

Provide Relief from Pain. As mentioned, when pain is present, a vicious cycle may have occurred, promoting greater muscular spasm. The self-help therapy program can be more effective and results obtained more quickly when pain is relieved. If spasm is minimal, pain relief may be obtained by such time-honored therapy as heat or cold applications, and aspirin prior to performing the self-help exercises. Intense muscle spasm can usually be relieved by injecting the "trigger point" with a long-acting corticosteroid-local anesthetic mixture. Similarly, such an injection for treatment of a suspected bursitis, tendinitis, or carpal tunnel syndrome can provide prompt pain relief, and may help establish a nonarticular rheumatic disease diagnosis.[56] Oral nonsteroidal anti-inflammatory drugs are often helpful but may require a trial and error routine in their selection. These agents should be used with caution in patients receiving diuretics, and in patients who have other diseases that can impair renal or hepatic function. If pain chronicity suggests a vicious pain-spasm-pain cycle, using tricyclic antidepressant drugs, such as amitriptyline, may be helpful even in patients without apparent depression. Used at night, in a dose sufficient to cause a mild dry mouth, amitriptyline or other tricyclics may help interrupt the pain-spasm-pain cycle.[57-62]

Project an Expected Outcome. The physician should be familiar enough with soft tissue rheumatic pain disorders that the expected outcome and duration until benefits become evident can be projected. Relief from carpal tunnel syndrome, bursitis, or tendinitis may require only a few days, whereas symptoms due to hypermobility syndrome or disorders of other structural deficits may require several months before moderate or great improvement is seen. This should be told to the patient at the outset. The patient should also understand that the physician's diagnosis may depend upon the patient achieving symptomatic relief; this in turn, often depends upon the patient performing the self-help program. The physician and the patient must work together.

AN OVERVIEW OF THE INJURED WORKER

Many facets of the problems surrounding a work-related injury must be considered:

1. The work effort: Does the worker have to do a repetitive task, remain in a fixed position for long periods of time, lift above or below a mechanically strainful height, or perform a tedious and monotonous task? What number of workers, performing the same job, have been disabled?

2. The workplace environment: Are lighting and temperature adequate? Are tools and machines adaptable to the physical features of the worker? Is the workplace safe?

3. Does the worker have a good relationship with co-workers and management? Is the milieu conducive to good work habits? How does the company manage the injured worker? How quickly is proper care given?

4. What personal physical characteristics, habits, and attitudes does the worker bring to the workplace? What is the worker's past experience in regard to time lost from work? Are physical characteristics of the worker important toward satisfactory job placement? Are there aggravating factors such as sports participation or a second job or hobby that contribute to so-called work-related injury?

These and other considerations are being assessed by experts in the medical field. Methods for educating management to consider these and other facets of occupational injury are proposed for further study.[63-66]

In a study of 584 injured workers, factors that related to length of disability were not the seriousness of the injury, but rather the age of the worker, lack of work skills, inadequate treatment, compensation neurosis, and worker motivation. These factors are difficult to measure.[67] Yet, in everyday practice, the clinician can consider the impact these factors might have on his patient, and provide appropriate advice in an effort to improve the worker's productivity and to prevent recurrences. Similarly, the psychologic status of the worker and its relation to "the accident process" may be an important consideration if disability persists beyond the expected duration. (See the next section.) Delay in referral to specialists correlates with longer periods of disability.[68-69]

THE PSYCHOLOGY OF INJURY

In a 3-year study of disability pensioning due to musculoskeletal disorders (in Denmark) it became evident that both medical and social factors are involved.[5] The interest in unconscious harmful motivation toward injury was crystallized by Hirschfeld and Behan in what they called "The Accident Process". From their study of the causes of accidents and injuries in the workplace (300 cases), the authors found that the accident process consisted of a state of conflict and anxiety within the patient; the worker then finds a self-destructive injury-producing act which causes the "death" of the person as a worker. Instead of presenting with a classical psychiatric syndrome, the patient presents with physical symptoms that defy medical solution.[70] This physical disturbance provides a solution to the original conflict. Others have found similar important psychologic factors in prolonged disability; they stress the importance of psychologic counseling and behavioral modification in treatment.[71-75]

Any person who suffers from disability beyond the expected duration should be considered for psychologic interview. Chronic pain (more than 6 months' duration) is thought to result from a complex adaptation and defense mechanism that has become operational. Pain then may serve to maintain the individual's psychic equilibrium.[72]

The occupational clinical psychologist may discover interpersonal conflicts, can measure the effects of environmental factors on behavior and performance, can detect psychologic stresses in the workplace, can measure prevailing attitudes, and can provide psychologic perspectives to the workers and management.[72a] The importance of conscious or unconscious motivation needs to be stressed. Some characteristics of the consciously motivated (or malingering) patient include extensive "documentation" of the problem, a defensive attitude, demands for surgery, anger, withholding of information, inconsistent behavior, "importance" of litigation to patient, and a relentless search for pain relief provided by someone else.[76]

Newer treatment methods utilize symptom control, stimulus control and social system modification. Results are encouraging.[77] Symptom control is obtained by relaxation training, biofeedback, and autohypnosis. Stimulus control involves behavior modification techniques which include changing

personal beliefs, identification of irrational thinking, and recognition of events and stresses that precipitate pain. Social intervention involves recognition of secondary gain such as attention from other persons, financial rewards, avoidance of work, sex and other responsibilities. In pilot studies, treatment resulted in significant reduction in pain, hopelessness, medication use, and depression from pretreatment levels.[73,77] Simply introducing an interview with questions concerning job stress, ambiguity of worker's role, overwork, and job suitability, resulted in a marked decrease in worker absenteeism in one controlled study.[78]

Motivation may be directed toward secondary gain. Finneson has recommended that in cases of low back pain, future psychologic and sociologic studies should compare compensated and noncompensated patients. Furthermore, compensation laws and insurance plans should encourage return to work with financial incentives favoring gainful employment.[79]

Neustadt[80] suggests consideration of the four "Rs" when a patient develops increasing disability despite apparently adequate management. These are:

1. *Roles*—the ability to carry on relationships as parent, spouse, student, or breadwinner. Look for loss of self esteem.
2. *Reactions*—the patient's emotional response to the disorder including anger, hostility, anxiety, discouragement, or defeat. Patient education is needed here.
3. *Relationships*—look for unsurmountable problems at work, in the family, in school, or with friends. The patient may be beating his head against such "brick walls."
4. *Resources*—has the patient tapped community programs, counselors, minister, or used simple joint protection methods that reduce stress?

Much more work is required on the preventive side. Industry and society must face the spiraling costs of disability. Recognition of a psychological motivation toward injury and disability may help prevent accidents in the workplace.

OUTCOME APPRAISAL TECHNIQUES

Because we currently lack reliable and reproducible methods to measure pain and spasm, or disability, we have few studies that compare therapeutic interventions in nonarticular and soft tissue disorders. What end point can be used? A number of techniques that use scales have been introduced.

The simplest tool is a visual analogue scale for pain determination. This subjective measurement consists of nothing more than a vertical line with cross lines. Huskisson's scale[81] stretches from "No pain" (at the bottom) to "Pain as bad as it can be" (at the top). Although suggestively sensitive as a measure, studies using this scale for repeated measurement of pain following treatment revealed declining reliability.[82] When patients could review their own initial scale scores, however, improved reliability was observed.[83]

In addition there are a battery of self-rating questionnaires that give reproducible results in the assessment of health status, functional ability or disability, and outcome. These questionnaires have been tested for reliability and validity. The answers are scaled as to severity and the scales used for outcome assessment. Clinimetrics, the study of the use of these types of scales to collect and analyze comparative clinical data, may provide a quantitative measurement of patient care.[84]

Scales under investigation that might be appropriate to the evaluation of medical care in soft tissue rheumatic disorders include the Toronto Activities of Daily Living questionnaire;[85] the Health Assessment Questionnaire (HAQ);[86,87] The Rand Health Perceptions;[88] the McGill Pain Questionnaire;[89] the Arthritis Impact Measurement Scales;[90] and the Sickness Impact Profile[91] and others. Critical appraisal of these is available to the interested reader.[87,92–99] Anyone considering an outcome study of the soft tissue rheumatic pain syndromes should have peer review before undertaking the study. There are many pitfalls to performing such a study. Nevertheless, a good outcome study with suitable controls is long overdue for physical therapy and occupational therapy modalities, soft tissue injections, and all surgical procedures.

Physicians concerned with cost effectiveness are recommending many of the treatment modalities described in this book.[100–102] We encourage the reader to try these measures, even though there is no proof of efficacy. Our 25 years of experience has established the safety of these measures in most disorders, and patient satisfaction that has resulted from the measures outlined here.

REFERENCES

1. Hench PK: Nonarticular rheumatism. Rheumatic Diseases: Diagnosis and Management. Edited by WA Katz. Philadelphia, JB Lippincott, 1977.
2. Cailliet R: Soft Pain and Disability. Philadelphia, FA Davis, 1977.
3. Reynolds MD: Prevalence of rheumatic diseases as causes of disability and complaints by ambulatory patients. Arthritis Rheum 21:377–382, 1978.
4. Kelsey JL, White AA III, Pastides H, Bisbee GE Jr.: The impact of musculoskeletal disorders on the population of the United States. J Bone Joint Surg 61A:959–963, 1979.
5. Jeune B, Mikkelsen S, Olsen J, Sabroe S: Epidemiological research in disability pensioning. Scand J Social Med. 16:5–7, 1980.
6. Department of Health, Education and Welfare, Pub. No. (NIH) 78-318, 70-73 (Tables 1, 2) 1977.
7. Lipscomb PR: Foreword. In Musculoskeletal Disorders. Edited by RD D'Ambrosia. Philadelphia, JB Lippincott, 1977.
8. Stonnington HH: Tension myalgia. Mayo Clin Proc 52:750, 1977.
9. Fanning D: Health Retirement as a Indicator of Morbidity. J Soc Occup Med 31:103–111, 1981.
10. Yelin E, Kramer J, Epstein W: A national study of medical care use by persons with four rheumatic conditions: effect of symptoms, social and demographic factors. (Abstract #A117) Arth Rheum 25 (No. 4) [Supp], 1982.
11. Epstein WV: Health Services Research in Rheumatology. Bull Rheum Dis 31:15–19, 1981.
12. Edeiken J, Wolferth CC: Persistent pain in the shoulder region following myocardial infarction. Am J Med Sci 191:201–210, 1936.
13. Travell J, Rinzler SH: The myofascial genesis of pain. Postgrad Med 11:425–434, 1952.
14. Bonica JJ: Management of myofascial pain syndromes in general practice. JAMA 164:732–738, 1957.
15. Travell J: Conferences on therapy: Management of

pain due to muscle spasm. New York St J Med 45:2085–2097, 1945.

16. Travell JG, Simons DG: Myofascial pain and dysfunction. The Trigger Point Manual. Baltimore, Williams & Wilkins, 1983.

17. Simons DG: Electrogenic nature of palpable bands and "jump sign" associated with myofascial trigger points. *In* Advances in Pain Research and Therapy, Vol I. Edited by JJ Bonica, D Albe-Fessard. New York, Raven Press, 1976; 913–918.

18. Bywaters EGL: Lesions of bursae, tendons and tendon sheaths. Clin Rheum Dis 5:883–918, 1979.

19. Raskin RJ, Lawless OJ: Articular and soft tissue abnormalities in a 'normal' population. J Rheum 9:284–288, 1981.

20. Raskin RJ, Rebecca GS: Posttraumatic sports-related musculoskeletal abnormalities: prevalence in a normal population. Am J Sports Med 11:336–339, 1983.

21. D'Ambrosia RD (ed): Musculoskeletal Disorders. Philadelphia, JB Lippincott, 1977.

22. Fowler WM, Taylor RG: Differential diagnosis of muscle diseases. *In* Musculoskeletal Disorders. Edited by RD D'Ambrosia. Philadelphia, JB Lippincott, 1977.

23. Kendall HO, Kendall FP, Boynton DA: Posture and Pain. Huntington, NY, Robert E. Krieger, 1970.

24. Sheon RP: Regional soft tissue pain syndromes. Postgrad Med 68(5):143–157, 1980.

25. Saper JR: Migraine I; classification and pathogenesis. JAMA 239:2380–2383, 1978.

26. Kozin F, Genant HJ, Bekerman C, McCarty DJ: The reflex sympathetic dystrophy syndrome. II. Roentgenographic and scintigraphic evidence of bilaterality. Am J Med 60:332–338, 1977.

27. Kozin F, Ryan LM, Carerra GF, et al: The reflex sympathetic dystrophy syndrome. III. Scintigraphic studies, further evidence for the therapeutic efficacy of systemic corticosteroids, and proposed diagnostic criteria. Am J Med 70:23–30, 1981.

28. Stodell MA, Sturrock RD: Frozen Shoulder. Lancet 2:527, 1981.

29. Yonker R, Webster E, Edwards NL, Katz P, Longley S, Panush RS: Pyrophosphate muscle scans in inflammatory muscle disease. (Abstract #A20) Arthritis Rheum 27:(No 4) [Supp.], 1984.

30. Arnold DL, Radda GK, Bore PJ, Styles P, Taylor DJ: Excessive intracellular acidosis of skeletal muscle on exercise in a patient with post-viral exhaustion/fatigue syndrome. Lancet 1:1367–1368, 1984.

31. Rothwell RS, Davis P, Lentle BC: Radionuclide bone scanning in females with chronic low back pain. Ann Rheum Dis 40:79–82, 1981.

32. Lotke PA, Ecker ML, Alavi A: Painful knees in older patients. J Bone Joint Surg 59A:617–621, 1977.

33. Schneider H, Yonker R, Longley S, Katz P, Carroll R, Panush RS: Diphosphonate bone scans in polyarthalgias. (Abstract #19) Arth Rheum 26: (No. 4) [Supp], 1983.

34. Raskin SP: Introduction to computed tomography of the lumbar spine. Orthopedics 3:1011–1023, 1980.

35. Raskin SP: Degenerative changes of the lumbar

spine: Assessment by computed tomography. Orthopedics 4:186–195, 1981.

36. Raskin SP: Computed tomographic findings in lumbar disc disease. Orthopedics 5:419–434, 1981.

37. Hashimoto I, Tak YK: The true sagittal diameter of the cervical spinal canal and its diagnostic significance in cervical myelopathy. J Neurosurg 47:912–916, 1977.

38. Kovarsky J, Davis R: Compression of obturator nerve by lipoma. Arth Rheum 23:871–872, 1980.

39. Zucker-Pinchoff B, Hermann G, et al: Computed tomography of the carpal tunnel radioanatomical study. J Comput Assist Tomography 5:525–528, 1981.

40. Hobbins WB: Thermography and pain. Progr Clin Biol Res 107:361–375, 1982.

41. Pochaczevsky R, Wexler CE, et al: Liquid crystal thermography of the spine and extremities. J Neurosurg 56:386–395, 1982.

42. Pochaczevsky R: The Value of Liquid Crystal Thermography in the Diagnosis of Spinal Root Compression Syndromes. Ortho Clin NA 14:271–289, 1983.

43. Rask MR: Thermography of the human spine: Study of 150 cases with back pain and sciatica. Orthop Rev 8:73–82, 1979.

44. Rothschild BM, Fisherwitz J, Reiss J, Prostic E, Abrams B, Carlson RA: Pathophysiology of carpal tunnel syndrome: electro-thermographic assessment. (Abstract #C2) Arth Rheum 28 (No. 4) [Supp], 1985.

45. Fischer AA: Thermography and Pain. Arch Phys Med Rehabil 62:542–543, 1981.

46. Binder A, Parr G, Hazleman B: Ultrasound in tennis elbow. Ann Rheum Dis 42:309, 1983.

47. Espiritu BR, Rothschild BM: Assessment of applicability of thermographic technique for identification of pedal pathology. (Abstract #77) Arth Rheum 26: (No. 4) [Supp], 1983.

48. Leroy PL, Bruner WM: Effects of electrical stimulation on the thermographic pattern in the human patient with chronic pain syndrome. Prog Clin Biol Res 107:389–395, 1982.

49. Abraham EA: Thermography: Uses and Abuses. Contemp Ortho 8:95–99, 1984.

50. Moon KL, Helms CA: Nuclear Magnetic Resonance Imaging: Potential musculoskeletal applications. Clin Rheum Dis 9:473–483, 1983.

51. Baker H, Berquist TH, Kispert DB, Reese DF, et al: Magnetic resonance imaging in a routine clinical setting. Mayo Clin 60:75–90, 1985.

52. Hull RG, Rennie JAN, Eastmond CJ, et al: Nuclear magnetic resonance (NMR) tomographic imaging for popliteal cysts in rheumatoid arthritis. Ann Rheum Dis 43:56–59, 1984.

53. Crawshaw C, Frazer AM, Merriam WF, Mulholland RC, Webb JK: A comparison of surgery and chemonucleolysis in the treatment of sciatica: a prospective randomized trial. Spine 9:195–199, 1984.

54. Modic MT, Pavlicek W, Weinstein MA, et al: Magnetic resonance imaging of intervertebral disk disease. Radiology 103–111, 1984.

55. Russell IJ: Clinical utility of acoustic arthrography and tendonography. (Abstract #9) Arth Rheum 28 (4) [Supp], 1985.

56. Kirsner AB, Sheon RP: Regional rheumatic syn-

dromes (including bursitis, tenosynovitis, tendinitis and ganglia). Primer on the Rheumatic Disease, 8th Ed; GP Rodnan and HR Schumacher, Editors. Arthritis Foundation, Atlanta; 1983, 161–163.

57. Raskin NH, Prusiner S: Carotidynia. Neurology 27:43–46, 1977.

58. Gomersall JD, Stuart A: Amitriptyline in migraine prophylaxis. J Neurol Neurosurg Psychiatry 36:684–690, 1973.

59. Halpern LM: Analgesic drugs in the management of pain. Arch Surg 112:861–869, 1977.

60. Duthie AM: The use of phenothiazines and tricyclic antidepressants in the treatment of intractable pain. S Afr Med J 51:246–247, 1977.

61. Beaumont G: The use of psychotropic drugs in other painful conditions. J Int Med Res 4:[Suppl (2)]56–57, 1976.

62. DeJong RH: Central pain mechanisms. JAMA 239:2784, 1978.

63. Sakata RT, Calvert CT, Patrone NA: Arthritis rehabilitation in industry—findings and conclusions. (Abstract #18) Arth Rheum 27:(No. 4) [Supp], 1984.

64. Waugh SE, Friedman CP, Lovelace, KA, Sadler JC: An arthritis training program for industrial managers. (Abstract #28) Arth Rheum 27:(No. 4) [Supp], 1984.

65. Mitchell DK, Chansky MS, McCarary KL, Waugh SE, Calvert CT, Slack D, Schuch C: Arthritis rehabilitation in industry—a model disability management program. (Abstract #220) Arth Rheum 25 (No. 4) [Supp], 1982.

66. Daltroy L, Eaton H, Pallozzi L: Application of the precede model of planning a health education program in the workplace: lessons from the Brigham back program. (Abstract #40) Arth Rheum 28 (No. 4) [Supp], 1985.

67. Woodyard JE: Injury, compensation claims and prognosis: Part II. J Soc Occup Med 30:57–60, 1980.

68. Lehmann TR, Brand RA: Disability in the patient with low back pain. Ortho Clin N Am 13:559–568, 1982.

69. Lehmann TR: Compensable back injuries and their management. J Iowa Med Soc 71:527–530, 1981.

70. Hirschfeld AH, Behan RC: The accident process: I. Etiological considerations of industrial injuries. JAMA 186:193–199, 1963.

71. Phillips AM, Weirton W: A study of prolonged absenteeism in industry. J Occup Med 575–578, 1961.

72. Maltbie AA, Cavenar JO Jr, Hammett EB, et al: A diagnostic approach to pain. Psychosomatics 19:359–366, 1978.

72a. Luoto K: The Role of Clinical Psychology in Occupational Medicine, Principles and Practice. Carl Zenz Ed., Year Book Medical Publishers, Chicago, 1975.

73. Khatami M, Rush AJ: A pilot study of the treatment of outpatients with chronic pain: Symptom control, stimulus control and social system intervention. Pain 5:163–172, 1978.

74. Diamond MD, Weiss AJ, Grynbaum B: The unmotivated patient. Arch Phys Med Rehab 49:281–284, 1968.

75. Cinciripini PM, Floreen A: An evaluation of a be-

haviour program for chronic pain. J Behav Med 5:375–389, 1982.

76. Florence DW, Miller TC: Functional overlay in work-related injury, a system for differentiating conscious from subconscious motivation of persisting symptoms. Postgrad Med 77 (No. 8):97–108, 1985.

77. Fordyce WE: An operant conditioning method for managing chronic pain. Postgrad Med 53:123–128, 1973.

78. Seamonds BC: Extension of research into stress factors and their effect on illness absenteeism. J Occup Med 25:821–822, 1983.

79. Finneson BE: Modulating effect of secondary gain on the low back pain syndrome. Advances in Pain Research and Therapy. Vol. 1. Edited by JJ Bonica, D Albe-Fessard. New York: Raven Press, 1976.

80. Neustadt DH: Commentary, psychosocial factors in rheumatic disease. Ortho Review 13:114–115, 1984.

81. Huskisson EC: Measurement of Pain. Lancet 2:1127–1131, 1974.

82. Carlsson AM: Assessment of Chronic Pain. I. Aspects of the Reliability and Validity of the Visual Analogue Scale. Pain 16:87–101, 1983.

83. Scott J, Huskisson EC: Accuracy of subjective measurements made with or without previous scores: an important source of error in serial measurement of subjective states. Ann Rheum Dis 38:558–559, 1979.

84. Feinstein AR: An additional basic science for clinical medicine: IV. The development of clinimetrics. Ann Intern Med 99:843–848, 1983.

85. Smythe HA, Goldsmith CH: 'Independent Assessor' and 'Pooled Index' as techniques for measuring treatment effects in rheumatoid arthritis. J Rheum 4:144–152, 1977.

86. Fries JF, Spitz P, Kraines RG, Holman HR: Measurement of Patient Outcome in Arthritis. Arth Rheum 23:137–145, 1980.

87. Pincus T, Summey JA, et al: Assessment of patient satisfaction in activities of daily living using a modified Stanford Health Assessment Questionnaire. Arth Rheum 26:1346–1353, 1983.

88. Ware JE, Davies-Avery A, Donald CA: Conceptualization and Measurement of Health for Adults in the Health Insurance Study. Volume V Gen Health Perceptions R-1978/5 HEW Rand Corp, 1980.

89. Melzack R: The McGill pain questionnaire: Major properties and scoring methods. Pain 1:277–299, 1975.

90. Meenan RF, Gertman PM, Mason JH: Measuring health status in arthritis: The arthritis impact measurement scales. Arth Rheum 23:146–152, 1980.

91. Bergner M, et al: The sickness Impact Profile: Validation of a health status measure. Med Care 14:57–67, 1976.

92. Liang MH, Cullen KE, Larson MG: Measuring Function and Health Status in Rheumatic Disease Clinical Trials. Clin Rheum Dis 9:531–538, 1983.

93. Liang MH, Cullen K, Larson M: In search of a more perfect mousetrap (health status or quality of life instrument). J Rheum 9:775–782, 1982.

94. Liang MH, Jette AM: Measuring functional ability in chronic arthritis. Arth Rheum 24:80–86, 1981.

95. Liang MH, Larson MG, Cullen KE, Schwartz JA: Comparative measurement efficiency and sensitivity of five health status instruments for arthritis research. Arth Rheum 28:542–547, 1985.

96. Meenan RF, Gertman PM, Mason JH, Dunaif R: The arthritis impact measurement scales. Arth Rheum 25:1048–1053, 1982.

97. Fries JF, Spitz PW, Young DY: The dimensions of health outcomes: the health assessment questionnaire, disability and pain scales. J Rheum 9:789–792, 1982.

98. Bombardier C, Tugwell P: Measuring disability; Guidelines for rheumatology studies. J Rheum [Supp] 10:68–73, 1983.

99. Brown JH, Kazis LE, Spitz PW, Gertman P, Fries JF, Meenan RF: The dimensions of health outcomes: a cross-validated examination of health status measurements. Am J Public Health 74:159–161, 1984.

100. Clark DD, Ricker JH, MacCollum MS: The efficacy of local steroid injection in the treatment of stenosing tenovaginitis. Plast Reconstr Surg 51:179–180, 1973.

101. Phalen GS: Soft tissue affections of the hand and wrist. Hosp Med 7:47–59, 1971.

101a. Otto N, Wehbé MA: Steroid injections for tenosynovitis in the hand. Orthoped Rev 15:290–293, 1986.

101b. Sonne M, Christensen K, Hansen SE, Jensen EM: Injection of steroids and local aneesthetics as therapy for low-back pain. Scand J Rheum 14:343–345, 1985.

102. Moskowitz RW: Clinical Rheumatology. 2nd Ed. Philadelphia, Lea & Febiger, 1982.

103. Sheon RP: Chapter 8. Non-Articular Rheumatism and Nerve Entrapment Syndromes. In Rheumatic Therapeutics, edited by Sanford H Roth, et al. New York, McGraw-Hill, 1985.

1

Etiology and Pathogenesis

Etiopathologic aspects of soft tissue rheumatic pain conditions to be discussed in this chapter include those pertaining to regional myofascial pain, bursitis, tendinitis, and nerve entrapment disorders. The etiology and pathogenesis of the more generalized conditions such as fibrositis, chronic persistent pain, and reflex sympathetic dystrophy are discussed in Chapter 13.

REGIONAL MYOFASCIAL PAIN AND FIBROSITIS

Whether persistent myofascial pain represents a psychophysiologic phenomenon or a localized pathologic state has been the subject of speculation for many years. The distinction between trigger points and tender points may be artificial but are presented in an effort to provide a clear separation between myofascial pain and fibrositis. See Table 1–1. Myofascial pain is a local disorder of muscle that usually occurs in one body region. The trigger point is the lesion of myofascial pain and is the result of injury. Trigger points may be latent, without symptoms; but they may be activated by acute muscle injury,

overuse, postural strain, or chilling. The pain is at a distance from the trigger point and occurs in specific locations known as target zones. Trigger points are palpable bands within muscle. Tender points, on the other hand, occur in muscle, fascia, fat, or periosteal locations, are seldom indurated, and are considered secondary phenomena at the site of referred pain. Tender points are found in fibrositis, a generalized pain disorder more fully described in Chapter 13. The trigger point, an indurated and tender zone within muscle, may represent sensitive areas over the site of innervation of the underlying muscle, where it is most accessible to percutaneous electrical stimulation.[1] A review of the world literature on trigger points has been published by Simons.[2-3] Perhaps the first reference to this subject was that of William Balfour in 1816.[4,4a]

Pathologic findings in tender points (fibrositis) are meager. Occasional reported findings include interstitial inflammatory changes,[5-7] necrosis and fibrosis,[4,8] and a metachromatic substance in interfibrillar spaces.[7]

No histopathologic changes have been re-

Table 1–1.   Features of Trigger Points and Tender Points

Feature	Trigger Point	Tender Point
Condition:	MYOFASCIAL PAIN	FIBROSITIS/FIBROMYALGIA
Tenderness and pain location:	Local tenderness variable but pain zone always distant	Tenderness and pain at same site
Local twitch after stroking:	Fiber twitch response	None
Aggravating factors:	Mechanical injury such as strain overuse, direct injury	Dampness, cold, fatigue, overuse
Local pathology:	None evident; local ischemia, or neurogenic factors suspected	Electron microscopic abnormalities: motheaten appearance; fiber atrophy, glycogen and fat deposition
Electrodiagnostic findings:	Measurable during twitch response	None reported

ported in trigger points. The "fasciitis" of myofascial pain has seldom been described histologically. The investing fascia of myofascial points was examined by Simon, Ringel, and Sufit[9] who reported normal findings in 8 of 9 patients biopsied. The one positive biopsy revealed marked lymphocytic and plasma cell infiltrates of the fascia with extension deep into the dermis. Skin and muscle was otherwise normal. In ten noninflammatory neuromuscular disease control patients, the investing fascia was histologically normal.

The presacral and gluteal fascia may be the site of trigger points and nodules. Episacroiliac lipomas or fibrofatty nodules located over trigger points about the dimple of Venus of the lower back, are common. Whether these conditions are part of myofascial pain or common accompaniments to myofascial low back pain is unclear. They may represent a fatty nodule that has herniated through the deep fascia[10] or fat encapsulated in a fibrous capsule.[11]

Fascia lata fasciitis, plantar fasciitis, and gluteal fasciitis are clinical diagnoses in which pathologic changes may be minimal or absent. This tissue has rarely been excised, biopsied, or studied. The relation of fasciitis to myofascial pain entities is unclear.

Local ischemia may play a role in *persistent* muscle induration and tenderness. The swollen muscle bundles may constrict the muscle's own blood supply. Ischemia as a cause for muscular pain has been suggested by findings of degenerated mitochondria and increased glycogen deposits in muscle fibers obtained from trapezius muscle biopsy and examined by electron microscopy.[12] However, in one study using ^{133}xenon clearance method to measure muscle blood flow, 12 patients with trigger points and matched controls were examined. Muscle blood flow results in the involved trapezius muscles were compared with controls; no difference was found.[12A]

Recently, Kalyan-Raman et al. biopsied the trapezius muscle tender points in 12 patients with fibromyalgia (fibrositis). They noted muscle fiber atrophy, segmental fiber necrosis with lipid and glycogen deposition, and subsarcolemmal mitochondrial accumulation on electron microscopy in all 12 cases. Papillary projections of sarcolemmal membrane were seen in 11/12 cases. The features were also interpreted to represent chronic muscle spasm and ischemia.[8] These findings were uncontrolled but are supported by another study.[12A] Whether findings in fibrositis can be construed as meaningful to regional myofascial pain remains to be proved.

Muscle fiber injury as a cause for the induration and abnormality of tender points is also supported by the report of Danneskiold-Samsoe et al. They measured plasma myoglobin (by radioimmunoassay) before, and after 45 minutes of massage to tender muscle areas and to control areas. A 10-fold increase in plasma myoglobin was found after tender point massage compared to the control area (quadriceps muscle) massage. Furthermore, as the measured area of tenderness receded with successive treatments, the plasma myoglobin "leakage" diminished.[13] These findings suggest inherent brittleness of muscle fibers at tender point locations. Immunologic deposits in vascular and cutaneous tissues in fibrositis/fibromyalgia will be discussed in Chapter 13.

We believe that both local and central nervous system factors operate together to create a pain-spasm-pain cycle, as discussed in later chapters. The etiology is thought to be of traumatic origin. The pathogenesis of myofascial pain may include, in addition to traumatic factors, other biochemical, metabolic, inflammatory, neurogenic, aging, and central nervous system contributions.

In many patients, a specific etiology is lacking, and the following are suggested pathogenetic mechanisms involved in perpetuating the myofascial pain disorder.

Traumatic Factors. Trauma to muscle will depend upon the state of conditioning, the degree of overuse, or in other instances, the type and severity of the injury. Injury often is associated with muscle spasm. Mechanical irritation of unmyelinated nerve fibers adjacent to intramuscular blood vessels gives rise to a dull ache and pain. Chemical changes (e.g., increase in lactic acid and potassium) in the interstitial fluid of muscle further enhances spasm and pain. These changes occur more rapidly in sedentary individuals than in athletes.[14]

Trauma must be considered more broadly than direct blows to muscle. In fact, most cases of persistent myofascial pain results from so-called "microtrauma of daily living" including many instances of improper body mechanics. Static work postures such as prolonged sitting or working bent over; frequent bending and twisting; forceful or sudden unexpected movements; repetitive work motions; and vibration exposure, such as working on trains or buses or riding tractors are potential forms of microtrauma.

Mild structural disorders may result in microtrauma. For example, in some patients with scapular-region myofascial pain, muscle injury results from such structural problems as scoliosis, round-shouldered posture, or from sagging of the upper limb as a result of neurologic diseases.[15]

Pain-induced inactivity might prolong myofascial pain. Conversely, the rate of healing has been thought to be hastened by early mobilization. Kvist and Jarvinen tested this hypothesis in rats and noted that histologic evidence of healing with scar formation and muscle regeneration occurred more rapidly and more intensively in mobilized than in immobilized rats. Microangiographic studies also showed faster revascularization and recovery of breaking strength of injured muscle in the mobilized group. Similar studies carried out in man are needed.[16]

Biochemical Factors. Local biochemical and metabolic factors may be important. Tissue damage results in the liberation of intracellular chemical substances (so-called pain substances) into the extracellular fluid surrounding nerve endings.[17] Prostaglandins E and F may be important. The former, if allowed to persist at the site of injury can render the area painful for several weeks.[18] Both substances are involved in increased vascular

permeability, edema, and fibrosis.[14,19] Use of magnetic resonance imaging to study muscle metabolism and disease is of increasing interest and may provide additional clues in a noninvasive fashion.[20-21] The rate of glycolysis during mild and severe muscle contraction can be estimated by this technique and subtle myopathies may thus be detected.

Specific metabolic or chemical etiologies for regional myofascial pain are often lacking but must be considered. For example, Mills and Edwards reported results of investigations, including biopsy of the muscle in 109 consecutive patients seen for the chief complaint of muscle pain. They found endocrine and enzymatic myopathies in 22 cases, inflammatory rheumatic disease in 8 cases, and neurogenic causes in 7 instances; in 72 patients they were unable to find any histologic diagnosis.[22] Whether these patients had myofascial pain is unclear. Trigger points and tender points are absent in most cases of myopathy. Thus, careful assessment for generalized myopathic disease states must be considered if trigger points are *not* detected. Other disorders to be differentiated include polymyalgia rheumatica and other inflammatory rheumatic diseases, alcoholism, metabolic bone diseases, defects in muscle energy metabolism, myoadenylate deaminase deficiency,[23-24] idiopathic paroxysmal myoglobinurias, muscle pain syndromes of unknown etiology, and drug induced myopathies. Drugs to be considered as pathogenic factors in myopathies include anticonvulsants, heroin, amphetamines, clofibrate, epsilon aminocaproic acid, vincristine, emetine, cimetidine, diuretics, laxatives, and licorice. Muscle cramp and fasciculation may further result from use of clofibrate, lithium, and cytotoxic drugs.[25] Thus the requirement for a careful history and examination, is stressed. The distinction between myofascial pain with trigger points and myopathies is usually not difficult.

Aging Factors. Muscle atrophy, an expected accompaniment of the aging process, is thought to result from progressive disuse, gradual neurotrophic (functional denervation) disturbances, environmental, and genetic factors. In one study comparing muscle biopsies in men whose age ranged from 22 to 65 years, findings showed a linear decrease in the proportion of type II fibers and decreased fiber diameter with increasing age; oxidative enzyme studies suggested an increased oxidative capacity per muscle unit with aging. The expected decrease in strength in old age was not accompanied by measurable changes in gross muscle size (e.g., thigh circumference). Rather the decrease in strength correlated to the type II fiber area.[26]

Slowing of the patellar reflex and nerve conduction velocity also occurs with aging.[26] Practical experience suggests that older patients do respond to conditioning programs; the results are similar to younger patients, but they just take a little longer before results are noted.

TENDINITIS

Tendon sheaths, like bursae, develop in response to motion. Tendons pull and transmit power. Some tendons are short and without sheaths. They are supplied with blood from their muscular origin and from the investing paratenon. Where there is excessive motion, the tendon is enveloped in a synovial sheath. The visceral sheath has a flat synovial lining, the parietal layer has vesicular and granular patches; there is no basement membrane, only a fatty or collagenous connective tissue.[27] Tendon healing is facilitated by an intact tendon sheath. Tendinitis was first described in 1763.[27a]

Tendon function can be impaired by local trauma, systemic disease, inflammation, fibrosis, impaired blood supply, atrophy or degeneration.[27–29] In most cases of chronic nonspecific tendinitis the upper limb is involved, and in 20% triggering occurs.[30] Snapping or "triggering" of joint movement can be due to nodular enlargement of the tendon, stenosis of the sheath, or both. Triggering—a momentary locking up of joint motion—can result from diverse etiologies, the most common of which is excessive repetitive hand use.

Other causes include anomalous muscles,[31] stenosing tenosynovitis at the wrist,[32] and as a familial disorder.[33] In most cases a stenosing tenosynovitis is found. Impingement of tendons between bone or ligamentous structures, most common at the shoulder, can result from repetitive motion of bone and a constricting second bone or ligamentous band.[35–36]

Inflammatory tendinitis may precede or accompany many systemic disorders ranging from tuberculosis, gonorrhea, and other infectious causes; rheumatic fever, rheumatoid arthritis, and other connective tissue diseases; gout, pseudogout, apatite deposition disease, hyperlipidemias, ochronosis and other metabolic disorders; giant cell tumors of tendon sheaths, and pigmented villonodular synovitis.[27,29,36]

Dystrophic calcareous deposits in tendons and bursae that develop after injury or inflammation, are of uncertain pathogenesis.[27] Amorphous calcium or urate do not provoke inflammation, whereas crystals do. Calcific tendinitis may result from apatite or calcium pyrophosphate (pseudogout) deposition disease after the calcific deposits erupt out of the tendon into the tendon sheath or bursa. Attacks of calcific tendinitis have a predilection for the shoulder, wrist and ankle. Other types of crystals deposited in soft tissues include monosodium urate, oxypyurinol, xanthine, hypoxanthine, calcium oxalate, and various other calcium and lipid crystals.[37] Hydroxyapatite, the most common type of calcification, is thought to precipitate as a result of a preceding degenerative process.

The enthesis, the site of attachment of a ligament or muscle into bone, is involved in a wide variety of diseases. Thirty-nine such sites have been described.[29] They have specialized nerve endings, and the bone is not covered by periosteum. The tendon fibers pass directly into Sharpey's fibers of bone. The tendon widens and attaches in a fanlike zone of attachment and hyaline cartilage is interposed at this site. The peritenon, perichondrium and periosteum are connected to each other and contain much of the blood supply. This site is vulnerable to inflammation and is the typical site of involvement in patients with HLA-B27 associated spondyloarthropathies. Osteoarthritis has a predilection for this site as does ochronosis, calcium apatite deposition disease, hypoparathyroidism, osteomalacia, fluorosis, and acromegaly. Ischemia also plays an important role in degenerative lesions at these attachment sites.[29]

Injury at these sites frequently is the result of conditioning and sport activities. A large gap exists between physiologic loads and the stress needed to cause tendon failure. Following a stress of as much as 17 times the body weight, a tendon can recover if given adequate time.[38] Reapplying the force before recovery may lead to tendon rupture. Tendons are most vulnerable when tension is applied quickly, when tension is applied obliquely, when the tendon is tensed before trauma, when the attached muscle is maximally innervated, when the muscle group is stretched by external stimuli, or when the tendon is weak in comparison to muscle. With increasing strains that elongate a tendon, some of the cross links between neighboring molecules break, and as more links break, the weakest fibers rupture. The load is then increased on the remaining fibers. Initial lesions are probably molecular, and with shearing force, the microvasculature is probably injured.[38] This leads to decreased oxygen, nutrition, and rupture of the cross links between tropocollagen molecules. Chronic strain results in marked degenerative changes with focal necrosis and hemorrhage into the tendinous and cartilaginous tissues, followed by reparative tissue changes.

The amount of acid mucopolysaccharides in small "lake-like accumulations" between fibers is distinctly different from that found in the aging process.[39] Vascular proliferation is a regular feature in these tendon lesions, and signifies reparative processes.[39–40]

Acute overuse tenosynovitis may be serous or fibrinous, the latter sometimes is referred to as "peritendonitis crepitans."[36] The basic feature is an inflammation due to changes in permeability of the cell membranes. Release of mediators of inflammation is followed by pain and edema, leading to impaired circulation. Fibrin deposits then become organized and are followed by adhesions.[16] Prolonged overstrain and inflammation results in similar pathologic changes. Electron microscopic findings suggest simultaneous degeneration and repair in chronic tendinitis.[40]

In summary, the pathologic findings of tendinitis are variable and may include features of degeneration, fibrin deposition, increased vascularity, edema, and occasionally, inflammation. The pathologic condition in typical lesions is presented in Figures 1–1 to 1–3. However, if the tenosynovitis is secondary to a systemic disease, then features characteristic of that disease are found.

BURSITIS

An atlas of the bursae was published by Monro in 1788.[27b] Bursae are formed in response to movement. They are lined by synovial cells that secrete collagen, proteoglycans, collagenases and other enzymes. Subcutaneous bursae, such as the olecranon, are formed after birth and develop in response to friction. Deep bursae develop in utero.[27,41] "Adventitious" bursae (superficial cutaneous bursae) form in response to shearing stress at the first metatarsophalangeal joint (bunion), over exostoses, and over prominent spinous processes.[27]

The normal bursa consists of a thin layer of sparse synoval cells supported by an adipose, reticular, and a fibrous layer. Synovianalysis of normal bursal fluid has not been reported; it consists of a thin fluid film. Traumatic fluid is hemorrhagic or xanthochromic, with fair to poor mucin clot. Glucose content may be 80% of serum levels. Mononuclear cells predominate.[41] Traumatic inflammation of the deep bursae results in the synovial cell lining becoming denuded in places with fibrin deposits, and the bursal walls become thickened. In some cases of metatarsal bursitis, the bursal wall showed fibrinoid necrosis.[42]

In addition to trauma or friction, other causes for inflammation of the bursae include

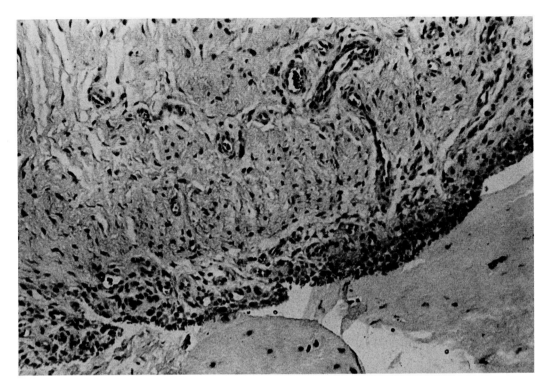

Fig. 1–1. DeQuervain's disease. Tenosynovium with slight synoviocyte hyperplasia and inflammation.

septic, metabolic, hematologic, and inflammatory connective tissue diseases. Also, villonodular synovial lesions may develop in bursae. Septic bursitis most often arises in the subcutaneous bursae (olecranon, bunion area, and prepatellar bursae); the inflammatory response in septic bursitis is less intense than that of joints. The septic bursal fluid white blood count may range from only 1200 cells upward and the bursal sugar content may not be as depressed as that of septic joint synovial fluid.[43–44] This is thought to be due to the lesser vascularity of bursae as compared to synovial membranes.[41]

Gout, pseudogout, and calcium apatite deposition disease frequently cause bursitis. Intense inflammation follows, resulting in local warmth, redness, and exquisite tenderness. Calcium apatite deposition disease may affect tendons, tendon sheaths, joint synovium, and bursae. Roentgenographic evidence of calcification is noted. Involvement of the shoulder, elbow, wrist, hip, knee, and ankle are well known.[45–46] The pathogenesis involves a number of inflammatory pathways. Severe destruction of the shoulder cuff in association with calcium apatite deposition, the "Milwaukee shoulder", results from collagenase and neutral protease activity. Enzymatic release of hydroxyapatite crystals from the synovium and endocytosis by synovial macrophage-like cells with subsequent crystal stimulated release of the enzymes complete a pathogenetic cycle.[47] Hydroxyapatite crystal deposition also occurs in patients with hyperlipidemia, gout, diabetes, and in association with HLA-BW35 and HLA-A2 genes.[37]

Villonodular synovitis and Gaucher's disease may result in a hemorrhagic bursitis.[48] Thus, in addition to trauma, the bursae may be afflicted by all the diseases that affect synovial joints, but the synovial fluid response is usually less intense.

NERVE ENTRAPMENT DISORDERS

Entrapment neuropathies[49] occur at many locations where neurovascular compression

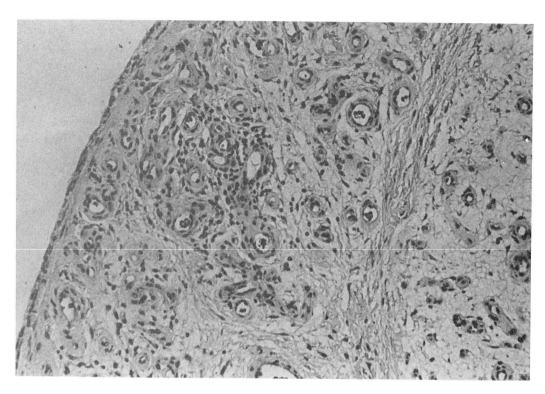

Fig. 1–2. DeQuervain's disease. Increased vascularity and slight perivascular cuffing by lymphocytes. (H&E × 100)

causes localized nerve damage. In addition, entrapment may result from direct external nerve compression or contusion from work, hobby, or sport activities including such entities as harp player's thumb, bowler's thumb; or by a constricting watch or belt.[50] Structural abnormalities such as a cervical rib, anomalous nerves, muscles, or bands may constrict adjacent nerves.[51–52] Stenosis of the cervical spinal canal[53] or lumbar spinal canal[54] results in both neurologic and vascular impairment. A peripheral neuropathy may coexist and create significant diagnostic confusion. The more common sites for nerve entrapment are the thoracic outlet, the cervical and lumbar spine, the coraco-acromial arch, the elbow, the wrist and hand, the pelvic region, the popliteal region, and the ankle and foot.[55–56]

The carpal tunnel syndrome is the most common entrapment neuropathy and was first reported in 1913.[56a] Median nerve impingement may result from diseases that invade the carpal tunnel, from swelling of the tendon sheaths within the tunnel, from stenosis of the tunnel by bone enlargement, or from thickening and degeneration of the volar carpal ligament. The elliptically shaped space enclosed by the inelastic flexor retinaculum ventrally and the carpal bones dorsally contains eight deep and superficial flexor tendons and their sheaths, the flexor pollicis longus tendon and sheath, and the median nerve. Occasionally, the space also contains the radial and ulnar palmar bursae, or the median artery.[57] The application of computed tomography to the carpal canal has suggested that the bony canal may become stenosed. Normal and affected women had significantly smaller carpal canals than healthy males and carpal size was inversely proportional to age. Hand size alone did not correlate with the development of a carpal tunnel syndrome.[58] A genetic propensity toward carpal tunnel stenosis has been suggested.[59]

The nerve compression may result from externally applied trauma or from factors within

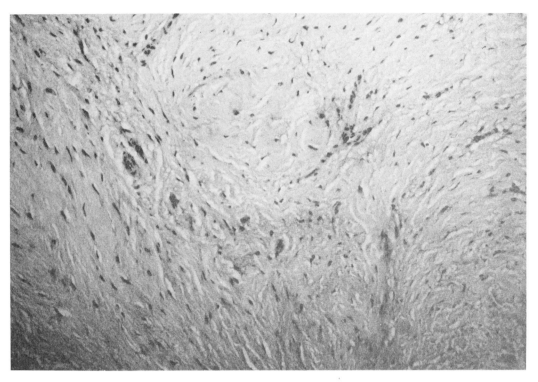

Fig. 1–3. Trigger thumb. Tenosynovium with marked collagenized fibrosis. Note lack of vascularity, inflammation or edema. (H&E ×100)

the canal such as tenosynovitis due to systemic rheumatic disorders, thickening of the retinaculum, hypertrophy of muscles, infiltrative diseases of the canal such as amyloid, myeloma, or myxedema, or bone involvement by disease or tumor. Nerve compression can result from synovitis of the long flexor tendons due to overuse,[60] fluid retention states, and systemic inflammation. Aberrant or hypertrophied muscles may also be found as contributing factors.[55] Overuse is thought to be a precipitating event rather than a primary etiologic factor in carpal tunnel syndrome.[61]

In cases of carpal tunnel syndrome, histologic examination reveals an increase in perineurial and endoneurial connective tissue and a marked reduction in the caliber of the nerve fibers.[61] Pathologic findings are so variable that they provide few clues to the mechanism responsible for impaired nerve conduction.

A complex pressure system operates within the canal.[61] Pressure within the carpal canal rises 3-fold during flexion or extension.[62] Once the carpal canal pressure rises, progressive nerve involvement occurs with edema of nerve tissue. Anoxia, caused by venous congestion and stasis, may be the end result.[61]

REFERENCES

1. Gunn CC, Milbrandt WE, Little AS, Mason KE: Dry needling of muscle motor points for chronic low-back pain. Spine 5:279–291, 1980.
2. Simons DG: Muscle pain syndromes—Part I. Am J Phys Med 54:289–311, 1975.
3. Simons DG: Muscle pain syndromes—part II. Am J Phys Med 55:15–42, 1976.
4. Reynolds MD: The development of the concept of fibrositis. J Hist Med & Allied Sci 38:5–35, 1983.
4a. Balfour W: Illustrations of the efficacy of compression and percussion in the cure of rheumatism and sprains, scrofulous affections of the joints and spine, chronic pains arising from a scrofulous taint in the constitution, lameness, and loss of power in the

hands from gout, paralytic debility of the extremities, general derangement of the nervous system; and in promoting digestion, with all the secretions and excretions. Lon Med Phys J 51:446–462; 52:104–115, 200–208, 284–291, 1824.

5. Abel O, Siebert WJ, Earp R: Fibrositis. J Missouri Med Assn 36:435, 1939.

6. Awad EA: Interstitial myofibrositis: Hypotheses of the mechanism. Arch Phys. Med Rehabil 54:449–453, 1973.

7. Brendstrup P, Jespersen K, Asboe-Hansen G: Morphological and chemical connective tissue changes in fibrositic muscles. Ann Rheum Dis 16:438–440, 1957.

8. Kalyan-Raman UP, Kalyan-Raman K, Yunus MB, Masi AT: Muscle pathology in primary fibromyalgia syndrome: A light microscopic histochemical and ultrastructural study. J Rheum 11:808–813, 1984.

9. Simon DB, Ringel SP, Sufit RL: Clinical spectrum of fascial inflammation. Muscle Nerve (Sept):525–537, 1982.

10. Singewald ML: Sacroiliac lipomata—an often unrecognized cause of low back pain. Johns Hopkins Med J 118:492–498, 1966.

11. Ries E: Episacroiliac lipoma. Am J Obst Gyn 34:490–494, 1937.

12. Fassbender HG, Wegner K: Morphologie und Pathogenese des Weichteilrheumatismus. Z Rheumaforsch 32:355, 1973.

12A. Klemp P, Nielsen HV, Korsgard J: Blood flow in fibromyotic muscles. Scand J Rehab 14:81–82, 1982.

12B. Henriksson KG, Bengtsson A, Larsson J, et al.: Muscle biopsy findings of possible diagnostic importance in primary fibromyalgia (fibrositis, myofascial syndrome). Lancet 2:1395, 1982.

13. Danneskiold-Samsoe B, Christiansen E, Lund B, Andersen RB: Regional Muscle Tension and Pain (Fibrositis). Scand J Rehab Med 15:17–20, 1982.

14. Hazelman BL, Laurin CA, Tremblay GR: Chapter 10. The injured joint with a 'normal' x-ray. Textbook of Rheumatology, edited by WH Kelley et al. Philadelphia, WB Saunders, 1985.

15. Cohen CA: Scapulocostal syndrome: Diagnosis and treatment. Southern Med J 73:433–437, 1980.

16. Kvist M, Jarvinen M: Clinical, histochemical and biomechanical features in repair of muscle and tendon injuries. Int J Sports Med 3:12–14, 1982.

17. Bonica JJ: Neurophysiologic and pathologic aspects of acute and chronic pain. Arch Surg 112:750–761, 1977.

18. Anderson NH, Ramwell PW: Biological aspects of prostaglandins. Arch Intern Med 133:30, 1974.

19. Muckle DS: Soft tissue trauma: sprains, strains, etc. Clin Rheum Dis 5:927–939, 1979.

20. Edwards RHT, Dawson MJ, Wilke DR, Gordon RE, Shaw D: Clinical use of nuclear magnetic resonance in the investigation of myopathy. Lancet 1:725–731, 1982.

21. Arnold DL, Radda GK., Bore PJ, Styles P, Taylor DJ: Excessive intracellular acidosis of skeletal muscle on exercise in a patient with post-viral exhaustion/fatigue syndrome. Lancet 1:1367–1368, 1984.

22. Mills KR, Edwards RHT: Investigative strategies for muscle pain. J Neuro Sci 58:73–88, 1983.

23. Valen PA, Nakayama DA, Veum JA, Wortmann RL: Myoadenylate deaminase deficiency: diagnosis by forearm ischemic exercise testing and oxypurine. (Abstract #A26) Arth Rheum 27:(4) [Supp], 1984.

24. Gertler PA, Jacobs RP: Myoadenylate deaminase deficiency in a patient with progressive systemic sclerosis. Arth Rheum 27:586–590, 1984.

25. Morgan-Hughes JA: Painful disorders of muscle. Br J Hosp Med 22:360–365, 1979.

26. Larrson L: Morphological and functional characteristics of the ageing skeletal muscle in man. A cross-sectional study. Acta Phys Scand ([Supp]) 457:3–36, 1978.

27. Bywaters EGL: Lesions of bursae, tendons and tendon sheaths. Clin Rheum Dis 5:883–926, 1979.

27a. DeSauvages de la Croix FB: Nosologia Methodica Sistens Morborum Classes, Genera et Species Juxta Sydenhami Mentum et Botanicorum Ordinem. Amsterdam, 1763.

27b. Monro A (Secundus): A Description of All the Bursae Mucosae of the Human Body. Edinburgh, Elliot, 1788.

28. Borgsmiller WK, Whiteside LA: Tuberculous tenosynovitis of the hand ("Compound palmar ganglion"): Literature review and case report. Orthopaedics 3:1093–1096, 1980.

29. Niepel GA, Sit'aj S: Enthesopathy. Clin Rheum Dis 5:857–863, 1979.

30. Lipscomb PR: Chronic nonspecific tenosynovitis and peritendinitis. Surg Clin N Am 24:780–797, 1944.

31. Aghasi MK, Rzetelny V, Axer A: The flexor digitorum superficialis as a cause of bilateral carpal-tunnel syndrome and trigger wrist. J Bone Joint Surg 62-A:134–135, 1980.

32. Parker HG: Dupuytren's Contracture as a cause of stenosing tenosynovitis. J Maine Med Assoc 70:147–148, 1979.

33. Weber PC: Trigger thumb in successive generations of a family. Clin Orthop 143:167, 1979.

34. Neer CS, II: The shoulder in sports. Orthop Clin N Am 8:583–591, 1977.

35. Hawkins RJ, Hobeika P: Physical examination of the shoulder. Ortho 6:1270–1278, 1983.

36. Moritz AR: The Pathology of Trauma. 2nd Ed. Philadelphia, Lea & Febiger, 1954.

37. Dieppe PA, Huskisson EC, Crocker P, Willoughby DA: Apatite deposition disease: A new arthropathy. Lancet 1:266–268, 1976.

38. Curwin S, Stanish WD: Tendinitis: its etiology and treatment. Lexington, Mass. The Collamore Press, 1984.

39. Merkel KHH, Hess H, Kunz M: Insertional tendopathy. Pathol Res Pract 173:303–309, 1982.

40. Sarkar K, Uhthoff HK: Ultrastructure of the common extensor tendon in tennis elbow. Virchows Arch A Pathol Anat Histol 386:317–330, 1980.

41. Canoso JJ, Yood RA: Reaction of superficial bursae in response to specific disease stimuli. Arth Rheum 22:1361–1364, 1979.

42. Bossley CJ, Cairney PC: The intermetatarsophalangeal bursa—its significance in Morton's metatarsalgia. J Bone Joint Surg 62B:184–187, 1980.

43. Thompson GR, Manshady BM, Weiss JJ: Septic bursitis. JAMA 240:2280–2281, 1978.

44. Ho G Jr, Tice AD: Comparison of nonseptic and septic bursitis: Further observations on the treat-

ment of septic bursitis. Arch Intern Med 139:1269–1273, 1979.

45. Pinals RS, Short CL: Calcific periarthritis involving multiple sites. Arth Rheum 9:566–574, 1966.

46. Fam AG, Pritzker KPH, Stein JL, Houpt JB, Little AH: Apatite-associated arthopathy: A clinical study of 14 cases, 2 with calcific bursitis. J Rheum 6:461–470, 1979.

47. Halverson PB, Cheung HS, McCarty DJ, et al.: "Milwaukee shoulder"—Association of microspheroids containing hydroxyapatite crystals with rotator cuff defects. II. Synovial fluid studies. Arth Rheum 24:474–476, 1981.

48. Gelfand G, Bienenstock H: Hemorrhagic Bursitis and Bone Crises in Chronic Adult Gaucher's Disease: A case report. Arth Rheum 25:1369–1373, 1982.

49. Kopell HP, Thompson WAL: Peripheral Entrapment Neuropathies. Huntington NY: RE Krieger, 1976.

50. Goldner JL: Symposium: upper extremity nerve entrapment syndrome. Contemp Ortho 6:89–112, 1983.

51. Levy M, Goldberg I: Four unusual causes of carpal tunnel syndrome. Orthop Rev 11:67–73, 1982.

52. Moss SH, Switzer HE: Radial tunnel syndrome: A spectrum of clinical presentations. J Hand Surg 8:414–420, 1983.

53. Hashimoto I, Tak YK: The true sagittal diameter of the cervical spinal canal and its diagnostic signifi-

cance in cervical myelopathy. J Neurosurg 47:912–916, 1977.

54. Choudhury AR, Taylor JC: Occult lumbar spinal stenosis. J Neuro Neurosurg Psych 40:506–510, 1977.

55. Wakefield G: Entrapment neuropathies. Clin Rheum Dis 5:941–956, 1979.

56. Sunderland S: The nerve lesion in the carpal tunnel syndrome. J Neurology, Neurosurg, Psych 39:615–626, 1976.

56a. Marie, Pierre, et Foix: Atrophie isolee de l'eminence thenar d'origine nevritique. Role du ligament annulaire anterieur du carpe dans la pathogenie do la lesion. Rev Neurol 26:647–649, 1913.

57. Zucker-Pinchoff B, Hermann G, et al: Computed tomography of the carpal tunnel radioanatomical study. J Comput Assist Tomography 5:525–528, 1981.

58. Armstrong TJ, Chaffin DB: Carpal tunnel syndrome and selected personal attributes. J Occup Med 21:481–486, 1979.

59. Dekel S, Papaioannou T, Rushworth G, Coates R: Idiopathic carpal tunnel syndrome caused by carpal stenosis. Br Med J 120:1297–1303, 1980.

60. Phalen GS: Soft tissue affections of the hand and wrist. Hosp Med 7:47–59, 1971.

61. Sunderland S: Nerve and Nerve Injuries. New York, Churchill Livingstone, 1978.

62. Werner CO, Elmqvist D, Ohlin P: Pressure and nerve lesion in the carpal tunnel. Acta Ortho Scand 54:312–314, 1983.

2

The Head and Neck

Pain in the head or neck region may be due to many different structures and etiologies. Sometimes a combination of these occur and complicate the evaluation. Physical examination maneuvers and trigger point identification often provide diagnostically useful information. The disorders described in this chapter can be recognized and treated satisfactorily in the office without time-consuming or expensive investigation in most cases.

If the physical examination reveals limitation of neck motion or loss of the normal cervical lordosis then roentgenographic examination should be carried out. The clinician should personally review the films to best determine if roentgenographic findings correlate with the patient's clinical presentation.[1] Table 2–1 details a list of danger signs and symptoms that should alert the clinician to conduct an especially detailed examination.

TEMPOROMANDIBULAR JOINT DYSFUNCTION SYNDROME

A common pain disorder, temporomandibular joint *dysfunction* syndrome (TMJDS) may result from anxiety or stress associated with unconscious jaw closing movements.[2,3] Less often, similar distressing pain can result from *organic* diseases of the temporomandibular joint. Organic etiologies incude sublux-

Table 2–1. Danger Signs

1. Fever and chills
2. Intense headache or spasmodic stabbing pains
3. Mental dullness
4. Visible swelling
5. Swollen lymph glands
6. Blood in the ear, nose, or mouth
7. Disturbed vision, smell, or taste
8. Numbness or weakness

ation and trauma, systemic inflammatory disease (e.g., rheumatoid arthritis, ankylosing spondylitis, or infection), and neoplasm.[4,5] As is often true of degenerative joint disease found elsewhere,[5-7] degenerative changes of the temporomandibular joint are poorly correlated with symptoms. Similarly, occlusal abnormalities correlate poorly with pain.[3]

Patients with temporomandibular joint dysfunction syndrome present with chronic pain in the jaw region with occasional pain radiating to the ear and neck. This syndrome is commonly seen in young to middle-aged females.[3,8] Temporomandibular joint noises, irregular mandibular movements, and limitation of jaw motion may accompany the pain. A sensation of pressure in the ear, or tinnitus sometimes delays recognition of the syndrome. Bruxism, grinding the teeth or clenching the jaw during sleep, is common. The pain is aggravated by chewing, by yawning, and sometimes by talking. Often the jaw deviates to one side during movement. In one study, migraine headaches were ten times more frequent in this patient population.[8a]

TMJ examination begins with inspection from the front. The patient is asked to open and close his mouth so that any jaw deviation may be noted. Then palpate over the joint as the mouth is opened and closed. To elicit joint tenderness, place the tips of the forefingers behind the tragi at each external acoustic meatus, and pull forward while the patient opens the mouth.[10]

Next, palpate the medial pterygoid muscles located at the back of the mouth within the tonsillar pillars. A gloved finger is introduced into the mouth and gentle palpation causes mild to exquisite pain (Fig. 2–1). Before attempting the examination, the clinician should warn the patient not to bite!

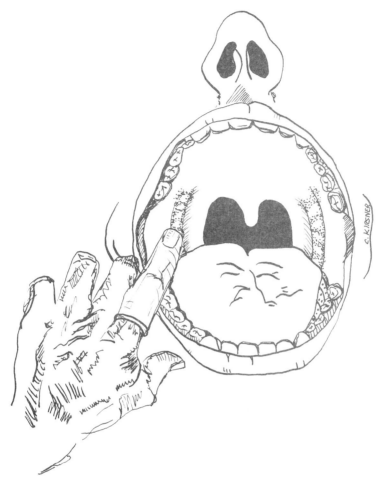

Fig. 2–1. Using a gloved finger, the examiner palpates the internal (medial) pterygoid muscle within the anterior pillar of the mouth. Each side is compared for pain reproduction. Tenderness is elicited on the symptomatic side.

Etiology. The temporomandibular joint dysfunction syndrome is often associated with malocclusion, which may be a cause for, or may result from, the chronic muscle tension compressing the joint.[5] Costen's syndrome (temporomandibular joint pain, limited joint excursion, hearing deficits, and headaches)[10] has been reassessed in the light of myofascial pain mechanisms,[11] and this eponym has been abandoned. The temporomandibular joint dysfunction syndrome may result from the use of cervical traction, dental manipulation, trauma, or most often, from muscle fatigue due to jaw clenching.[5]

In a controlled study in which direct measurements of nocturnal tooth contact were taken by continuous computer monitoring, Trenouth demonstrated that most patients with TMJDS had bruxism at night, whether they were aware of it or not. Tooth contact occurred an average of 360 times per night in normal volunteers (n = 10), 1325 times in patients with known bruxism (n = 9), and 999 times in patients (n = 6) without known bruxism. In addition, the duration of nocturnal tooth contact was 5.4 minutes per night for the control group, 38.7 minutes in the bruxism group, and 11.5 minutes in those without bruxism. Overall, evidence for tooth grinding was found in 78% of patients.[12]

Jaw clenching, in turn, is often due to anxiety and leads to a myofascial syndrome with a trigger point in the pterygoid musculature. However, psychologic investigation has yielded conflicting information.[13,14] Although these patients usually suffer from anxiety, the psychoneurosis apparently does not interfere with the response to treatment. One exception appeared to be those with a severely disturbed capacity for interpersonal relationships; they were found least likely to gain from therapy.[15]

Radiographic changes, including erosions of the mandibular condyle or degenerative arthritis are difficult to relate to symptoms. Toller found no correlation of erosions to symptoms.[7] After 5 years of follow-up, 52% of patients with temporomandibular joint pain and *erosions* had relief from pain and radiographic *improvement*. This radiographic improvement of the erosion followed treatment that included a single corticosteroid injection of the temporomandibular joint. The relief from chronic joint compression may have allowed healing to occur.

The most severe degenerative joint changes were found in those patients who had the poorest results from therapy.[7] Persistent joint compression by the temporomandibular joint dysfunction syndrome may lead to degenerative arthritis.[5]

Laboratory and Radiographic Examination. Radiographic examination of the temporomandibular joint should be obtained if symptoms are persistent (rather than intermittent) or other features suggest tumor or infection. Erosions are not of prognostic significance.[7] Arthrography of the temporomandibular joint is an expensive and invasive procedure, not without risk. It should be used with careful patient selection. Evaluation of articular disc disease and its clinical significance is still the subject of more definitive study. The erythrocyte sedimentation rate is normal in the temporomandibular joint dysfunction syndrome. Leukocytosis, anemia, or an abnormal sedimentation rate suggests organic disorders.

Differential Diagnosis. Exclusion of organic disease as a cause for symptoms is essential. Inflammatory rheumatic diseases affecting the temporomandibular joint (such as rheumatoid arthritis or ankylosing spondylitis) rarely cause joint swelling.[6] Looking at the patient as a whole for evidence of other joint swelling is important to exclude systemic inflammatory disease and arthritis. Examination of the neck, teeth, tonsils, and cervical lymph nodes to exclude regional infection is necessary, but only a minority of patients have underlying organic disease.[17]

Management. Treatment obviously requires the exclusion of mechanical and inflammatory diseases. Patients with temporomandibular joint dysfunction syndrome may require dental evaluation for occlusive abnormalities and possible correction. Furthermore, a joint spacer (also called a bite plate or bite plate appliance) is helpful when used during sleep.[3,6,8,18] The acrylic bite plate appliance acts to gently stretch the pterygoid muscles and prevents jaw clenching during sleep (Fig. 2–2). Its use should be continued for at least several months. Although some dentists think these retainers are nothing more than placebos, others feel they prevent damage to the joint.[12] The use of an occlusal splint in patients with clicking provided relief in 40% of patients, improvement in 85% with TMJ pain and improved symptoms in 88% with pain primarily of muscular origin. The splint was used over periods of 1 to 12 months.[19] Our experience has been similar. Some patients with accompanying neck pain can be helped by proper sleep instructions. The patient should sleep with a thin pillow that holds the neck in a neutral position. A neck contour pillow or a Jackson pillow (a soft tubular pillow) may assist the patient in attaining the proper sleep position. Isometric jaw exercises are helpful. See Jaw-Balancing exercises, Table 2–5 and Figure 2–3. Jaw relaxation during the day may be provided by the acrylic bite plate appliance. Nocturnal sedation is helpful during the first few weeks.

Outcome and Additional Suggestions. The outcome is satisfactory in most patients with temporomandibular joint dysfunction syndrome.[3,20,21] The bite plate appliance should

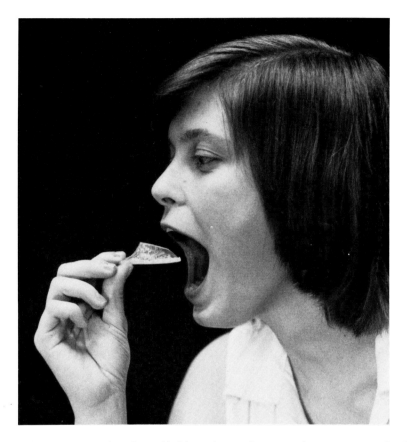

Fig. 2–2. One of several types of acrylic molded bite plate appliances used to prevent jaw clenching and to provide gentle stretching of the pterygoid muscle. (Courtesy Dr. Richard M. Klein.)

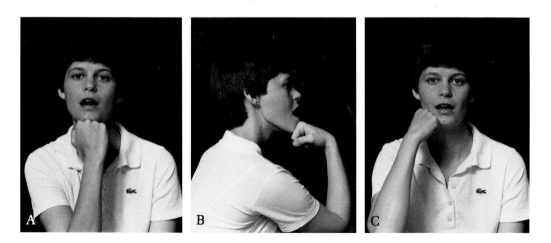

Fig. 2–3. Isometric jaw exercises: The jaw is opened an inch, then thrust against the immovable fist placed *(A)* under the jaw, *(B)* in front of the mandible, and *(C)* to each side of the jaw. The mandible is held with medium effort for 20 seconds and repeated three times in each direction.

be worn for some time after symptoms are relieved.

If, in follow-up, the patient has not responded, a single injection of a corticosteroid-local anesthetic mixture into the temporomandibular joint (Fig. 2–4) may provide pain relief with subsequent relaxation of the pterygoid muscles and allow the rest of the treatment program to take hold. Biofeedback has been advocated by some for patients without depression, and in whom symptoms have been less than 2 or 3 years' duration.[22] For the few patients who fail to benefit after these measures have been applied, reassessment of the patient, both from a mechanical and psychological standpoint, is indicated. The patient, obviously, will be concerned with coping with the chronic pain. Often, the addition of a tricyclic antidepressant is helpful (see Chapt. 13).

A special situation exists when temporomandibular joint pain occurs in a patient with previously established rheumatoid arthritis.

Rheumatoid synovitis of the temporomandibular joint produces constant muscle spasm, and the patient cannot fully open the jaw. The joint should be injected with a steroid-local anesthetic mixture on the first visit. Instead of an acrylic bite plate appliance, the patient should be instructed to obtain 3 or 4 corks, ranging in size up to 1½ inches in diameter. Several times a day the patient should insert the series of corks between the front teeth, beginning with the smallest cork. Each is held in place for 1 minute. Relief from pain and return to normal function is expected within 10 days.[6]

ANTERIOR NECK AND FACE PAIN

Pain about the face and anterior neck and throat may arise in any of the soft tissues including vessels, nerves, ligaments and muscles. See Anatomic Plate I.

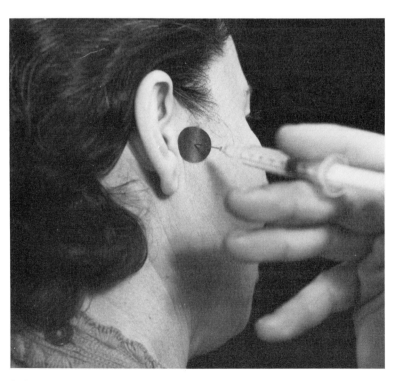

Fig. 2–4. With the mouth open, the temporomandibular joint may be injected using a No. 25 or No. 27 short needle with 1 ml of medication.

Table 2–2. Management of Temporomandibular Joint Dysfunction Syndrome

1. Exclude infections and inflammatory diseases.
2. Recognize aggravating factors (e.g., spasm, jaw muscle fatigue, dental malocclusion, anxiety, or stress).
3. Eliminate nocturnal jaw clenching with an acrylic bite plate appliance.
4. Provide dental care if indicated.
5. Provide jaw exercises.
6. Provide muscle relaxants, sedatives, and amitriptyline or similar tricyclic compounds at bedtime.
7. Perform local anesthetic-corticosteroid joint injections for persistent symptoms.

Vascular Neck and Face Pain (Carotidynia)

Young and middle-aged men and women with this disorder, often with a past history or family history of migraine, present with persistent or intermittent aching pain over one temporomandibular joint, radiating forward along the mandible, up to the temple and into the ear.[23] The pain is described either as a dull ache or as an intermittent throbbing. Often, these patients have seen a dentist and otolaryngologist to no avail. Muscle contraction headache may coexist. Visual abnormalities do not occur. Jaw motion is normal. Physical examination reveals tenderness and sometimes palpable swelling of the external carotid artery.[24] Gentle pressure upon the external carotid artery often reproduces and intensifies the neck and facial pain (Fig. 2–5). Examination and comparison of the carotid vessels on each side of the neck may reveal unilateral swelling or tenderness of the involved vessel. Trigger points within the trapezius and posterior neck muscles commonly coexist. Tenderness and fullness within the temporal and masseter muscles may be found.[23–26]

Etiology. An elongated stylomastoid process probably is *not* a cause for this syndrome. Most current opinion suggests that carotidynia is a migraine equivalent.[24–26] Often, drugs useful in migraine prophylaxis appear effective in vascular neck and face pain.

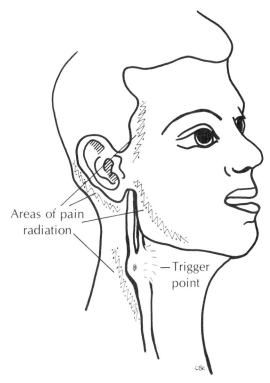

Areas of pain radiation

Trigger point

Fig. 2–5. Palpation of the carotid artery just below the bifurcation accentuates pain referral forward along the mandible, up toward the temple, and occasionally into the ear.

Laboratory and Radiographic Examination. Laboratory and roentgenographic findings are not revealing. The normal Westergren sedimentation rate should exclude underlying sepsis or polymyalgia rheumatica or giant cell arteritis in the elderly. Radiographic evidence of cervical degenerative arthritis does not relate to this syndrome and should be considered a coincidental abnormality.

Differential Diagnosis. Differential diagnosis includes occult infection within the oropharyngeal structures, giant cell arteritis (only to be considered in the elderly), neoplasm, carotid body tumors, and the temporomandibular joint dysfunction syndrome.[27]

Treatment. Treatment begins with telling the patient to keep her hands off her neck. Once a patient realizes the pain is originating

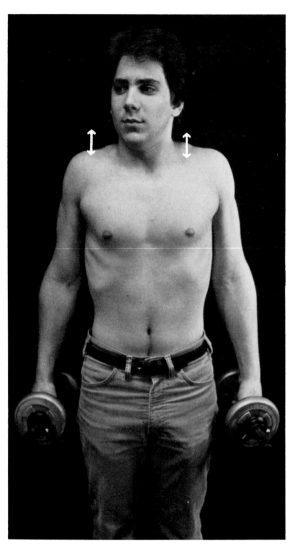

Fig. 2–6. Active-resistance shoulder shrugging: Using 5 to 10 pounds of weight placed upon each shoulder or held in each hand, the shoulders are shrugged and rotated upward and backward, and then slowly let down; the movement is repeated for 1 to 2 minutes.

from the carotid artery, she has a tendency to stroke the area, thus exacerbating the condition. Often, we have found that these patients have coexisting myofascial trigger points in the trapezius and posterior neck muscles. In these cases, relaxing the trapezius muscle with a steroid-local anesthetic injection (see pages 297–298), performing exercises including shoulder shrugging and

neck erector strengthening (Figs. 2–6, 2–7), and using a tricyclic antidepressant (amitriptyline) have been helpful.[24,25] Occasionally, ergot preparations or propranolol useful in the treatment of migraine are helpful.[24,26,28,29]

Outcome and Additional Suggestions. Most patients will be greatly improved following this treatment regimen. Therapy is continued for at least 3 months, and the exercises should be continued twice daily for several months. Patients should be instructed to avoid sleeping on their stomachs because neck hyperextension may intensify distress. The recently introduced calcium channel blocking agents, such as verapamil and nefedipine, may be of value for patients with resistant pain.[30]

Eagle's Syndrome

An elongated styloid process (normal length = 2.5 cm) can compress the carotid vessels; this results in pharyngeal pain and referred otalgia. Abnormalities of the stylohyoid ligament with resulting stretching of the muscles that attach to the hyoid bone may cause similar pain. The trigger point may be palpated within the tonsillar crypt. Intralesional injection with a local anesthetic will provide immediate temporary relief. Another source for the pain may be tendinitis adjacent to muscular attachments to the hyoid bone. This "hyoid syndrome" can be alleviated with intralesional corticosteroid/local anesthetic injection (10 mg methylprednisolone plus 1 ml 1% procaine) near the cornua of the hyoid bone in the lateral anterior neck between the mandible and the larynx.[31]

Myofascial Face Pain

Travell[32] describes a number of potential myofascial sources for head and face pain.

The sternocleidomastoid muscle may have trigger points with the following pain referral: the clavicular division refers pain to the forehead, deep in the ear, and to the posterior auricular region; the sternal division refers pain to the face, orbit, occiput, top of the scalp, throat, and the sternum. A gentle pinch-grasp examination of the muscle will

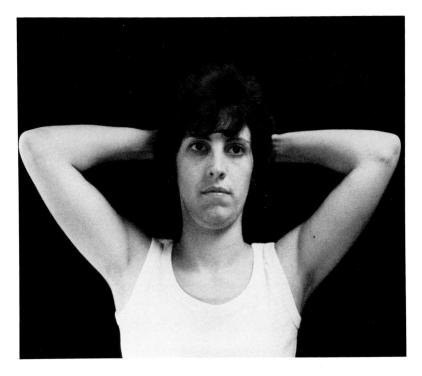

Fig. 2–7. Neck-erector strengthening: In isometric fashion, preferably while sitting or standing with back to wall, the head is pressed progressively into the hands, which act as a passive cushion.

reveal the indurated tender trigger point and reproduce the pain. Treatment with a spray and stretch routine is performed by spraying with fluorimethane from the trigger point toward the pain zone while the muscle is passively stretched. With the patient seated, and the head leaning back, the clavicular end of the sternocleidomastoid is stretched by having the patient's head tilted away from the painful side. For the sternal division, the head is rotated toward the same side and the face is tilted downward. Spray is applied slowly in one direction while the muscle is stretched. Usually only one or two sprayings is performed in order not to cool the muscle itself. If twice daily spray and stretch does not afford benefit, then intralesional injection of the trigger point with a local anesthetic and corticosteroid (10 mg methylprednisolone and 1 ml 1% procaine using a #25 one inch needle) will often provide relief. Exercise B3 in Table 2–5 may be helpful.

Trigger points in the masseter, orbicularis oculi, trapezius, temporalis, and external pterygoid muscles may refer pain to facial areas and present as atypical neuralgia. Palpation of the involved muscles will discern the trigger points; treatment of the lesion with either spray and stretch or intralesional injections is usually helpful.[32]

A trigger point in the inferior belly of the omohyoid muscle located adjacent to the sternal division of the sternomastoid muscle has been described as a cause for pain in the shoulder, neck, arm, and mandible.[33] The etiology may be trauma, intense vomiting, or inflammation from regional or systemic disease. Local injection can be helpful.

Neuralgias

Glossopharyngeal neuralgia presents with a cluster of lancinating, burning, stabbing pains in the region of the tonsil and radiates to the ear, neck, or anterior jaw. Swallowing may trigger the attack. The attacks may provoke cardiac arrhythmias due to irritation of the carotid sinus. Superior laryngeal neuralgia is characterized by similar paroxysms of unilateral pain above the lateral thyroid cartilage with radiation to the angle of the jaw and the ear. Direct nerve block into the pyriform sinus provides diagnostic relief. Lesions of the larynx may involve the nerve, so careful examination is important to exclude other causes of the syndrome. Use of dilantin or carbamazepine (Tegretol) is often helpful. Surgical intervention may require posterior cranial fossa root sections as last resort therapy.[29]

Other conditions to be considered include trigeminal neuralgia, postherpetic neuralgia, and temporal arteritis. A careful neurologic examination, tests of inflammation, and consultation with an otolaryngologist may be needed.[34]

THE CERVICAL SYNDROME: SPRAIN (WHIPLASH); MYOFASCIAL NECK PAIN

Whiplash, a lay term, signifies a flexion-extension injury to the neck. Because such injuries may range from mild muscle tears to vertebral fractures and dislocations, the term should not be used for diagnosis. This chapter considers the conditions that can be managed by the personal physician (see Table 2–3 for diagnostic considerations). See Anatomic Plates II and III.

Cervical Sprain

The patient with an acute neck injury requires immediate expert care. Following sudden forceful hyperextension of the neck, with flexion recoil, as in automobile accidents, the ligamentum nuchae may be ruptured, or rarely the spine of C7 may be fractured. Neck muscle spasm and a torticollis may result (chin is tilted toward the lesion) and tenderness is elicited over the lower cervical spinous processes. Sometimes edema with soft crepitus can be felt over the lower portion of the ligamentum nuchae. During the acute phase, the patient should lie with the head and shoulders raised up. Very gentle exercises can be tried, as detailed in B4, Table 2–5.[35]

Tension Neck Syndrome

Another syndrome is the tension neck syndrome, or simply, the cervical syndrome. This has the added findings of bilateral diminished upper limb reflexes and evidence of cervical degenerative disc disease with limitation of neck motion.[36] These patients may have root sleeve fibrosis. They may respond to cervical traction applied twice daily and followed by mobilizing and strengthening exercises. (Exercises B1 + B2, Table 2–5.) Ibuprofen seems helpful in our experience. Causative factors include frequent lifting of heavy objects on the job, cigarette smoking (coughing), and frequent diving from a board.[37] Frequent twisting or turning of the neck did not appear related. If the patient considers the job as a cause, and if review of joint protection principles (Table 2–4) has not been of value, then referral to an occupational therapist should be considered. More often than not, factors outside of the workplace can be significantly aggravating. Then the job just is a corollary to the problem.

Cervical Myofascial Pain

Chronic pain in the muscles of the posterior neck worsens when sitting or upon arising in the morning. This pain improves with motion and may occur as an isolated complaint or as part of a more generalized fibrositis syndrome.[38] The aggravation of the pain *after rest* is a cardinal feature. Muscle contraction headaches often coexist. Numbness, tingling, weakness, and scotomata do not occur. Active neck motion may be restricted, but passive neck motion is normal. Clicking noise is common. No neurologic abnormalities are noted. Trigger points within the trapezius and neck erector muscles are easily found by palpation. Sometimes a tight, tender ligamentum nuchae is noted during neck flexion (Fig. 2–8). When the cervical myofascial pain occurs after trauma, several weeks often elapse before the onset of chronic diffuse neck pain.[39]

The sternomastoid muscle should always

Table 2–3. Decision Chart, The Head and Neck

Problem	Action	Other Actions	Further Actions
A. Chronic Neck Pain Trigger points present No limitation of motion No neurologic signs	CONSERVATIVE CARE Correct aggravating factors (joint protection) Provide pain relief; NSAIDS, vapo- coolant spray, trigger point injec- tions, TENS, antidepressants, relaxants, mild analgesics Prescribe exercises	Tests for inflammation Roentgenographic studies Bone scan → CT scan Electrodiagnostic tests Review exercises and Joint protection measures	Repeat physical examination Consultation with: → Orthopedist/Neurosurgeon Physiatrist Rheumatologist
B. Subacute Neck Pain Minor injury Limitation of movement No neurologic signs			
C. Acute Neck Injury Soft tissue tenderness No swelling No neurologic signs Normal passive motion Normal roentgenograms			
D. Danger List Present Neurologic findings present Bleeding from any orifice Fever, chills, swelling Meningismus	URGENT CONSULTATION Orthopedist/Neurosurgeon Emergency medicine specialist Oral examination Spinal tap		

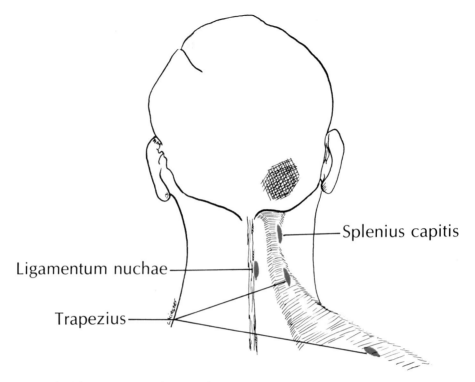

Fig. 2–8. Myofascial trigger points in the cervical region.

be examined for trigger points when neck pain is associated with postural dizziness, and painful neck motion. Multiple trigger points give rise to widely referred pain. Activation of the autonomic nervous system has been described.[40]

Laboratory and Radiographic Examination. Proper radiographic assessment must be obtained. Upright anteroposterior and lateral neck roentgenograms, in the neutral, flexion, and extension positions, and open-mouth odontoid views should be obtained to exclude cervical spine disease. Oblique views of the cervical spine are obtained for evaluation of the neuroforamina. Muscle spasm may lead to loss of the normal forward curve; skeletal injuries can be identified. Osteoporosis, neoplasm, and other diseases can also be ruled out. Degenerative changes, consistent with age, are often unrelated to symptoms. Computed tomography (CT) of the neck is of value also, particularly for studying soft tissue masses within the neck.[41] In addition, CT of the C1–C2 region following trauma to the neck may detect odontoid fracture.

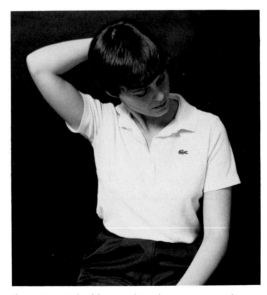

Fig. 2–9. Method for stretching the sternomastoid muscle.

Differential Diagnosis. Neck pain and stiffness that follow rest and improve during movement seldom result from more serious disease. However, a careful history and physical examination, with exclusion of referred pain from the temporomandibular joint, diaphragm, and hiatus hernia, and with consideration for neurologic or cardiovascular disease, are necessary.[39]

Sometimes spinal enthesopathies can cause chronic neck discomfort and stiffness. They can affect the paraspinal ligaments with degeneration and calcification. Involvement of the anterior longitudinal ligament, Forestier's disease, also involves other segments of the spine. Characteristic flowing ossifications are usual roentgenographic findings. Ossification of the posterior longitudinal ligament may result in a cervical myelopathy with added complaints of altered sensation and motor function in the upper and lower limbs. Most cases occur among Japanese persons.[42–44] Calcific tendinitis of the longus colli muscle tendon can result in a self-limited condition with neck and throat pain and dysphagia. Pain is aggravated by neck motion and neck motion is severely restricted.[45–46]

Psychogenic neck pain tends to occur episodically and does not improve with activity; pain is out of proportion to the physical findings, and palpation during the physical examination often reveals tenderness in excess of usual trigger point tenderness. Treatment of psychogenic pain requires the addition of helpful solutions to life problems. The floppy head syndrome, consisting of severe neck weakness and associated fatigue, strongly suggests hypothyroidism or polymyositis.[47]

Management. Treatment includes avoiding activities in which the head is held motionless for prolonged periods. Tasks requiring sitting or standing still should be interrupted every 30 minutes. Lying on a sofa with the head propped up on the sofa arm induces neck strain, and should be avoided. Sleep position with the head preferably in a neutral position (with the patient lying on his back with legs elevated) is helpful[48] (see Fig. 8–10, p. 188). See Table 2–4: Joint protec-

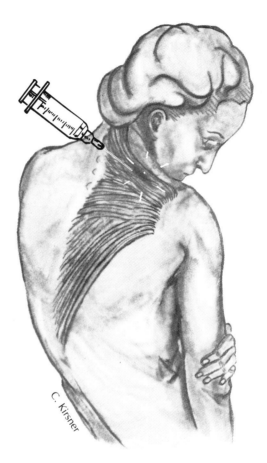

Fig. 2–10. Injection of trapezius trigger point with a 1-in. No. 23 needle.

tion. Structural abnormalities such as adult round back or scoliosis, and alterations in head and neck motion in patients with unilateral loss of vision or hearing may be associated with myofascial neck pain. Joint protection advice will help these people also. If work requires that both hands be free when on the phone, then use of a headphone or speaker phone is helpful. Users of computer video display terminals may develop musculoskeletal complaints. These may result from such factors as surface screen glare, poor screen and keyboard heights relative to the user, inappropriate seating, and the type of tasks being performed. Tasks consisting of high volume work, those under rigid control and continuous performance can produce sig-

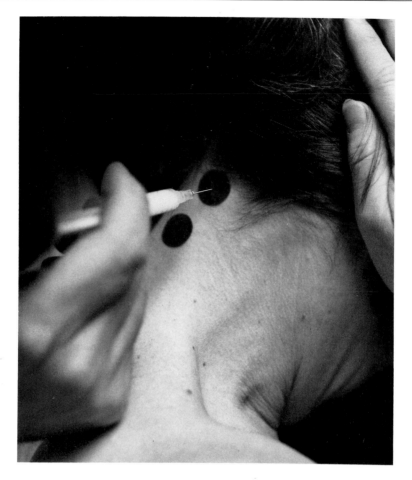

Fig. 2–11. Injection of cervical myofascial trigger points in the splenius capitus and upper cervical muscles using a No. 25 short needle and 1 to 2 ml of medication.

nificant job stress, and health complaints.[49] The "bird watcher's neck" is a frequent strain. The neck is jutted forward as if looking through a pair of binoculars.[40]

Injection of trigger points in the trapezius (Fig. 2–10) and neck erector (Fig. 2–11) muscles with a steroid-anesthetic combination may be performed on the first visit.[38]

Neck mobilizing and strengthening exercises are helpful in our experience. Exercises are selected for posture control, stretching and strengthening. They must be performed gradually and repeated twice daily. Begin with the milder gentle motions (Exercise B4 a to d, Table 2–5, and progress to the strengthening movements (Exercise B1 and B2, Table 2–5, Figures 2–6 and 2–7).

Generally the exercises are performed with 3 to 10 repetitions each held for 10 to 20 seconds, and for 1 or 2 minutes for each exercise. When the sternomastoid is tender, the muscle can be stretched as detailed in Exercise B3, Table 2–5. See Figure 2–9.

Individual muscles that are tender and tight should be stretched, then contracted. For example, for the trapezius, Exercise B2 and B4d followed by B1 could be recommended. Using this combination of stretch followed by contraction of the muscle resulted in pain relief in 63% of patients (n = 244).[50]

Cervical manipulation is controversial. In addition to being only of questionable value,[51] cervical manipulation has allegedly caused

Table 2–4. A Joint Protection Guide for the Head and Neck[71-78] (After Sheon[71])

AGGRAVATING FACTORS	HELPFUL PRACTICES
■ Sitting or standing for more than 30 minutes can induce more neck strain than lifting heavy objects	■ Alternate tasks in which the body does not move (e.g., knitting) with tasks that allow the body greater movement (e.g., sweeping).
■ Lying on a sofa with the head propped forward, falling alseep in a chair and allowing the head to drop forward, or lying on more than one thin pillow stretches the muscles at the back of the neck. Hours later, these muscles may go into spasm, resulting in headache, stiff neck, or limited neck movement.	■ Align the entire trunk, chest, and head on a slanted wedge or a very large pillow to watch television or read in a reclining position. Anyone with hiatus hernia, sinus trouble, or heart disease who has been told to sleep in a propped-up position should elevate the entire mattress or the head of the bed rather than simply putting two or three pillows under the head.
■ Sleeping on the stomach can strain the neck.	■ Sleep on the side or the back, keeping the arms below the level of the chest.
■ Clenching the jaw can cause muscle spasm in the neck.	■ Use a bite spacer, relaxation techniques, or muscle relaxants.
■ Storing items in the kitchen at a level that is too high or too low can strain the neck.	■ Store items that are used daily no higher than shoulder height or lower than knee level. If storage is a problem, use a step stool to avoid tilting the head excessively.
■ Working too close to work materials can strain the neck.	■ Maintain the proper hand-to-eye distance of 16 in. (abut 40 cm). Position work materials in such a way that the neck remains straight. Place a computer screen at eye level.
■ Incorrectly using the telephone can cause neck pain.	■ If both hands must be free during phone conversations, use a speaker phone or a shoulder holder briefly.

cerebral infarction.[52] Using an amnesic dose of diazepam, a controlled study of manipulation showed no consistent favorable response.[51] Four patients who suffered cerebral infarction following chiropractic neck manipulation were reported.[52] The cost of chiropractic treatment of the neck was determined to be no less than that of other methods of care in patients with work-related neck pain.[53]

The local application of heat is of proved value,[54] as is the use of cervical pillows.[55] We have used the Jackson pillow and the Walpilo (a commercial foam pillow designed to provide a beneficial cervical position during rest) with generally good results.

Overhead cervical traction is frequently necessary (Fig. 2–12). Cervical traction should never be prescribed without first obtaining roentgenograms of the cervical spine. Note that 10 pounds of cervical traction produce no visible distraction of the vertebrae; 25 to 35 pounds of traction do distract the vertebrae, and furthermore, may free adhesions between dural sleeves.[39] Cervical traction should be performed at least twice daily (morning and evening) for 5 to 10 minutes. Beginning with 8 to 15 pounds, the weight is increased gradually until benefit results. Home traction of up to 20 pounds is usually well tolerated. Traction is then followed by neck strengthening exercises.

Outcome and Additional Suggestions. After these therapeutic measures, relief from cervical myofascial pain should begin within a week or two in the majority of patients.

Table 2–5. Exercises for the Head and Neck Region

A. *JAW BALANCING EXERCISES*

1. With the mouth opened an inch, place a fist in front of the lower jaw and try to jut the jaw forward against the immovable fist. No motion actually occurs.
2. Place the fist to one side of the jaw and similarly thrust the lower jaw against the fist. Then move to the other side and finally place the fist beneath the lower jaw and thrust against the fist. In each instance hold the thrust for 10 seconds and repeat 6 times in each direction. Perform the exercise morning and evening (see Fig. 2–3).

B. *NECK EXERCISES*

1. Back up to a wall with feet about 6 inches from the wall. Place hands behind head and push buttocks against the wall; then push head and shoulders back against the wall. The hands act as a cushion between the head and the wall; now begin a gradual forceful thrust of the head backward to the wall, keeping the chin tucked in like a military soldier at attention. As the head is thrust backward the arms are loose, just allowing the hands to act as a cushion behind the head. There should be a sensation of muscle tension in the back of the neck. This thrust is maintained for up to 30 seconds and then relaxed for a second and repeated for one to two minutes (see Fig. 2–7).
2. Shoulder shrugging: Mobilize the neck and shoulder muscles with two weights, each 2- to 10-pounds. These can be made from socks stuffed with a plastic freezer bag and then filled with gravel, sand, or dirt. The weights can be held at the sides of the body or draped over each shoulder. Arms are held down along the sides of the body while seated or standing. Then the shoulders are slowly drawn upward, then backward, then slowly let down. The shoulder blades are thus brought toward each other as the shoulders are raised. This movement is repeated slowly for 1 to 2 minutes twice daily (see Fig. 2–6).
3. Stretch the muscles on the side of the neck behind the ear. Take the right arm, swing it behind the neck, and grasp the left ear. Now bend the head forward and pull the head to the right with the right hand and arm, thus pulling the ear away from the shoulder. There should be a pulling sensation in the muscles radiating at the left side of the neck. Similarly, reverse and use the left arm, swung behind, and grasp the right ear. Draw the head to the left, with the head tilted forward and there should be a pulling sensation in the muscles behind the right side of the neck (see Fig. 2–9).
4. Mobilizing exercises for a stiff painful neck can be done with a rolled towel and performed on the bed.[35]
   a. Lie face down, towel under forehead; push down with forehead to towel firmly for 6 seconds, repeat 3 times.
   b. Lie face up, towel under back of head, push down hard for 6 seconds, repeat 3 times.
   c. Lie on side and ear to towel. Press down on towel for 6 seconds, repeat 3 times. Repeat on opposite side.
   d. Sit upright, rotate head and neck with a firm steady circular motion. Lift and lower head during the rotation for 12 seconds.
   These exercises should be performed twice a day and for at least 1 to 2 minutes' duration.

Whenever cervical traction is prescribed, the patient may have to continue the twice daily traction therapy for a prolonged period. Supervision by a physical therapist is desirable. A tricyclic antidepressant (amitriptyline), given at bedtime to relieve a pain-spasm-pain cycle, may be helpful. Biofeedback relaxation has also been advocated[56,57] (see Chapt. 14).

TORTICOLLIS

Wryneck, a contracted state of the cervical muscles, with the head drawn to one side, may result from congenital, infectious, or inflammatory diseases of the sternocleidomastoid muscle. Rarely the condition is hysterical in origin. Most cases will subside in a few roid (10 mg methylprednisolone and 1 ml 1% procaine using a #25 one inch needle) will usually be helpful. When psychogenic factors are suspected, biofeedback and psychologic counseling have proved helpful in some cases. Spasmodic torticollis, a neurologic disorder, should not be confused with a self-limited torticollis of traumatic origin.[58]

IMPINGEMENT OF THE FIFTH CERVICAL NERVE ROOT

Compression of the lower cervical nerve roots may result in shoulder region pain and disability. Dull aching about the shoulder, intermittent at first, later persistent, may be due to C-5 nerve root irritation resulting from such entities as disc degeneration, root sleeve injury, or trauma. Coughing, sneezing, or neck hyperextension may aggravate the pain. Neck and arm motion often are normal. Two helpful examinations are the Spurling maneuver and determination of vibratory sensation. The Spurling maneuver is an attempt to reproduce the pain by direct compression of the nerve.[59] The examiner places his hands on the seated patient's head, and rotates the head slightly to the painful side. In addition to turning the chin, the head is also slightly angled so that the patient's ear is tilted toward the painful shoulder. Pressure is then exerted downward on the patient's head with perhaps 20 pounds of force for 10 seconds (Fig. 2–13). Pain is reproduced or accentuated in the shoulder region if the Spurling test is positive. Vibration sense and pinprick sensation are usually diminished over the involved deltoid region, Atrophy is rare. Strength is usually preserved if the patient is seen soon after onset. Passive motion of the shoulder joint is normal. Swelling or the sensation of swelling does not occur.

Cervical spine roentgenograms must include oblique views to demonstrate the neuroforamina. Radiographic changes may not correlate with clinical features in some patients. Electrodiagnostic studies may not reveal abnormality, especially if performed within the first month of onset of symptoms.

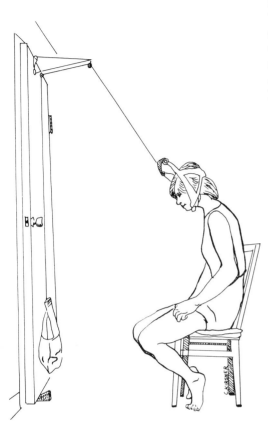

Fig. 2–12. Cervical traction is performed with the head flexed forward 15 to 25 degrees. Duration ranges from 5 to 15 minutes and traction is usually performed twice daily.

weeks. Painful spasm of the muscle results in the head being tilted away from the painful side. Careful examination is needed to exclude pathologic processes in the neck. When injury is the cause, treatment with a spray and stretch routine is performed by spraying with fluorimethane from the trigger point toward the pain zone while the muscle is passively stretched. Spray is applied slowly in one direction while the muscle is stretched. Usually only one or two sprayings are performed in order to avoid irritation. If twice daily spray and stretch does not afford benefit, then intralesional injection of the trigger point with a local anesthetic and corticoste-

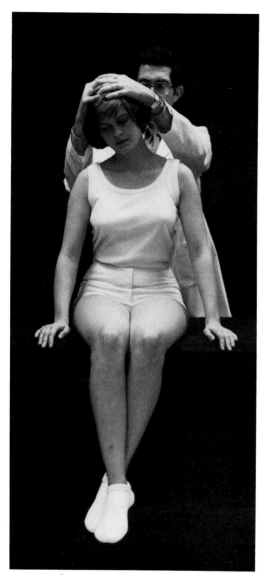

Fig. 2–13. The Spurling maneuver: Downward force for 10 seconds' duration is used to reproduce symptoms resulting from cervical nerve impingement.

Treatment begins with instructing the patient in proper sleep and sitting positions and avoidance of hyperextension of the neck.[60] A helpful sleep position is to have the patient lie flat on his back with thighs elevated on pillows, thus flattening the long spinal muscles. A rolled-up towel under the neck may be used.[48] Some patients prefer the use of a soft neck collar or neck pillow. Reducing cer-

vical erector muscle spasm is imperative. Measures to do this include the application of local moist heat, the injection of cervical muscle trigger points with a local anesthetic-corticosteroid mixture, and the use of neck-erector strengthening exercises. Cervical traction performed several times a day with a motorized intermittent traction machine or with a home traction kit is helpful (Fig. 2–12).[39,61] Use of a mild muscle relaxant-analgesic preparation is beneficial only when used in conjunction with physical therapy measures. If cervical traction is necessary, the patient may need to use it daily for several months. Isometric neck exercises following each traction treatment can be helpful. Cervical collars are of value for protecting the neck from further injury especially while driving.

Most patients respond quickly and do not require electrodiagnostic (EMG) studies or consideration for a surgical procedure. As a rule, we treat patients initially with local heat and exercises, and if no benefit occurs in the first few weeks, we then add cervical traction. Never order cervical traction without performing a cervical spine radiographic examination to exclude malalignment or fractures. If traction fails, we then proceed to EMG and surgical consultation. In our experience, fewer than 1% of these patients require surgical intervention.

CERVICOTHORACIC INTERSPINOUS BURSITIS

Midline posterior cervical pain may result from formation of a bursa between the posterior spinous processes.[62,63] The pain is dull, usually constant, and localized in the region between the posterior processes of C-7 and T-1. The patient usually has a dorsal kyphosis with a forward inclination of the neck in relation to the shoulders. The pain is worse with resting or sitting, but improves during movement. Often, the provoking cause is an activity requiring hyperextension of the neck and head, such as cleaning the upper shelves of a cupboard.

Physical examination reveals point tender-

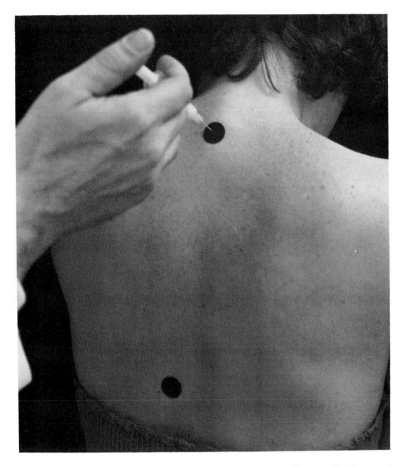

Fig. 2–14.   Injection of intraspinous bursitis: A 1-in. No. 25 or No. 23 needle is used with a 45-degree angulated approach. Up to 2 ml volume is used.

ness directly at the midline of the lower cervical or upper thoracic spine. Rubbery swelling of the soft tissues may be palpated. Passive range of motion is normal. Roentgenographs to exclude osteoporosis and an erythrocyte sedimentation rate to exclude sepsis should be obtained.

Treatment includes injection of the interspinous space, approached from a lateral point of entry about ½ inch from the midline. A long-acting steroid-local anesthetic mixture is injected into each side of the bursa (Fig. 2–14). Proper sleep position, with the neck in a neutral position, is advised, and neck erector strengthening and shoulder shrugging exercises are provided. The patient is instructed to avoid hyperextension of the neck.

MUSCLE CONTRACTION HEADACHE

These patients describe a dull, aching, or occasionally throbbing pain in regions of the ocular orbit, forehead, temple, or scalp, preceded by a sensation of tightness in the neck erector muscles. Unlike migraine, these patients state that the headaches last for days or weeks. Similar headache may result from intense bearing down during prolonged labor (postpartum headache).[64] Musculoskeletal symptoms consisting of pain in the neck and at the back of head, with a sensation of tightness and pressure, can usually be differentiated from headache of intracranial origin.[65] Attributes of pain, as determined by history, can follow the *PQRST* questioning:[9]

   Provocative factors: head position, coughing, straining, emotion
   Quality: burning, aching, throbbing, continuous, superficial
   Region: location of pain
   Severity: On a scale from none to terrible
   Timing: duration and periodicity

Danger Signs, as detailed in Table 2–1, should be sought in the examination of any patient with significant headache complaints.

Often the headaches have been precipitated by working on a project while sitting for several hours at a time, going for a long drive or falling asleep in a chair and allowing the head to fall forward. These patients often sleep on their stomachs, hyperextending their heads if a pillow is used.[48] Less often, nuchal muscles are strained during neck hyperextension from working overhead, such as painting a ceiling. Visual symptoms, if present, are described as a sensitivity to bright lights or foggy vision, but never scotomata.

Physical examination reveals a normal range of passive neck motion (when the examiner moves the patient's head laterally, forward, and backward, with the patient relaxed). Trigger points within the trapezius as well as the neck erector muscles are uniformly present. Other physical findings and tests for inflammation are normal.

Radiographic examination of the neck may reveal degenerative changes expected for age, but abnormalities are often unrelated. A Westergren sedimentation rate should be performed in elderly patients to exclude giant cell arteritis.[27]

Treatment includes instruction in proper sleep position, preferably with the patient lying on his back with a thin pillow or towel rolled up behind the neck.[48] Activities or tasks performed while sitting or standing should be paced, with no longer than 30 minutes at a time spent in sedentary activities. Exercises include neck erector strengthening and shoulder shrugging (to loosen the trapezii) performed twice daily. (See Exercises B1 and

B2, Table 2–5.) Women with pendulous breasts should use bras with wide elastic straps that prevent tugging on the trapezius (Figs. 2–15, 2–16). Injection of the cervical and trapezius trigger points with a steroid-local anesthetic mixture may be performed on the first visit.[38] Usually a relaxant or sedative is provided at bedtime for a few weeks.

The expected result is relief within a few days, but the exercises and preventive measures to avoid neck strain are continued for a prolonged period. Therapeutic failure is uncommon, but two additional helpful modalities are use of flexion cervical traction (Fig. 2–12) and amitriptyline.[28,66,67] Biofeedback relaxation may also be helpful.[56]

OCCIPITAL NEURALGIA

Pain at the base of the skull posteriorly, with occasional burst of pain and paresthesia traveling up the occiput, sometimes to the entire scalp, can be due to irritation of the sensory root of the second cervical nerve (the greater occipital nerve). Neck strain, from working with the head hyperextended, may have precipitated the pain. Occipital neuralgia may occur as a result of trauma, often in association with degenerative disease of the atlantoaxial joint.[68] Palpation at the base of the skull may reproduce or exacerbate the sensation.

Injection of splenius capitus trigger points with a steroid-local anesthetic mixture, instructions in sleep position (head and neck in line with trunk), and neck erector strengthening exercises should provide prompt relief. Proper radiographic assessment of the upper neck region should be obtained if symptoms persist. Lateral flexion and extension views and open-mouth odontoid views can identify underlying abnormalities, which may rarely require surgery.

Spinal stenosis with bilateral neurologic impairment may be a devastating result of osteoarthritis and spur formation;[38,69] fortunately it is not common. Upper limb weakness and impairment, and limitation of neck motion are the usual presenting features.

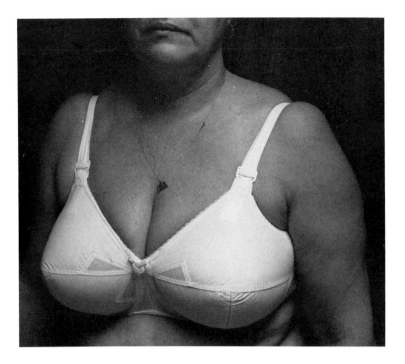

Fig. 2–15. Improper brassiere providing inadequate support and creating excessive traction on the shoulders.

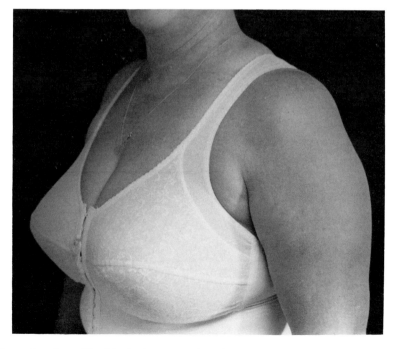

Fig. 2–16. Proper brassiere with wide elastic straps and good support.

Careful diagnostic assessment using computed tomography[70] and, if required, myelography should be performed before surgical decompression is considered. Only a surgeon with wide experience and conservative judgment should be involved.

REFERENCES

1. Kattan KR: Reading cervical spine films. Hospital Med 83:32e–32v, 1983.
2. Schwartz L.: Disorders of the Temporomandibular Joint: Diagnosis, Management, Relation to Occlusion of Teeth. Philadelphia, WB Saunders, 1959.
3. Zarb GA, Speck JE: The treatment of temporomandibular joint dysfunction: a retrospective study. J Prosthet Dent 38:420–432, 1977.
4. Sharav Y: The myofascial pain dysfunction syndrome—a common expression to various etiologies. Israel J Dent Med 26:11–15, 1977.
5. Guralnick W, Kaban LB, Merrill RG: Temporomandibular-joint afflictions. N Engl J Med 299:123–129, 1978.
6. Mayne JG, Hatch GS: Arthritis of the temporomandibular joint. J Am Dent Assoc 79:125–130, 1969.
7. Toller PA: Use and misuse of intra-articular corticosteroids in treatment of temporomandibular joint pain. Proc Roy Soc Med 70:461–463, 1977.
8. Pinals RS: Traumatic Arthritis and Allied Conditions. In Arthritis and Allied Conditions, 10th Ed. Edited by Daniel J. McCarty. Philadelphia, Lea & Febiger, 1985.
8a. Berry DC: Mandibular dysfunction, pain and chronic minor illness. Br Dent 3 127:170–175, 1969.
9. DeGowen EL, DeGowen RL: Bedside Diagnostic Examination. 4th Ed. New York, Macmillan Pub Co, 1981.
10. Costen JB: A syndrome of ear and sinus symptoms dependent upon disturbed function of the temporomandibular joint. Ann Otol Rhinol Laryngol 43:1–15, 1934.
11. Freese AS: Costen's syndrome: A reinterpretation. AMA Arch Otol 70:309–314, 1959.
12. Trenouth MJ: The relationship between bruxism and temporomandibular joint dysfunction as shown by computer analysis of nocturnal tooth contact patterns. J Oral Rehab 6:81–87, 1979.
13. Small EW: An investigation into the psychogenic bases of the temporomandibular joint myofascial pain dysfunction syndrome. Advances in Pain Research and Therapy, ed by Bonica and Albe-Fessard I. 889–894, 1976.
14. Stein S, Loft G, Davis H, Hart DL: Symptoms of TMJ dysfunction as related to stress measured by the social readjustment rating scale. J Prosthetic Dent 47:545–548, 1982.
15. Heloe B, Heiberg AN: A follow-up study of a group of female patients with myofascial pain-dysfunction syndrome. Acta Odontol, Scand 38:129–134, 1980.
16. Marbach JJ, Varoscak JR: Treatment of TMJ and other facial pains: A critical review. NYS Dent J 80:181–188, 1980.

17. Marbach JJ: Arthritis of the temporomandibular joints. Am Fam Phys 20:131–139, 1979.
18. Greene CS, Laskin DM: Splint therapy for the myofascial pain-dysfunction (MPD) syndrome: a comparative study. JADA 84:624–628, 1972.
19. Goharian RK, Neff PA: Effect of occlusal retainers on temporomandibular joint and facial pain. J Prost Dent 44:206–208, 1980.
20. Hall LJ: Physical therapy treatment results for 178 patients with temporomandibular joint syndrome. Am J Otol 5:183–196, 1984.
21. Greene CS, Laskin DM: Long-term evaluation of treatment for myofascial pain-dysfunction syndrome: a comparative analysis. JADA 107:235–238, 1983.
22. Scott DS, Gregg, JM: Behavioral-relaxation therapy. Pain 9:231–241, 1980.
23. Lovshin LL: Carotidynia. Headache 17:192–195, 1977.
24. Lovshin LL: Vascular neck pain—A common syndrome seldom recognized: Analysis of 100 consecutive cases. Cleve Clin Q 27:5–13, 1960.
25. Fay T: Atypical facial neuralgia, a syndrome of vascular pain. Ann Otol 41:1030–1062, 1932.
26. Raskin NH, Prusiner S: Carotidynia. Neurol 27:43–46, 1977.
27. Goodman BW Jr: Temporal arteritis. Am J Med 67:839–852, 1979.
28. Couch JR, Ziegler DK, Hassanein R: Amitriptyline in the prophylaxis of migraine. Neurology 26:121–127, 1976.
29. Karlan MS, Beroza L, Cassisi NJ: Anterior cervical pain syndromes. Otol Head Neck Surg 87:284–291, 1979.
30. Meyers-Stirling J: Calcium channel blockers in the prophylactic treatment of vascular headache. Ann Intern Med 120:395–397, 1985.
31. Krespi YP, Shugar JMA, Som PM: Stylohyoid Syndromes: an uncommon cause of pharyngeal and neck pain. Am J Otolaryngol 2:358–360, 1981.
32. Travell J: Identification of myofascial trigger point syndromes: A case of atypical facial neuralgia. Arch Phys Med Rehabil 62:100–106, 1981.
33. Rask MR: The omohyoideus myofascial pain syndrome: Report of four patients. J Cranioman Prac 2:256–262, 1985.
34. Asher SW: Headache and facial pain. Hosp Med 16:33–40, 1980.
35. Murtagh JE: Patient education: exercises for the neck. Australian Fam Phys 10:947, 1981.
36. Waris P, Kuorinka I, et al: Epidemiologic screening of occupational neck and upper limb disorders. Scand J Work Environ and Health 5:25–36, 1979.
37. Kelsey JL, Githens PB, Walter SD, Southwick WO, et al: An epidemiological study of acute prolapsed cervical intervertebral disc. J Bone Joint Surg 66A:907–914, 1984.
38. Moskowitz RW: Clinical Rheumatology. 2nd Ed. Philadelphia, Lea & Febiger, 1982.
39. Jackson R: The Cervical Syndrome. Springfield, Charles C Thomas, 1978.
40. Travell JG, Simons DG: Myofascial Pain and Dysfunction. The Trigger Point Manual. Baltimore, Williams and Wilkins, 1983.
41. Reede DL, Whelan MA, Bergeron RT: CT of the

soft tissue structures of the neck. Radiol Clin N Am 22:239–250, 1984.

42. Norman A: Roentgenologic Diagnosis. *In* Osteoarthritis: Diagnosis and Management. Edited by Roland W. Moskowitz et al. Philadelphia, WB Saunders, 1984.

43. Resnik D: Hyperostosis and ossification in the cervical spine. Arth Rheum 27:564–569, 1984.

44. Williamson PK, Reginato AJ: Diffuse idiopathic skeletal hyperostosis of the cervical spine in a patient with ankylosing spondylitis. Arth Rheum 27:570–573, 1984.

45. Sarkozi J, Fam AG: Acute calcific retropharyngeal tendinitis: an unusual cause of neck pain. Arth Rheum 27:708–710, 1984.

45A. Karasick D, Karasick S: Calcific retropharyngeal tendinitis. Skel Radiol 7:203–205, 1919.

46. Newmark H, Zee CS, Frankel P, et al: Chronic calcific tendinitis of the neck. Skel Radiol 7:207–208, 1981.

47. Katz AL, Pate D: Floppy head syndrome. Arth Rheum 23:131–132, 1980.

48. Kraus H: Clinical Treatment of Back and Neck Pain. New York: McGraw-Hill, 1970.

49. Cohen A: Trends in human factors research. Occupational Health and Safety (June):30–36, 1982.

50. Lewit K, Simons, OG: Myofascial pain: relief by post-isometric relaxation. Arch Phys Med Rehabil 65:452–456, 1984.

51. Sloop PR, Smith DS, Goldenberg E, Dore C: Manipulation for chronic neck pain—a double-blind controlled study. Spine 7:532–535, 1982.

52. Sherman DG, Hart RG, Easton JD: Abrupt change in head position and cerebral infarction. Stroke 12:2–6, 1981.

53. Greenwood JG: Work-related back and neck injury cases in West Virginia. Ortho Review 14:51–63, 1985.

54. Lewith GT, Machin D: A randomized trial to evaluate the effect of infra-red stimulation of local trigger points. Acupunc Elec Therap 6:277–284, 1981.

55. Melvin JL: Effectiveness of a cervical pillow for management of neck pain: a survey of patient use. Arth Rheum (Abst. 29) 27 (No. 4) [Supp], 1984.

56. Peck CL, Kraft GH: Electromyographic biofeedback for pain related to muscle tension: A study of tension headache, back, and jaw pain. Arch Surg 112:889–895, 1977.

57. Jacobs A, Felton GS: Visual feedback of myoelectric output to facilitate muscle relaxation in normal persons and patients with neck injuries. Arch Phys Med Rehab 50:34–39, 1969.

58. Lee MC: Spasmodic torticollis and other idiopathic torsion dystonias. Postgrad Med 75:139–146, 1984.

59. Spurling RG, Scoville WB: Lateral rupture of the cervical intervertebral discs. Surg Gynecol Obstet 78:350–358, 1944.

60. British Association of Physical Medicine: Pain in the neck and arm: A multicentre trial of the effects of physiotherapy. Br Med J 1:253–258, 1966.

61. Honet JC, Puri K: Cervical radiculitis: Treatment and results in 82 patients. Arch Phys Med Rehabil 57:12–16, 1976.

62. Bywaters EGL: Lesions of bursae, tendons and tendon sheaths. Clin Rheum Dis 5:883–918, 1979.

63. Bywaters EGL: Rheumatoid and other diseases of the cervical interspinous bursae, and changes in the spinous processes. Ann Rheum Dis 41:360–370, 1982.

64. Hubbell SL, Thomas M: Postpartum cervical myofascial pain syndrome: Review of four patients. Obst Gyn 65(3) Supp: 56s–57s, 1985.

65. Kaganov JA, Bakal DA, Dunn BE: The differential contribution of muscle contraction and migraine symptoms to problem headache in the general population. Headache 21:157–163, 1981.

66. Gomersall JD, Stuart A: Amitriptyline in migraine prophylaxis. J Neurol Neurosurg Psych 36:684–690, 1973.

67. Saper JR: Migraine: classification and pathogenesis: JAMA 239:2380–2382, 1978.

68. Turek SL: Orthopaedics: Principles and Their Application. 4th Ed. Philadelphia, JB Lippincott, 1984.

69. Hinck VC, Sachdev NS: Developmental stenosis of the cervical spinal canal. Brain 89:27–40, 1966.

70. Hashimoto I, Tak YK: The true sagittal diameter of the cervical spinal canal and its diagnostic significance in cervical myelopathy. J Neurosurg 47:912–916, 1977.

71. Sheon, RP: A joint protection guide for nonarticular rheumatism. Postgraduate Medicine 77 (No. 5):331–337, 1985.

72. Bjelle A, Hagberg M, Michaelson G: Occupational and individual factors in acute shoulder-neck disorders among industrial workers. Br J Ind Med 38:356–363, 1981.

73. Fraser TM: Ergonomics and the office. JRSH 5:196–200, 1983.

74. Grandjean E, Hunting W, Pidermann M: VDT workstation design: preferred settings and their effects. Human Factors 25:161–175, 1983.

75. Hayne CR: Ergonomics and back pain. Physiotherapy 70:9–13, 1984.

76. Ignatius J: Saccadic eye movements—use in ergophthalmology. Acta Opthal 161:149–152, 1984.

77. Maeda K, Hunting W, Grandjean E: Localized fatigue in accounting machine operators. J Occup Med 22:810–816, 1980.

78. Saari KM: Occupational ophthalmology and ergonomics of vision. Acta Opthalmologica, Ergo Symposium Finland August 6–7, 1983.

3

The Thoracic Outlet Region

When the classic triad of numbness, weakness, and a sensation of swelling occurs in one or both upper limbs, a diagnosis of a neurovascular entrapment disorder is strongly suggested. More often, symptoms are vague and physical findings are lacking. Physical examination maneuvers often clarify the disorders that arise in the thoracic outlet. Sometimes a therapeutic trial of the treatment measures described in this chapter assists in diagnosis by providing symptomatic relief. Surgical procedures should be considered only after the diagnosis has been established and conservative measures have failed.[1,2]

THE THORACIC OUTLET AND RELATED SYNDROMES

Intermittent obstruction of the neurovascular bundle of the upper extremity results in both neurologic and vascular symptoms. Paresthesia, pain, and often a *sensation* of swelling of the arm and hand on one or both sides occur. Occasional complaints include weakness of the hands, chest wall pain,[3] and less often, discomfort of the entire shoulder girdle. Intermittent pain and paresthesia occur in nearly all patients, and usually follow the ulnar nerve distribution, or involve the entire hand and lower arm.[4,5] Vascular disturbances, which accompany neurologic symptoms, include a sensation of coldness, congestion of the entire hand (rings feel tight in the morning), and distension of the veins of the hand. The symptoms represent compression of the neurovascular bundle as it traverses the cervico-axillary canal, comprising three potential spaces. These are the triangular space between the scalene muscles, the costoclavicular space, and the pectoralis minor space under the pectoralis minor muscle[6,7] (Fig. 3–1). Sir Ashley Cooper

was probably the first to describe the features of thoracic outlet syndrome in 1821.[8] In the past, multiple terms were used for this syndrome. Terminology was based upon a presumed site of obstruction, and included the costoclavicular syndrome,[9] the hyperabduction or Wright's syndrome,[10–11] the scalenus anticus syndrome, and the cervical rib syndrome. In recent years, observations made at the time of operation demonstrated *multiple sites* of obstruction in individual patients.[5,10] Therefore, the more general term, thoracic outlet system, is preferred.

Etiology. By far the most common cause is sagging musculature related to aging, obesity, heavy breasts and arms. Swift and Nichols have aptly designated this condition "the droopy shoulder syndrome."[12] Anatomic anomalies include cervical ribs with or without radiolucent cervical bands, first rib anomalies, elongation of a cervical transverse process, hypertrophy of the omohyoid or the scalenus anticus muscles, and poststenotic aneurysms of the subclavian artery.[10] Roos described surgical findings in 232 patients who required surgical decompression.[13] Of these, 27 cases were associated with cervical ribs or clavicle anomalies; other anatomic anomalies found included cervical bands (22 cases), and hyperplastic first ribs (3 cases). Roos found no anatomic anomalies in the remaining 81% of his cases.

Cervical ribs are common, and may, or may not, contribute to thoracic outlet syndrome. Often, the cause is a functional change in the thoracic outlet due to aging (sagging muscles from sedentary activities) with no significant anatomic fault.[5,6,11]

A carpal tunnel syndrome may coexist.[5,14] Retrograde neurologic symptoms from a carpal tunnel syndrome are common and may

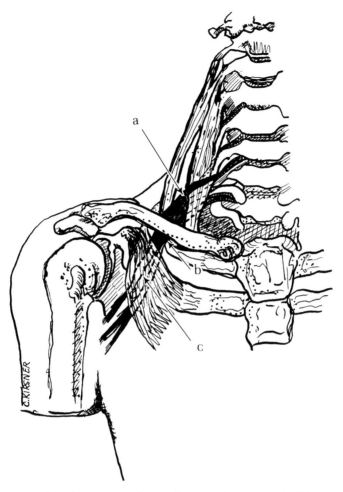

Fig. 3–1. The thoracic outlet: The neurovascular bundle passes through 3 potential spaces, which are (a) the triangular space between the scalene muscles, (b) the costoclavicular space, and (c) a space beneath the pectoralis minor muscle.

be confusing diagnostically. Patients may complain of hand congestion, arm weakness, shoulder pain, and nocturnal paresthesia relieved only by elevating and hyperabducting the arm—all due to a carpal tunnel syndrome.[14] Positive tests for median nerve compression at the wrist, or relief following a corticosteroid injection into the carpal tunnel, will help resolve the cause of symptoms in most patients. Thus, the carpal tunnel syndrome can accompany a thoracic outlet syndrome, or can cause similar symptomatology. Chest pain often results from thoracic outlet syndrome but this syndrome may be overlaid upon coronary artery disease or reflux esophagitis. In fact, it is not uncommon for all three conditions to be present at the same time.

The Examination. A careful history and physical examination are essential. Of 149 patients reviewed by Dale and Lewis,[5] all had reported painful upper extremities; 58% suffered intermittent paresthesia, 23% reported motor incoordination, and only 16% had edema of the upper extremities. In two large series, over 80% of patients had neurologic complaints of intermittent paresthesia or motor incoordination; less than 20% had vascular symptoms or edema.[5,15]

Occupational and other aggravating causes should be elicited. Painters, welders, mailmen, and auto mechanics who frequently work with their arms overhead may acquire the syndrome during hyperabduction. Poor sleep position, with the arms hyperabducted, leads to neurovascular compression. Sedentary activities that allow the shoulders to drop down and forward may provoke symptoms.

The important factor in the physical examination is to *look at the patient*. Is there a postural problem? In the female with heavy pendulous breasts, tight brassiere, and deep strap marks, drooping shoulders will be evident (Fig. 1, p. 5). Is the patient's thorax unusually narrow at the apex? Does the patient have poor muscle tone with drooping clavicles? Palpation and auscultation of the costoclavicular space for the presence of a cervical rib, tumor, aneurysm, or malformation of the body structures are quick, simple, and necessary procedures.[5] The scalene muscles and brachial plexus may be tender to palpation or percussion, and if the condition is unilateral, the tenderness of the involved side should be compared with the uninvolved side.[16] Therefore, laying on of hands is essential in the art of dealing with nonarticular rheumatism.

Physical maneuvers, to determine the presence of compression of the neurovascular bundle, include the Adson test, the costoclavicular maneuver,[17] and the hyperabduction maneuver.

The Adson test is performed by having the patient sit with pronated forearms on the knees, chin raised high and pointed toward the side being examined, holding his breath during inspiration; determine whether the radial pulse is abolished or diminished; then repeat with head pointed straight forward. The latter position should not cause compression.[18]

The modified *Adson test* is performed with the patient seated, arms at her side; the pulse is palpated at the wrist, and auscultated for a bruit in the supraclavicular space.[15,19] During the Adson maneuver, the patient performs a Valsalva maneuver with the neck fully

extended, arm elevated and the chin turned toward the side being examined, or away from the involved side[10,11] (Fig. 3–2). The purpose of this test is to tense the scalenus anticus muscle. A positive test results in diminished pulsation of the radial artery and a bruit over the axillary vessels; the patient becomes aware of increased paresthesia.

The *costoclavicular maneuver* is performed by having the patient's shoulder rotated backward and downward, with neurovascular features similar to Adson's test becoming evident (Fig. 3–3). Yet another technique is as follows: Patient stands with elbows flexed at 90 degrees. In the coronal plane of the body (arms in 90 degrees abduction), the arms are placed in three positions: at 45 degrees, 90 degrees, and 135 degrees (arms on top of head); at each position the radial pulses are palpated and the examiner auscultates inferior to the midpoint of the clavicle for a bruit. Pulse diminution and bruit occur in cases of obstruction by the first rib.[18] The *hyperabduction maneuver* reproduces symptoms when the patient laterally circumducts the arms and clasps the hands over the head (Fig. 3–4). This results in compression of the neurovascular bundle beneath the insertion of the tendon of the pectoralis minor muscle at the coracoid process.

The *Spurling maneuver*, discussed in Chapter 2, helps to exclude the presence of a cervical nerve root impingement as a cause of symptoms[20] (Fig. 2–13). Of normal asymptomatic persons, 38% have a positive Adson's test, 68% have a positive costoclavicular maneuver, and 54% have a positive hyperabduction maneuver.[14] The reproduction of the patient's symptoms with these tests is valuable in making the diagnosis.

Taking a complete history, observing for neurovascular compression, reproducing symptoms with one or another of the test maneuvers, and determining any occupational or positional aggravating causes for thoracic outlet compression certainly helps the clinician.[5] A good response to therapy is excellent support for the diagnosis.

Laboratory and Radiographic Examina-

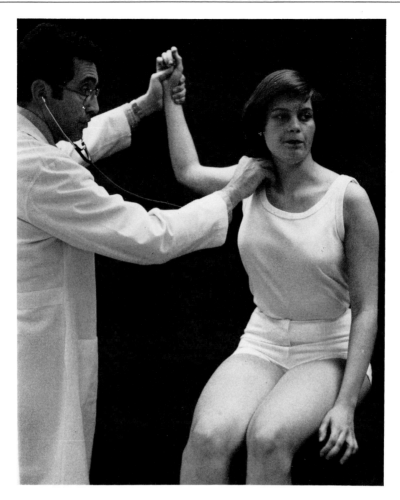

Fig. 3–2. The modified Adson maneuver for neurovascular compression by scalenus anticus muscle. A positive test includes reproduction of symptoms, diminution of the pulse at the wrist, and the development of a bruit over the axillary vessels.

tion. Roentgenographs of the chest and cervical spine are necessary to exclude the presence of tumors, cervical ribs, or other skeletal anomalies. An erythrocyte sedimentation rate should be performed to exclude inflammatory and neoplastic conditions. Special tests, including nerve conduction or invasive vascular studies, can be withheld as long as vascular features are not objectively present at the time of the first visit. Stress electrocardiograms may be necessary to exclude other causes if chest pain is a prominent feature.[5] If the patient does not respond to initial therapy, nerve conduction velocities can sometimes provide prognostic information. In nor-

mal persons, the ulnar nerve conduction velocity ranges from 68 to 75 m/sec; however, patients with thoracic outlet syndrome usually have delayed conduction levels. Urschel reported that patients whose ulnar nerve conduction velocity was less than 60 m/sec generally required surgical intervention.[4] Recently the value of electrodiagnostic study was re-evaluated;[21–23] electrodiagnostic testing was found useful only in order to exclude cervical nerve root compression or a carpal tunnel syndrome.[5,15] The cost:benefit ratio of the test is poor in our experience as well as that of others.[16] Vascular studies, including arteriography and venography, are indicated

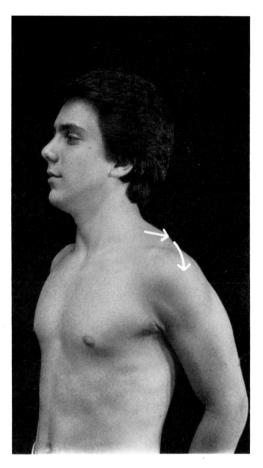

Fig. 3–3. The costoclavicular maneuver (arrows) reproduces symptoms and decreases the pulse amplitude at the costoclavicular space. Backpacking is a common cause for the costoclavicular syndrome.

Diagnostic Workup for Thoracic Outlet Syndrome

History
1. Intermittent pain, paresthesia, and swelling of part or all of an upper extremity.
2. Aggravating factors, such as hyperabducting arms, at work or during sleep.
3. Absence of specific features of carpal tunnel syndrome, cervical disc disease, or other systemic disease.

Physical Examination
1. Check for masses in supraclavicular fossa.
2. Perform special maneuvers (e.g., Adson's, hyperabduction, costoclavicular maneuvers).
3. Absence of objective swelling or atrophy in most patients.

Routine Tests
1. Cervical spine and chest roentgenograms.
2. Tests for inflammation.
3. Electrocardiogram if chest pain coexists.

A beneficial response to treatment may be the best test

Special Tests (rarely needed)
1. Electrodiagnostic studies.
2. Vascular studies, incuding venography, venous flow rates, or angiography.

---

when physical findings suggest a vascular disorder, such as an aneurysm or venous thrombosis,[14] but otherwise help little in making the diagnosis. When symptoms suggest the presence of a carpal tunnel syndrome, nerve conduction tests of the ulnar and median nerves can be helpful. Cervical myelography may have to be considered in order to exclude cervical disc disease. We must emphasize that all tests may be normal and careful assessment of each patient is essential.

Differential Diagnosis. Conditions outside of the thoracic outlet rarely cause intermittent neurologic and vascular symptoms in the upper extremity. One should consider the possibility of tumors of the superior pulmonary sulcus (Pancoast's syndrome; see "Pancoast's Syndrome" in this chapter), impingement of a cervical nerve, cervical cord tumor, brachial plexus paralysis, carpal tunnel syndrome with retrograde symptomatology, peripheral neuropathies, syringomyelia, progressive muscle atrophy, reflex sympathetic dystrophy, and thrombosis or inflammation of the vascular tree.[4,24]

A review of those features that should warn of more serious disease is listed in Table 3–1.

Complaints of a purely vascular obstruction, with objective swelling of the upper

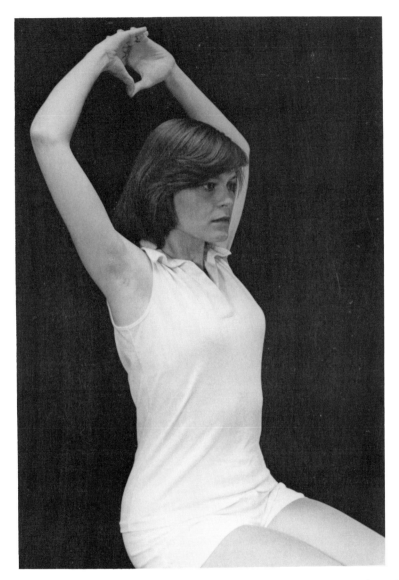

Fig. 3—4. The hyperabduction maneuver reproduces symptoms when compression occurs beneath the insertion of the pectoralis minor tendon at its insertion upon the coracoid process.

limb or Raynaud's phenomenon, are rare. Inflammatory diseases, such as giant cell arteritis, Takayasu's arteritis, and thrombosis of the subclavian vein (also called effort thrombosis or Paget-Schroetter's syndrome) must be considered.[4,6]

Management. On the first visit, if the examination is suggestive of a thoracic outlet syndrome, the patient may be told that the diagnosis is probably a benign neurovascular compression syndrome. Aggravating factors can be remedied. For example, women with heavy pendulous breasts should obtain brassieres that support properly. Sleep position should be reviewed with each patient. Patients should avoid sleeping with their arms hyperabducted or elevated. Some patients can be trained to avoid hyperabduction by tying their wrists with a stocking. This, in turn, is safety-pinned to the bed sheet to

Table 3–1. Danger Signs for Thoracic Outlet Region

1. Fever and chills
2. Horner's syndrome
3. Night pain in the limbs
4. Axillary pain
5. Ischemic limb appearance
6. Absent pulses
7. Arm claudication
8. Atrophy

allow some arm motion, but will restrict hyperabduction of the arms during sleep. (If the patient maintains her sanity, this can work. Most patients break the hyperabduction habit quickly.) During sedentary activities, patients should learn to roll their shoulders up and backward to prevent drooping of the clavicle. Hyperabduction required by employment may necessitate consultation with an occupational therapist. Other jobs that may require modification include letter carriers, painters, welders, who carry heavy loads on their shoulders, or who work overhead as when painting a ceiling or welding. Repetitive abduction and adduction may result in hypertrophy of the subclavius and pectoral muscles and in the susceptible person, this may compress the neurovascular bundle. Crane operators who push and pull can be at risk for thoracic outlet syndrome.[25]

Trigger points are frequently present along the trapezius ridge, and if palpable, can be relieved with injection of a nonaqueous steroid-anesthetic mixture (see Fig. 2–10). Of paramount importance are exercises to strengthen and correct postural deficits.[5,26] The following exercises should be prescribed: shoulder elevation with resistance, isometric neck strengthening, and if symptoms of chest-wall pain are evident, chest-wall stretching. These exercises correct the forward inclination of the neck and stretch the pectoral musculature.

The exercises for shoulder elevation can be performed with a 5- to 10-pound weight in each hand or across each shoulder; the patient may be seated or standing. The shoulders are rotated backward, and shrugged slowly up

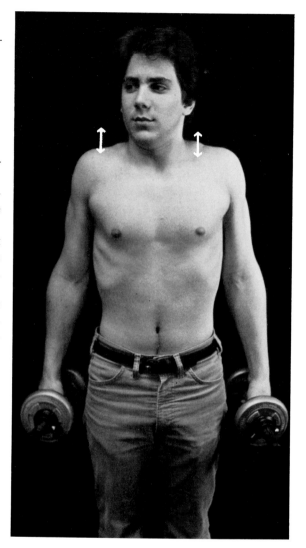

Fig. 3–5. The shoulder shrugging exercise: Using 5 to 10 pounds of weight placed upon each shoulder or held in each hand, the shoulders are shrugged and rotated upward and backward, and then slowly let down; the movement is repeated for 1 to 2 minutes.

and down while the arms hang at the sides (Fig. 3–5). This exercise is repeated slowly for a few minutes twice daily. An isometric neck-strengthening exercise that seems helpful is performed with the patient backed up to a wall. The patient's heels are 6 to 8 inches out from the wall, the torso lies back against the wall, and the hands are placed loosely behind the vertex of the head. The elbows may be pointed at a 45 degree forward angle from the wall, and the chin is kept neutral (face held perfectly vertical, parallel to the wall). The patient presses her head backward with increased vigor, and feels a stretching and contracting of the neck musculature (Fig. 3–6). This position is held for 10 to 30 seconds, with 3 to 10 repetitions, and is performed twice daily. Chest-wall stretching is accomplished by having the patient stand facing a corner of a room. The patient stands approximately 2 feet out from the corner and places her hands on each wall with the fingers pointed toward the corner. The shoulder,

arm, elbow, and hand are held at shoulder height. She then thrusts her chest slowly into the corner with her head held in the neutral position (the chin neither raised nor lowered).[27] The patient should experience a feeling of stretching in the pectoral muscles (Fig. 3–7). This position is held for 10 to 30 seconds and repeated 3 to 10 times at least twice daily. If sleep is disturbed, a relaxant or sedative

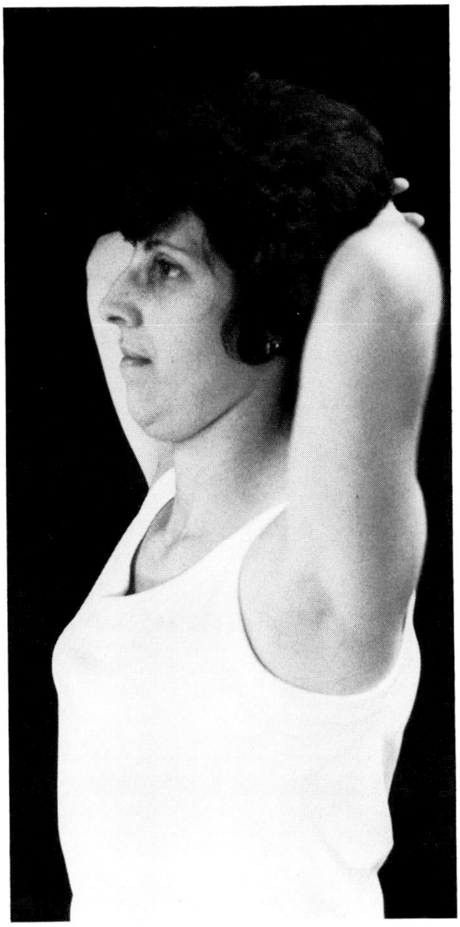

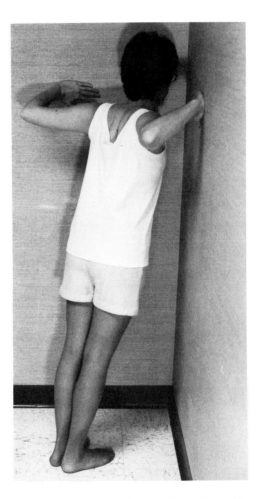

Fig. 3–7. The corner "push up": Chest wall stretching is easily accomplished by standing 2 feet out from a corner, with each hand approximately 18 to 24 inches away from the corner, hands pointed toward the corner and held at shoulder height. With the chin held neutral, the chest wall is gently forced in toward the corner, until a stretching sensation is perceived in the pectoral muscle region.

Fig. 3–6. Isometric neck exercise with the chin kept neutral. The hands should *not* press the head forward, but should only meet the backward thrust of the head and hold it from further motion.

may be prescribed at bedtime for the first week or two.[5]

Outcome and Additional Suggestions. Physical therapy and exercise, instructions in proper sitting, and proper work and sleep positions, should provide relief in 50 to 90% of patients[5,10,13–15] usually within 6 weeks.[5] Morning stiffness, hand congestion, paresthesia are the first symptoms to improve. Fewer than 5% of our patients require surgical treatment.

Before surgical exploration, check out the following:

1. Has carpal tunnel syndrome or cervical disc lesion been excluded?
2. Has chest roentgenogram for tumor been reviewed recently?
3. Were aggravating factors eliminated (sleep position, sitting positions, improper work habits)?
4. Did the patient comply with the exercise program?

Vascular studies and nerve conduction tests may be normal, yet surgical intervention is still undertaken because of persistent symptoms. At operation, compression has been found as low as the second rib,[13] and the current surgical procedure of choice is resection of the first rib to provide more space for the neurovascular bundle. Unfortunately, we have seen surgical failures. The symptoms have returned when the patient resumed work requiring hyperabduction. A change in jobs should have preceded operation. We have found that if cases are properly selected, first rib resection through the transaxillary approach gives good results in 85% of operated patients.[28] Others reported somewhat less surgical success.[29,30] Failure following first rib resection may result from surgical inexperience[31] or coexisting reflux esophagitis, coronary artery disease, or carpal tunnel syndrome.[15] Whenever a carpal tunnel coexists, we would treat the carpal tunnel more aggressively before considering thoracic outlet surgery, and reassess the thoracic outlet symptoms after relief from median nerve entrapment has been effected.

REFLEX SYMPATHETIC DYSTROPHY (RSD)

The essential features of reflex sympathetic dystrophy (RSD), which may occur in either the upper or lower extremity, include *throbbing, burning pain*, diffuse uncomfortable aching, sensitivity to touch or cold, altered color or temperature of the involved extremity, localized edema, and erythema. Three stages in the course of RSD may occur. In the earliest stage, the presentation consists of hyperesthesia, hyperalgesia, localized edema, erythema, and altered skin temperature. In the second stage, 3 to 6 months from the time of onset, progression of the soft tissue edema, thickening of the skin and articular soft tissues, muscle wasting, and brawny skin develop. In the third and most severe stage, the shoulder-hand syndrome manifestations of limitation of movement, contractures of the digits, waxy trophic skin changes, and brittle, ridged nails appear.[32–36]

Classic trophic skin changes include skin atrophy or pigmentary changes, hypertrichosis, hyperhidrosis, and nail changes.[37]

Terminology has included causalgia, minor causalgia, shoulder-hand syndrome, shoulder-hand syndrome variant, Sudeck's atrophy, and acute atrophy of bone. Often the syndrome follows injury, surgical intervention, or vascular accidents, such as heart attack or stroke. Pak, in a study of 140 patients, reported that 40% of cases of RSD occurred following soft tissue injury, 25% followed fractures, 20% occurred postoperatively, 12% followed myocardial infarction, and 3% followed cerebral vascular accidents.[38] Of patients with RSD, 37% had significant emotional disturbances at the time of onset.[38] Myofascial trigger points are common in the area of trauma or about the shoulder girdle and trapezius.[39,40] Although only one extremity may appear involved, careful inspection may reveal symmetric synovitis.[35,40] The elbow is usually spared.

Etiology. The probability that central nervous system (CNS) disturbance plays a role in RSD causation is supported by the finding that unilateral sympathetic nerve blocks result in improvement in bilateral skin potential variations (pain thresholds).[39] This improvement lasts 48 hours, long after the pharmacologic effect of the anesthetic has worn off. Furthermore, myofascial trigger points also disappear (even in the limb contralateral to the sympathetic nerve block). A feedback loop with involvement of skin, afferent input into the CNS, then feeding back via a sympathetic output to the skin is proposed as the method for CNS involvement.[39] Nine patients with RSD were studied with ^{133}Xe washout technique to measure blood flow, using the normal side as control. Changes in flow with the arm first elevated and then dangling were compared. The patients were found to have increased flow at rest but normal vasoconstriction responses. The authors concluded that patients with RSD have normal function of peripheral vascular mechanisms, increased resting blood flow, and therefore a decreased sympathetic activity.[41] Changes in the "gate controls" of Melzack and Wall are probable[33,34,42,43] (see Chapt. 14). A self-perpetuating "short circuiting" between pain fibers and sympathetic nerves is then established. Histologic findings in one study of three children with reflex sympathetic dystrophy revealed skin capillary endothelial swelling and basement membrane thickening and reduplication. Muscle findings suggest ischemic changes.[44] Synovial changes include synovial edema, proliferation and disarray of synovial lining cells, proliferation of capillaries, fibrosis of the subsynovium, and slight perivascular infiltration with lymphocytes. The synovitis was more marked in the small finger joints of the affected side.[37,45,46]

The occurrence of RSD following vascular or surgical insults has been mentioned. Reflex dystrophy of a lower extremity in adolescents[47] and following knee surgery were reported.[48] The presentations were typical, often post-traumatic; pain was disproportionate to physical findings and typical skin changes occurred. Management consisted of sympathetic nerve blocks or sym-

pathectomy.[49] One case of RSD complicating polymyalgia rheumatica was reported.[50]

Laboratory and Radiographic Examination. In the early stage, reflex sympathetic dystrophy may reveal no abnormal findings on laboratory testing. After 6 weeks' duration, scintigraphy, using technetium 99m pertechnetate (99m TcO_4), may reveal increased uptake in the peripheral joints of the involved extremity.[45,51] In patients studied soon after onset of symptoms, scintigrams taken immediately post-injection usually show decreased perfusion of the affected areas.[44] Sedimentation rate and other tests of inflammation may increase in the later stages. In the third stage, roentgenographs of the involved extremities may reveal patchy osteoporosis, presumably due to increased blood flow to the involved extremity.[45] A valuable test is the use of regional sympathetic nerve blocks, for both therapy and diagnosis. Abrupt relief from pain and dysesthesia, although transient, is suggestive of a diagnosis of reflex dystrophy. Tests to rule out insidious onset of a connective tissue disease should include rheumatoid and antinuclear factor determinations. A chest roentgenogram for an occult neoplasm at the apex of the lung, on the involved side, should be performed. EMG with nerve conduction velocity may be helpful if thoracic outlet syndrome or carpal tunnel syndrome is a consideration.

Differential Diagnosis. In the earliest stages, reflex sympathetic dystrophy is a difficult diagnosis. However, the quality of *throbbing, burning* pain, *paresthesia*, and *altered skin temperature* is suggestive. Cervical nerve root impingement, Pancoast's syndrome, vasculitis, rheumatoid arthritis, peripheral neuropathy, migratory osteolysis, venous thrombosis, arteriovenous fistulae, progressive systemic sclerosis, and angioedema might be confused with early features of various presentations of RSD.

Management. Four modes of therapy are available, depending on the stage of the dystrophy at the time of the first visit. These are (1) myofascial trigger point injection and physical therapy, adrenergic blocking agents (guanethidine) or alpha-receptor blocking agents (phenoxybenzamine),[52,53] (2) sympathetic nerve blocks, (3) oral corticosteroids, and (4) sympathectomy.[54] The best treatment is prevention. Early mobilization of the shoulder and arm after injury, and following myocardial infarction or stroke needs to be encouraged. Prolonged use of intravenous therapy should be accompanied by intermittent passive shoulder motion. In the first stage, trigger-point injections with a corticosteroid-local anesthetic mixture, followed by physical therapy, including heat and exercise, may abort progression of the dystrophy. Guanethidine or phenoxybenzamine should be considered in first and second stage dystrophy. The dosage of either medication can begin with 10 mg tid, orally.[52,53] Regional intravenous infusion of reserpine may be tried if patients fail to respond to oral medication.[49] The value of physical therapy is anecdotal but all agree that it appears beneficial. However, it must be individualized and supervised. Hand splinting while at rest is useful to prevent contractures. Active stretching with use of wand exercises, range of motion exercises, and in the acute stage, gentle passive motion should be started. Deep friction massage may dampen the autonomic nervous system and relieve pain. Transcutaneous electric nerve stimulation (TENS) has been described as of value.[55] In our experience, local steroid injections have been helpful in alleviating the throbbing burning pain that interferes with any active exercise plan. Use of a TENS unit can be initiated after the initial visit; it is a noninvasive treatment and is worth trying before more complex treatment measures are utilized. Use of sedation or antidepressive medication may be helpful. Consideration for any possible missed diagnosis (e.g., a missed fracture) is important.

In second stage dystrophy, with beginning induration of the skin of the hand, resting hand and wrist splints may be helpful. At this point, stellate ganglion blocks performed at intervals of 1 to 4 days and repeated 6 to 12 times have been useful. If an immediate response (improved temperature, lessened pain) does not occur following the first or second nerve block, this treatment is abandoned.[34,37] An alternative therapy is using oral corticosteroids in divided doses, ranging from 30 mg per day[37] to 80 mg per day.[36] Steroid treatment was of most benefit in patients in whom positive [99]technetium bone scans suggested an active inflammatory lesion.[37] The dose of corticosteroids is tapered quickly as the patient responds; continued low-dose corticosteroid treatment may be necessary for a prolonged period in severe cases. In all patients, at all stages of the disease, physical therapy should be performed twice daily at home, and use of resting splints should be maintained. Sympathectomy is indicated if progression is apparent, and a positive response to sympathetic nerve blocks occurs. A new noninvasive technique using equipment that emits high frequency radio waves, radiofrequency, to perform upper thoracic sympathectomy may be applicable to the treatment of RSD.[56] Patients with advanced dystrophic hands should have consultations with physical and occupational therapists. Patients, on occasion, have both reflex sympathetic dystrophy and thoracic outlet syndrome, and may require surgical treatment for both conditions (resection of the first rib and cervical sympathectomy).[5]

Outcome and Additional Suggestions. Our experience with treatment of reflex dystrophy prior to contracture has been excellent with either stellate ganglion blocks or corticosteroid therapy. As mentioned, if seen early after onset, trigger-point injections may break the cycle. We have seen patients have an exacerbation several months after treatment, either upon exposure to cold or following emotional trauma. Small doses of amytal (30 to 60 mg qid) for several weeks, or use of tricyclic antidepressants (amitriptyline) for a recurrence has been helpful in our experience. In late-stage dystrophy, with a practically immobilized hand, aggressive physical therapy is essential, and sympathectomy must be considered. We have seen late-stage dystrophy significantly improve without resorting to sympathectomy. Oral corticoste-

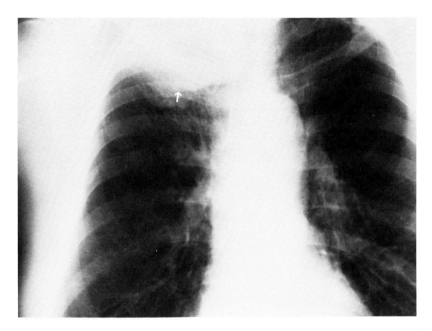

Fig. 3–8. A lung tumor (arrow) associated with Pancoast's syndrome. Although such lesions may be clinically silent until late, chest roentgenograms with apical lordotic views should be performed if symptoms are at all suggestive.

roids have not proven as helpful in late-stage dystrophy.

PANCOAST'S SYNDROME

Tumors within the superior pulmonary sulcus that compress the lower roots of the brachial plexius, the intercostal nerves, the stellate ganglion, and the sympathetic nerve chain comprise Pancoast's syndrome. Features include constant pain, at first in the shoulder region, and later along the ulnar distribution to the arm and hand. Still later, Horner's syndrome and anhidrosis of the ipsilateral face and upper extremity occur, and atrophy of the intrinsic muscles of the hand may be noted.[57]

Careful study of the superior pulmonary sulcus with standard and apical lordotic roentgenographs is essential (Fig. 3–8). Treatment obviously depends upon finding the nature of the mass, since the vast majority are malignant.

We must again emphasize that discomfort of the thoracic outlet syndrome is intermit-

tent, whereas Pancoast's syndrome of pain, burning, and numbness is constant. The constancy of symptoms (present day and night) must stimulate the physician to order appropriate roentgenographs and study them carefully. In one report, 34% of patients treated surgically for superior sulcus tumors survived 5 years, and 29% survived 10 years.[58]

REFERENCES

1. Wakefield G: Entrapment neuropathies. Clin Rheum Dis 5:941–956, 1979.
2. Hope T: Pinpointing entrapment neuropathies in the elderly. Geriatrics 35:79–89, 1980.
3. Urschel HC, Razzuk MA, Hyland JW, et al: Thoracic outlet syndrome masquerading as coronary artery disease (Pseudoangina). Ann Thoracic Surg 16:239–248, 1973.
4. Urschel HC, Razzuk MA: Management of the thoracic-outlet syndrome. N Engl J Med 286:1140–1143, 1972.
5. Dale WA, Lewis MR: Management of thoracic outlet syndrome. Ann Surg 181:575–585, 1975.
6. Bertelsen S: Neurovascular compression syndromes of the neck and shoulder. Acta Chir Scand 135:137–148, 1969.
7. Keshishian JM, Smyth NPD: Thoracic outlet syndrome: Diagnosis and management. Ann Thorac Surg 9:391–400, 1970.

8. Carroll RE, Hurst LC: Relationship of thoracic out-let syndrome and carpal tunnel syndrome. Clin Orthop 164:149–153, 1982.

9. Winsor T, Brow R: Costoclavicular syndrome. JAMA 196:109–111, 1966.

10. Tyson RR, Kaplan GF: Modern concepts of diagnosis and treatment of the thoracic outlet syndrome. Ortho Clin N Am 6:507–519, 1975.

11. Steinbrocker O, Argyros TG: The shoulder-hand syndrome: present status as a diagnostic and therapeutic entity. Med Clin No Am 42:1533–1553, 1958.

12. Swift TR, Nichols FT: The droopy shoulder syndrome. Neurol 34:212–215, 1984.

13. Roos DB: Experience with first rib resection for thoracic outlet syndrome. Ann Surg 173:429–442, 1971.

14. Conn J Jr: Thoracic outlet syndromes. Surg Clin N Am 54:155–164, 1974.

15. McGough EC, Pearce MB, Byrne JP: Management of thoracic outlet syndrome. J Thorac Cardiovasc Surg 77:169–174, 1979.

16. Crawford FA: Thoracic outlet syndrome. Surg Clin N Am 604:947–957, 1980.

17. Roos DB, Owens JC: Thoracic outlet syndrome. Arch Surg 93:71–74, 1966.

18. DeGowen EL, DeGowen RL: Bedside Diagnostic Examination. 4th Ed, New York Macmillan Pub Co., 1981.

19. Jackson R: The Cervical Syndrome. Springfield, Charles C Thomas, 1978.

20. Spurling RG, Scoville WB: Lateral rupture of the cervical intervertebral discs. Surg Gynecol Obstet 78:350–358, 1944.

21. Wilbourn, AJ: Evidence for conduction delay in thoracic-outlet syndrome is challenged. N Engl J Med 310:1052–1053, 1984.

22. Urschel HC Jr: Letter to the editor. New Engl J Med 310:1053, 1984.

23. Relman AS: Responsibilities of authorship: where does the buck stop? N Engl J Med 310:1048–1049, 1984.

24. Duthie RB, Ferguson AB: Mercer's Orthopedic Surgery. 7th Ed. Baltimore, Williams & Wilkins, 1973.

25. Feldman RG, Goldman R, Keyserling WM: Peripheral nerve entrapment syndromes and ergonomic factors. Am J Indus Med 4:661–681, 1983.

26. Peet RM, Henriksen JD, Anderson TB, et al: Thoracic outlet syndrome: Evaluation of a therapeutic exercise program. Proc Staff Meet Mayo Clin 31:281–287, 1956.

27. Swezey RL: The modern thrust of manipulation and traction therapy. Seminars Rheum Dis 12:321–331, 1983.

28. Goldberg VM: The results of first rib resection in thoracic outlet syndrome. Orthopedics 4:1025–1029, 1981.

29. Spittell JA Jr: Raynaud's phenomenon and Allied Vasospastic Disorders. Peripheral Vascular Diseases. Edited by John L. Juergons et al. Philadelphia, WB Saunders, 1980.

30. Derkash RS, Goldberg VM: The results of first rib resection in thoracic outlet syndrome. Orthop 4:1025–1029, 1981.

31. Roos DB: Recurrent thoracic outlet syndrome after first rib resection. Acta Chirurgica Belgica 79:363–380, 1980.

32. Homans J: Minor causalgia: A hyperesthetic neurovascular syndrome. N Engl J Med 222:870–874, 1940.

33. deJong RH, Cullen SC: Theoretical aspects of pain: Bizarre pain phenomena during low spinal anesthesia. Anesthesiology 24:628–635, 1963.

34. Bonica JJ: Causalgia and other reflex sympathetic dystrophies. Postgrad Med 53:143–148, 1973.

35. Steinbrocker O, Argyros TG: The shoulder-hand syndrome: Present status as a diagnostic and therapeutic entity. Med Clin North Am 42:1533–1553, 1958.

36. Mowat AG: Treatment of the shoulder-hand syndrome with corticosteroids. Ann Rheum Dis 33:120–123, 1974.

37. Kozin F, McCarty DJ, Sims J, Genant H: The reflex sympathetic dystrophy syndrome. I: Clinical and histologic studies: response to corticosteroids and articular involvement. Am J Med 60:321–331, 1976.

38. Pak TJ, Martin GM, Magness JL, Kavanaugh GJ: Reflex sympathetic dystrophy. Minn Med 53:507–512, 1970.

39. Procacci P, Francin F, Zoppi M, et al: Role of sympathetic system in reflex dystrophies. In Advances in Pain Research and Therapy. Vol. 1. Edited by JJ Bonica, D Albe-Fessard. New York, Raven Press, 1976.

40. Edeiken J. Wolferth CC: Persistent pain in the shoulder region following myocardial infarction. Am J Med Sci 191:201–210, 1936.

41. Christianssen K, Henriksen O: The reflex sympathetic dystrophy syndrome—an experimental study of blood flow and autoregulation in subcutaneous tissue. (Abstract #E42) Arth Rheum 25(No. 4) [Supp], 1982.

42. Bonica JJ: Neurophysiologic and pathologic aspects of acute and chronic pain. Arch Surg 112:750–761, 1977.

43. Melzach R, Wall PD: Pain mechanisms: A new theory. Science 150:971–979, 1965.

44. Nickeson R, Brewer E, Person D: Early histologic and radionuclide scan changes in children with reflex sympathetic dystrophy syndrome. (Abstract #C38) Arth Rheum 28(No. 4) [Supp], 1985.

45. Kozin F, Genant HK, Bekerman C, McCarty DJ: The reflex sympathetic dystrophy syndrome. II. Roentgenographic and scintigraphic evidence of bilaterality and of periarticular accentuation. Am J Med 60:332–338, 1976.

46. Kozin F, Ryan LM, Carerra GF, et al: The reflex sympathetic dystrophy syndrome. III: Scintigraphic studies, further evidence for the therapeutic efficacy of systemic corticosteroids, and proposed diagnostic criteria. Am J Med: 70:23–30, 1981.

47. Wettrell G, Hallbook T, Hultquist C: Reflex sympathetic dystrophy in two young females. Acta Paediat Scand 68:923–924, 1979.

48. Kim HJ, Kozin F, Johnson RP, Hines R: Reflex sympathetic dystrophy syndrome of the knee following meniscectomy: report of three cases. Arth Rheum 22:177–181, 1979.

49. Benzon HT, Chomka CM, Brunner ED: Treatment of reflex sympathetic dystrophy with regional intra-

venous reserpine. Anesth Analgesia 59:500–502, 1980.

50. Wysenbeck AJ: Reflex sympathetic dystrophy syndrome complicating polymyalgia rheumatica. Arth Rheum 24:863–864, 1981.

51. Carlson DH, Simon H, Wegner W.: Bone scanning and diagnosis of reflex sympathetic dystrophy secondary to herniated lumbar disks. Neurology 27:791–793, 1977.

52. Tabira T, Shibasaki H, Kuroiwa Y: Reflex sympathetic dystrophy (Causalgia) treatment with guanethidine. Arch Neurol 40:430–432, 1983.

53. Ghostine SY, Comair YG, Turner DM, Kassell NF, Azar CG: Phenoxybenzamine in the treatment of causalgia. J Neurosurg 60:1263–1268, 1984.

54. Moskowitz RW: Clinical Rheumatology, 2nd Ed. Philadelphia, Lea & Febiger, 1982.

55. Schutzer SF, Gossling HR: The treatment of reflex sympathetic dystrophy syndrome. J Bone Joint Surg 66A:625–629, 1984.

56. Wilkinson HA: Radiofrequency percutaneous upper-thoracic sympathectomy. N Engl J Med 311:34–48, 1984.

57. Hepper NGG, Herskovic T, Witten DM, et al: Thoracic inlet tumors. Ann Intern Med 64:979–988, 1966.

58. Paulson DL: Carcinomas in the superior pulmonary sulcus. J Thoracic Cardiovasc Surg 70:1095–1104, 1975.

4

The Shoulder Girdle Region

When presented with a shoulder problem, the physician must take a careful history to determine whether the complaint is an *intrinsic* shoulder problem (e.g., osteoarthritis, bursitis), an *extrinsic* shoulder problem reflecting pain from other structures (e.g., reflex dystrophy, referred pain arising from cholecystitis), or part of systemic disease.[1-3] A *pain pattern* may delineate the nature of the specific shoulder problem.[1] Furthermore, the clinician should seek aggravating factors that might cause recurrences.

The History. Pain quality, location, duration, and frequency are important. For example, axillary pain of a constant undulating quality should raise suspicion of a mediastinal lesion. Pain over the deltoid region is frequently referred from the subacromial bursa, but can also arise from a myofascial trigger point in the infraspinatus muscle; and pain in the triceps area may be referred from the serratus posterior superior muscle.[4]

Intermittent pain and disability suggest tendon injury or myofascial disturbances. Pain that is present both day and night suggests capsular involvement, true shoulder synovitis, or tumor. Pain that is intermittent, throbbing, or burning suggests reflex sympathetic dystrophy (shoulder-hand syndrome). Abrupt onset of pain accompanied by limitation of movement suggests tissue disruption, such as a capsular tear or a shoulder joint dislocation.

What about the rest of the body? Are there complains in other parts of the same extremity, or is there a history of systemic inflammatory rheumatic disease? For example, a patient with carpal tunnel syndrome occasionally has retrograde nerve involvement to the shoulder,[5] and cervical radicular pain is often noted at the shoulder. Knowledge of the patient's past history may suggest intra-abdominal or intrathoracic problems with referral of pain to the shoulder or scapular regions. Diaphragmatic irritation from intrathoracic or intra-abdominal structures has specific patterns of pain referral. For example, irritation of the anterior portion of the diaphragm may refer pain to the clavicle or to the front of the shoulder, pain from the posterior diaphragm may refer to the supraspinatus region of the shoulder, pain from the dome of the diaphragm may refer to the acromioclavicular joint area, and irritation of the central portion of the diaphragm may refer pain into both shoulder regions.[6] Danger signs and symptoms are listed in Table 4–1.

Therefore, systemic rheumatic diseases, metabolic disorders (e.g., hyperparathyroidism, hypothyroidism, hyperthyroidism, diabetes), neurologic disturbances, and cardiovascular diseases involve the shoulder.[7-9] Fortunately, fewer than 5 to 10% of shoulder afflictions are due to true arthritis.[3,10]

Aggravating factors (Table 4–2) can range from activities on the job, sports, hobbies, or sleep position. Most important are activities

Table 4–1. Danger List: Shoulder

1. Any visible swelling.
2. Fever and chills.
3. Constant and progressive pain.
4. Pain in the axilla.
5. Numbness or tingling.
6. Inability to maintain active arm elevation.
7. Shoulder pain that is aggravated by neck motion.
8. Shoulder pain unrelated to arm movement.
9. Bruit over subclavian vessels.
10. Other features of vascular impairment.

Table 4–2. Aggravating Factors for the Shoulder[15,16]

Harmful	Helpful
Repetitively moving the shoulder to and fro while holding the elbow out to the side pinches tendons inside the shoulder.	■ Frequently interrupt such tasks as washing windows, vacuuming, and working on an assembly line. Keep the elbow close to the body during to-and-fro movement. When raking or sweeping, hold the rake or broom out in front of the body. Doing so changes the angles of shoulder motion.
Sleeping with the arms overhead can pinch muscles and nerves in the shoulder region.	■ Sleep with the arms below the level of the chest.
Similarly, working with the arms overhead for prolonged periods can be injurious.	■ Take frequent breaks when working with the arms overhead.
Using the shoulder as a weight-bearing joint (e.g., when leaning on crutches or canes or pushing off from chairs) can lead to shoulder injury.	■ See that crutches fit 2 in. (about 5 cm) below axillae; carry weight on ribs. A forearm cane may be preferred. When arising from a chair, push off with thigh muscles, not the hands.
Reaching sideways and backward into the back seat of a vehicle to bring a briefcase, grocery bag, or other object forward is a common cause of pain in the shoulder-blade region.	■ Face the object and draw it forward.
Repetitively reaching behind for a kitchen utensil and bringing it forward has a similar effect.	■ Turn the body, not just the shoulder, and grasp the utensil.
Placing the hands on top of the steering wheel for long periods can be irritating to nerves and muscles in the shoulder region.	■ Keep the hands below the 3- and 9-o'clock positions on the wheel. If possible, use a steering wheel that tilts.

in which the arm is held in close to the body for prolonged periods (e.g., typing or needlepoint). Next in importance are work habits with repetitive motions, particularly while the arm is raised over the head. A middle-aged person taking up tennis, carpentry, or starting a new calisthenic program may become symptomatic. Sleeping with the arms held overhead may be a factor in developing shoulder pain. Sports that are commonly associated with shoulder problems include swimming, baseball, tennis, football, and gymnastics. In swimmers, the condition more often occurs on the side on which the swimmer breathes, and after sprinting. Tennis players may develop the "King Kong arm" with shoulder girdle droop in association with unilateral muscle hypertrophy.[11]

Persons with a compulsive "I'm going to finish this if it kills me!" attitude are prone to tendinitis from overuse. When shoulder pain arises from employment, it is important to consider underlying congenital malformations and diseases which predispose to symptoms, the contribution of joint stress from outside the workplace, as well as excessive joint movement and loading.[12,13] Shoulder pain might result from prolonged videogame use![14]

The Shoulder Examination. Examining a patient with a shoulder problem is an art. The examiner must know the accepted normal ranges of shoulder motion, something about the dynamics of shoulder function, and something about innervation of the shoulder structure. Shoulder function depends on a scapulohumeral rhythm, an unhampered gliding motion, integrity of the musculotendinous cuff, normality of the bursae, integrity of the long head of the biceps, and mobility of the joint capsule.[3] The sternoclavicular joint is the pivot on which the shoulder girdle moves on the trunk.[17] See Anatomic Plates IV and V.

It is important that the clinician examines the whole patient. We have already demonstrated the importance of postural disturbances, and have stressed that shoulder problems arising from involvement of distant structures (e.g., the neck, the carpal tunnel, or systemic inflammatory disease) may be apparent on gross inspection. Note the *symmetry* of acromioclavicular joints of the scapulae and muscle bulk, and observe scapular movement during active shoulder and neck motion.

When the patient performs a movement, the movement is called *active movement;* when the examiner moves the patient's arm, it is called *passive movement;* and when the patient attempts active movement against the examiner's resistance, the movement is called *active resistive motion.*

First, the patient performs an active motion, shoulder abduction, which should be observed from the rear. The patient swings his arm away from his side, out and up. *Abduction* occurs from zero degrees (arm hanging dependently at the side) outward and upward to 90 degrees; *elevation* proceeds from 90 to 180 degrees. Next, the shoulder, used as a hinge, is observed from the side view as *forward* and *backward extension.* Motion is next observed with the shoulder used as a rotary or ball-and-socket joint. With his arm at his side, the patient bends his elbow to 90 degrees and rotates his elbow internally (hand to chest), or externally (hand away from chest). This rotation may also be observed with the arm abducted to 90 degrees; this time external rotation brings the hand up, and internal rotation brings the hand down. Thus, *internal* and *external rotation* refer to the direction of movement of the humerus (Figs. 4–1, 4–2, 4–3).[18]

Active shoulder motion may be limited either from pain or from intrinsic shoulder disturbances. With the patient as relaxed as possible, *passive* shoulder motion is attempted by the examiner to determine the presence of intrinsic shoulder disease. The

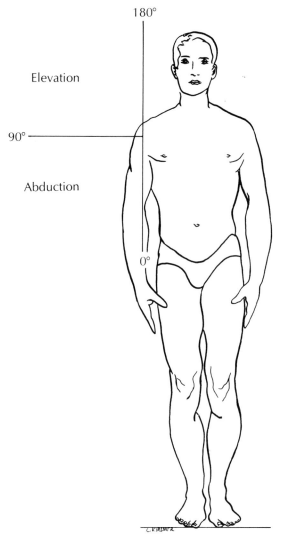

Fig. 4–1. Active shoulder motion *abduction* from 0 to 90 degrees. Further raising of the arm, *elevation,* proceeds from 90 to 180 degrees.

examination should be performed slowly in each direction to prevent muscle guarding. The examination for passive range of movement includes abduction-elevation and internal-external rotation, while keeping scapular movement to a minimum. The examiner should keep a hand upon the suprascapular ridge, to identify scapular movement and to demonstrate true glenohumeral motion, while performing passive arm motion.

There is a gradual loss of passive range of

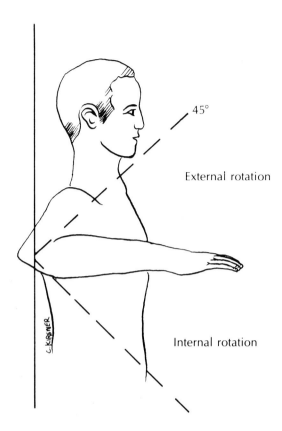

Fig. 4–2. Rotation of the humerus, internally and externally.

motion with aging and females lose more motion than males; no differences have been noted between dominant and non-dominant sides.[19]

Bursitis and tendinitis may interfere with active movement, but usually allow passive movement. Adhesive capsulitis restricts both active and passive shoulder motion. Furthermore, loss of motion in only one direction suggests a single tendon injury or bursitis, whereas loss of passive motion in two or more planes suggests capsule or true shoulder joint disease. Severe shoulder pain, with loss of active range of motion, is often called "the painful arc syndrome".[20] A painful arc between 60 and 120 degrees of abduction usually indicates some disorder within the subacromial region, whereas a painful arc which becomes increasingly severe at full elevation

of the arm suggests a disorder of the acromioclavicular joint area. Identification of the source of pain requires careful palpation to detect the point of maximum tenderness. Generally, myofascial disorders or nerve root impingement interfere little, if at all, with passive shoulder motion.

The examiner palpates for synovitis, bicipital tenosynovitis, acromioclavicular joint swelling, sternoclavicular joint swelling, and shoulder joint crepitus. The examiner palpates posteriorly for myofascial trigger points in the serratus, rhomboid, trapezius, teres minor, and supraspinatus muscles, and along the medial border of the scapula while the scapula is drawn laterally (by having the patient adduct the arm across the chest to rotate the scapula laterally) (Fig. 4–4). Firm pressure over these structures in obscure shoulder pain problems may establish the presence of a myofascial trigger point, which will then reproduce the pain in the "target zone." A common example is an infraspinatus trigger point with a target zone over the deltoid area of the shoulder (Fig. 4–5).

We have already mentioned performing the Spurling maneuver in patients with suspected cervical nerve root impingement (see Chapt. 2). Patients with bicipital tenosynovitis may have palpable swelling of the biceps tendon sheath; tenderness and swelling are detected by rolling a finger across the biceps tendon and comparing this with the uninvolved biceps tendon of the opposite shoulder (Fig. 4–6). Active resistant motion is performed by having the patient abduct and elevate the arm from 80 to 100 degrees against the examiner's resistance.[1,21] The examiner searches particularly for a tear of the shoulder capsule. Shoulder pain in a patient with a normal shoulder examination should raise the suspicion of referred shoulder pain. The physician should develop a patterned habit of shoulder examination, and should no longer simply label a shoulder problem "arthritis."

MUSCULOTENDINOUS ROTATOR CUFF DISORDERS

Shoulder injury and morbidity are second only to back injury in industrial-related in-

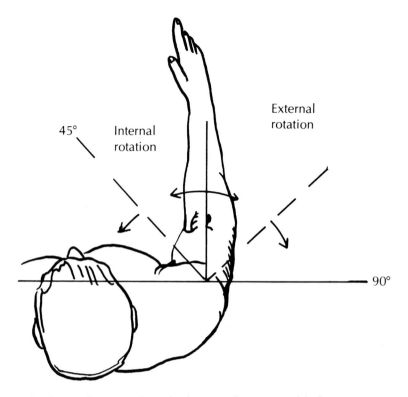

Fig. 4–3.   Internal and external rotation refer to the direction of movement of the humerus.

juries.[22] The conditions included as "rotator cuff" disorders are often overlapping, and are initially the result of tendon injury and degeneration. The musculotendinous rotator cuff portion of the shoulder capsule is the conjoint tendon of the supraspinatus, infraspinatus, and teres minor muscles, which insert onto the greater tuberosity, and the subscapularis, which inserts onto the lesser tuberosity.[1] Injury generally occurs in patients over the age of 40, following stressful activities of the shoulder, or in young patients after a severe injury.

Types of Rotator Cuff Disorders. The most common rotator cuff disorders are supraspinatus tendinitis, the impingement syndrome, calcific tendinitis, subacromial and subcoracoid bursitis, and rotator cuff tears. Rotator cuff tendinitis is seldom isolated to a single musculotendinous structure, and unless promptly recognized and treated, the tendinitis can progress to a frozen shoulder. The *impingement syndrome* refers to supra- spinatus tendinitis or bicipital tendinitis, which results from these tendons being pinched between the head of the humerus and the acromion[23] (Fig. 4–7).

The Impingement Syndrome. The supraspinatus muscle and tendon are the most common sites of shoulder disease.[7] Disorders of these structures may cause painful limitation of active motion, but with the arm held limp, full passive range of motion is possible in most cases. The site of injury often is against the coracoacromial arch, an unyielding structure, consisting of the coracoid anteriorly, the strong coracoacromial ligament running from the coracoid to the anterior leading edge of the acromion, and the acromion itself.[24,25] The impingement involves the coracoacromial ligament and the anterior part of the acromion because of their close relationship to the tendon of the long head of the biceps, and the supraspinatus muscle during overhead elevation of the arm (Figs. 4–7, 4–8). Repetitious overhead motion can lead

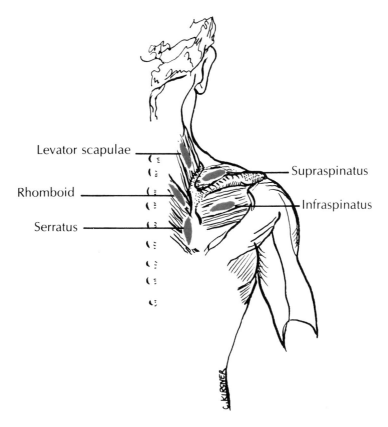

Fig. 4–4. While the scapula is drawn laterally by having the patient bring his arm across the chest, palpation in the region of the supraspinatus, infraspinatus, serratus, rhomboideus, and levator scapulae muscles may establish the presence of myofascial trigger points with reproduction of pain in the "target zone."

to inflammation of the rotator cuff, reduction in shoulder motion, trauma to the acromion, and formation of an osteophyte. In one study of this syndrome[29] a subacromial spur was found in 23% of patients. The spur was located at the insertion site of the coracoacromial arch on the anteroinferior aspect of the acromion. Another radiographic feature reported was flattening and sclerosis of the greater tuberosity of the humerus. The patient complains of painful motion of the shoulder in an arc from 60 to 75 degrees of abduction. Forward motion is generally unimpaired. Night pain is usually troublesome. This pain is distributed generally throughout the shoulder region, and may vary from day to day or become constant. The impingement sign is produced by having the arm brought to a position of maximum for-

ward elevation by one of the examiner's hands, while the scapula is held down with the other hand. (The examiner stands behind the seated patient.) If pain is produced by this maneuver, the presence of subacromial impingement is suggested.[18] Another diagnostic technique consists of forcibly forward flexing the humerus, compressing the greater tuberosity against the anterior inferior acromial surface. The examiner then rotates the patient's arm internally (with the arm forward, the humerus is forcibly rotated clockwise)[30,31] (Fig. 4–8B). Pain relief with injection of a local anesthetic agent beneath the acromion is a helpful diagnostic sign.[23] The impingement syndrome usually results from injury to the supraspinatus and upper-end of the biceps tendons, during repetitious elevation and forward motion of the arm, in work

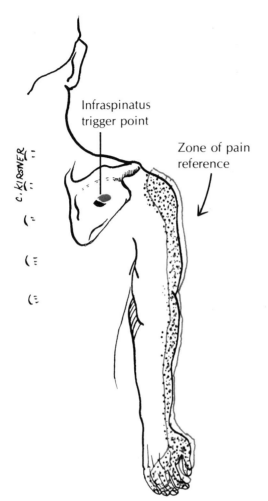

Infraspinatus
trigger point

Zone of pain
reference

C. KIRSNER

Fig. 4–5. Infraspinatus trigger point with target zone radiating from the deltoid region down as far as the hand.

or sports. Occasionally, the neurovascular bundle can also be impinged at this site,[32] in an area of relatively decreased blood supply. At this point, ischemic degenerative disruption of the rotator cuff can occur.[33]

Pathologically, the syndrome has been classified into Stage I: edema and hemorrhage; Stage II: fibrosis and tendinitis; and Stage III: tendon degeneration, bony changes, and tendon rupture.[23] Calcific tendinitis is not usually associated with impingement syndrome.[31,34] In one study, subacromial spurs, degenerative changes, and inferior acromioclavicular joint spurs did not correlate with short term treatment results.[35]

Rotator Cuff Tendinitis. Supraspinatus tendinitis may occur as an isolated shoulder problem. When acute, it may result from calcific tendinitis, usually involves the supraspinatus or biceps muscles and tends to occur in younger individuals, and in particular, white collar workers.[17,36] Calcific tendinitis can mimic gout with acute attacks not only in the shoulder, but in other periarticular sites.[8,37] Calcific tendinitis tends to have an acute onset that reaches maximum severity within several days, and then has a rapid spontaneous improvement as the calcum ruptures into the subacromial bursa. Calcium deposits, as seen on roentgenograms, frequently correlate poorly with shoulder symptoms. Only 35% of patients with radiographic evidence of soft tissue shoulder calcification develop symptoms (Fig. 4–9). However, if the deposits are greater than 1.5 cm in diameter, most patients develop shoulder symptoms.[8,38]

Radiographic features of the calcification, whether fluffy or more sharply defined, were also unrelated to outcome. In most cases, calcium apatite was detected within the supraspinatus tendon sheath.[39]

The supraspinatus muscle has to provide leverage for shoulder stabilization during external rotation, initiation of abduction, and it provides strength when carrying heavy objects with the arm abducted. This work load results in early degeneration of the tendon at its insertion. This site can be palpated if the examiner's index fingertip is placed in a triangle bounded laterally by the acromion, anteriorly by the clavicle, and posteriorly by the spine of the scapula. Tenderness on palpation that is aggravated by active abduction of the arm against resistance supports a diagnosis of supraspinatus tendinitis.[40]

Bicipital tendinitis may occur as an isolated condition. The patient notices discomfort in the anterior upper area of the bicipital tendon. Often the tendinitis results in palpable swelling of the biceps tendon sheath. This area is frequently injured during forced resistance to the flexed elbow while the forearm is supinated (palm turned upward).[6] Repeti-

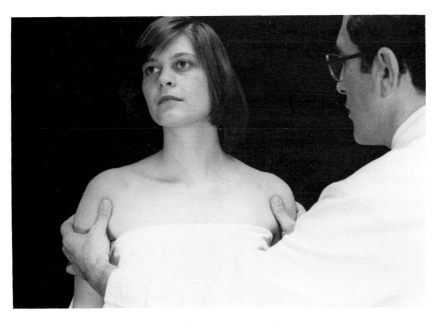

Fig. 4–6. Detection of bicipital tendinitis by rolling across the long head of the biceps and comparing one side to the other.

Table 4–3. Differential Diagnosis of Shoulder Pain (After Goodman CE and Serebro LH[104])

Neurologic disorders	*Rheumatic disorders*
Brachial plexus neuritis	Aseptic necrosis humeral head
Cervical nerve root compression	Crystal deposition diseases
Herpes zoster	Polymyalgia rheumatica
Nerve entrapment syndromes	Polymyositis
Shoulder hand syndrome	Rheumatoid arthritis
(Reflex sympathetic dystrophy)	
Spinal cord lesions	
Musculoskeletal disorders	*Referred pain*
Adhesive capsulitis	Heart
Bursitis, tendinitis	Lung
Myofascial pain disorders	Stomach
Fractures and dislocations	Aortic aneurysm
Infection	Gallbladder
Metabolic disorders	Diaphragm
Neoplasia	
Osteoarthritis	
Rotator cuff tear	
Thoracic outlet syndrome	

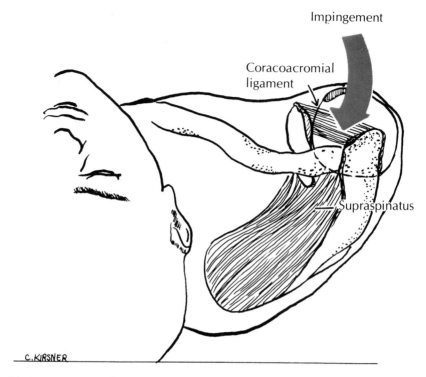

Fig. 4–7. The impingement syndrome: Pinching the supraspinatus or bicipital tendons between the head of the humerus and the acromion.

tive movement, as in tightening jar lids, is a common cause. Bicipital tendinitis may be a part of the *impingement syndrome,* and the patient may complain of pain in the anterior shoulder and over the coracoacromial ligament. Impingement of the biceps in sports results in symptoms during the serve and overhand strokes of tennis, and in the follow-through stages of a golf swing. A painful catching sensation may be noted. This painful catching sensation may be relieved by internal rotation of the shoulder which clears the biceps tendon from under the coracoacromial arch.[24]

Physical examination of patients with supraspinatus tendinitis may reveal tenderness over the greater tuberosity while the arm is hanging downward (Dawbarn's sign). Pain elicited while the examiner pulls downward on the patient's arm may also suggest supraspinatus tendinitis. Scapulohumeral rhythm (see "Scapular Region Disorders" on p. 88) during active shoulder movement may

be altered as the patient splints the glenohumeral joint and uses the scapula to provide shoulder motion. This results in a shrugging-type motion of the shoulder.[1] Bicipital tendinitis is usually accompanied by swelling of the biceps tendon sheath; the enlargement is palpable as the examiner rolls his fingers across both the involved and uninvolved biceps tendons at the same time, and compares the two sides (Fig. 4–6). Tenderness is usually exquisite over the involved biceps tendon. The test for Yergason's sign for bicipital tendinitis is performed by flexing the elbow and having the patient forcefully supinate (turn the palmar aspect upward) the forearm against resistance (Fig. 4–10). In the presence of bicipital tendinitis, the patient feels pain in the area of the bicipital groove. Most important, in tendinitis of the long head of the biceps or the musculotendinous cuff, *passive range of movement is normal.* Examination of the muscles of the rotator cuff is important in evaluating injuries in young ath-

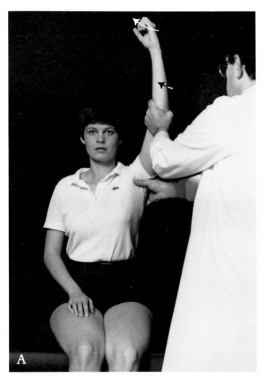

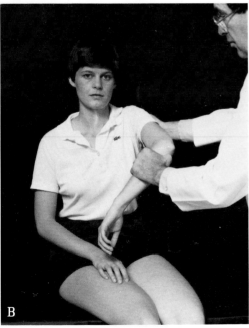

Fig. 4–8. *A.* Test for impingement syndrome. Note arm is internally rotated at maximum elevation. *B.* Similar maneuver using compression of the greater tuberosity against the acromion.

letes. The strength of the infraspinatus, teres minor and subscapularis muscles can be tested with the subject in the sitting position, with the elbow flexed 90 degrees. The patient is tested for external rotation against resistance (infraspinatus/teres minor) or internal rotation against resistance (subscapularis). The involved side should be compared with the uninvolved side. The supraspinatus can be tested with the arm in 90 degrees of abduction, held horizontally, and then rotated into full internal rotation so that the back of the hand is rotated upward, then forward.[41] See Figure 4–11.

Arthroscopic examination of the shoulder may provide direct inspection of the biceps tendon, the humeral head, the glenoid labrum, the glenohumeral ligaments, the scapularis tendon and recess, the rotator cuff muscles, and the superior recess.[42,43] In patients with rotator cuff tears studied by arthrography and then examined by arthroscopy, the latter procedure did not provide additional new information.[43]

Rupture of the biceps tendon, following a fall on the shoulder, results in visible swelling of the biceps muscle belly rolled up in the distal one third of the arm, and weakness of elbow flexion is apparent.[17] Subluxation of the biceps tendon may result from rupture or stretchng of the fascial covering overlying the bicipital groove.

To test for the impingement syndrome, the examiner attempts to force the humerus against the anterior acromion while elevating the arm to reproduce impingement pain. Pain relief with injection of a local anesthetic agent beneath the acromion is a helpful diagnostic sign.[23]

Bursitis. The onset of subacromial bursitis may be acute or chronic. The attack often follows injury to the musculotendinous cuff, particularly the supraspinatus tendon. The pain is often exquisite, may be present day and night, and is aggravated by active abduction of the arm. *The pain frequently is referred to the insertion of the deltoid muscle at the junction of the upper third and middle*

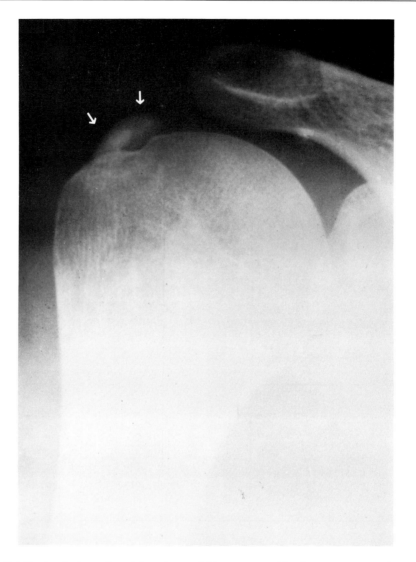

Fig. 4–9. Calcification in the region of the subacromial bursa as noted by the arrows. (From the ARA Clinical Slide Collection, 1972. Used by permission of the Arthritis Foundation.)

third of the arm,[6] and may be the prominent site of the patient's complaint.

Subacromial and subcoracoid bursitis are frequently secondary to adjacent tendon injury.[1] Bursitis may occur following tendinitis of the musculotendinous cuff, biceps tendon, or impingement of the bursa. A tear of the musculotendinous cuff may involve the floor of the subacromial bursa with a buildup of pressure by the fluid.[1] The subcoracoid bursa, which is between the coracoid process and the joint capsule, may be irritated by pressure from the coracoid against the head of the humerus during excessive arm use. Pain is noted over the coracoid process and medial shoulder.[6] The presenting symptom of bursitis is seldom swelling, unless a systemic disease has caused true joint synovitis with spread to the communicating bursae. Physical examination of patients with acute bursitis requires absolute patient relaxation before *passive* range of movement can be determined to be normal. If muscle splinting prevents passive range of movement in a patient with bursitis,

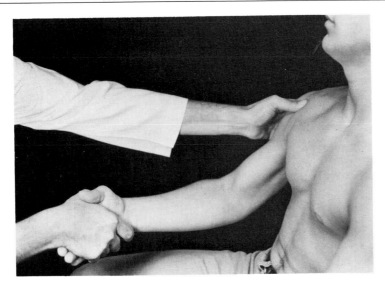

Fig. 4–10. Yergason's sign for bicipital tendinitis: Patient forcefully turns the palmar aspect of the hand upward (supination) while the elbow is held in a flexed position. Supination is performed against the examiner's resistance. Pain is produced if bicipital tendinitis is present.

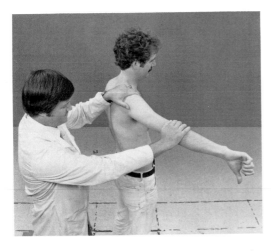

Fig. 4–11. Examination of the supraspinatus muscle. (From Jobe and Moynes.[41])

the loss of range of movement occurs in only one plane, *abduction.*

Rotator Cuff Tear. In the younger individual, rupture or tear of the musculotendinous cuff causes acute pain following trauma; it is less noticeable and easily missed in the elderly.[17] A history of falling on the shoulder joint or on the outstretched arm should raise suspicion of a tear of the musculotendinous cuff. Physical examination to elicit a shoulder cuff tear is important in evaluating any patient with shoulder pain. In a cuff tear, the patient may be able to actively abduct the arm to slightly less than 90 degrees. When the patient attempts further abduction and elevation against the examiner's resistance, the arm gives way and drops (the Moseley test), yet the shoulder is capable of normal passive motion.[1,17] This discrepancy should quickly raise concern for a musculotendinous tear.

McCarty et al. have recently described rotator cuff tear in association with the presence of hydroxyapatite crystals, a syndrome referred to as "Milwaukee shoulder". Aged women with or without soft tissue calcification, who suffered complete tears of the shoulder cuff had hydroxyapatite crystals within microspheroids, along with activated collagenase and neutral proteases.[44] The enzymatic release of hydroxyapatite crystals from the synovium, endocytosis by synovial macrophages, and subsequent further release of collagenases and neutral proteases is thought to complete a pathogenetic cycle.[45]

In summary, examination of the shoulder joint requires the following rules: (1) think of the whole patient, (2) consider aggravating factors, such as poor posture or injurious work habits, activities, hobbies, or sports, (3) examine the entire arc of shoulder motion actively, passively, and against resistance, (4) inspect scapulohumeral "rhythm" during active motion of the shoulder. "Laying on of hands" is essential.

Etiology. The etiology of soft tissue shoulder disturbances is obscure, but probably is biochemical and traumatic in origin.[34] Some degeneration of the musculotendinous cuff occurs in all of us after the fifth decade.[17] The "critical zone" of the musculotendinous cuff at its insertion on the humerus is vulnerable to injury. Ischemia of the cuff in this region may play a role in rupture. Incomplete tears of the musculotendinous cuff have been noted in 30% of cadavers.[6] The supraspinatus tendon is under constant friction against the acromion during motion, and degeneration of this tendon is a constant feature of shoulder cuff disorders.[6,46] The biceps tendon is often noted to be eroded at operation; it can completely disappear or remain fixed and scarred in the bicipital groove in patients over the age of 50.[17]

In an electromyographic study of workers with shoulder pain of 1 year or longer duration, the findings revealed that the patients had significantly greater signs of fatigue (amplitude increase and mean power frequency decrease) than other workers and the patients had no increase in motor activity at rest or with endurance. Furthermore the patients demonstrated diminished endurance. The findings suggest localized muscle fatigue rather than neurogenic mechanisms for persistent shoulder pain in these patients.[47]

Dislocation of the biceps brachii may occur when the joint capsule is stretched, allowing the tendon to slip over the lesser tuberosity, resulting in bicipital tendinitis.[6] The biceps tendon is covered by a transverse humeral ligament that crosses the bicipital groove, and the tendon is enveloped by a synovial extension from the true joint capsule. A supratubercular ridge of Meyer or a shallow bicipital groove (both of which are congenital) may be found in patients with chronic bicipital tendinitis. Tenosynovitis of the biceps may occur

in systemic disease, particularly rheumatoid arthritis. Any shoulder joint inflammation may communicate with the bicipital tendon sheath, and cause tenosynovitis, as may infection of the true shoulder joint.[17]

Patients with a shallow glenoid are subject to subluxation or dislocation following trauma. In contact sports, acute subacromial bursitis may result from hemorrhage into the bursa from adjacent tendon tears; rupture of the musculotendinous cuff must be considered.[23] Impingement syndrome frequently occurs in sports enthusiasts over 40 years of age; biceps tenosynovitis may be the presenting problem. Bicipital tendon subluxation can also occur in the older athlete when the musculotendinous cuff is torn.

In calcific tendinitis, histopathologic studies reveal calcific deposits, infiltration with chronic inflammatory cells, and giant cells in dystrophic fibrillation of tendons. This suggests that calcification is secondary to dystrophic changes within the tendon.[22] Tendon rupture is rarely seen in surgical examination of patients with calcific tendinitis. Calcium deposits with a toothpaste consistency commonly occur about the tendocapsular structures and tendon insertions.[48] Specific identification of the calcific deposits, as hydroxyapatite, may be difficult due to their small crystal size, but shiny, globular coin-like bodies, which appear to represent crystals in clumps, provide a clue to their presence.[8,49,50] Electron microscopic and electron probe analysis techniques can corroborate crystal identification as apatite.[48–50] If the calcium deposit is deep in the tendon body, no symptoms result; pain occurs when the deposit irritates the bursa, and is relieved when the deposit ruptures into the bursa.[6] A metabolic disorder resulting in calcium hydroxyapatite deposition may be primary to the etiology of calcific tendinitis. Radiographic examination for deposits in other periarticular structures is helpful.

In summary, the etiology of musculotendinous rotator cuff disorders is mechanical and biochemical. Impingement of bony structures upon tendons may occur, and degenerative change is a constant finding. Biochemical processes, particularly those involving hydroxyapatite deposition, may be involved. Consideration of aggravating repetitious microtrauma should be in the clinician's mind. Occupational factors include awkward positions and repetitive tasks.[51] Sport, hobby, and domestic activities that involve repetitive abduction, and to-and-fro motions are also implicated (Table 4-2). When the aggravating factors are alleviated, most patients enjoy longstanding improvement. The history of job, sports activities, hobbies, and sleep position must be considered to recognize and prevent future repetition of the musculotendinous injury.

Laboratory and Radiographic Examination. Erythrocyte sedimentation rate, roentgenograms of the chest, and routine, rotational, trans-scapular, or axillary roentgenographic views of the shoulder should be obtained. These may be deferred if the problem appears straightforward and the patient agrees to obtain roentgenograms on the first follow-up visit if relief has not occurred. Radiographic examination of the chest, with lateral view and with particular reference to the mediastinum, should be obtained in every patient with axillary pain.

Roentgenograms of the shoulder may reveal the presence of calcification with a "skull cap" appearance in the soft tissues about the lateral shoulder tip (Fig. 4–9). This is suggestive of calcium that has ruptured into the subacromial bursa,[34,52] and which, as a rule, will be absorbed spontaneously. However, if the calcium deposit is greater than 1.5 cm in diameter, irrigation of the bursa should be considered. This will be discussed under "Management," in this chapter.

The roentgenogram may reveal osteoporosis or patchy cysts of the head of the humerus in the presence of supraspinatus tendinitis. The outer border of the clavicle may have disappeared in patients with malignancy. Degenerative arthritis of the glenohumeral joint or the acromioclavicular joint may be seen. Oblique views may be needed. Further roentgenographic studies include

using contrast media injected at this site and anteroposterior and axial radiographs taken with the shoulder in the degree of abduction and rotation which had been most painful. Oblique views and tangential roentgenographs of the acromioclavicular joint, and tangential views of the bicipital sulcus are taken when indicated. Kessell and Watson[20] reported findings in 97 patients using this technique. The patients could be divided into those with lesions in the posterior part of the rotator cuff, lesions in the subscapularis tendon, and those with lesions of the supraspinatus tendon associated with arthritis of the acromioclavicular joint. The first two groups benefited from local corticosteroid injections, whereas most of the last group required excision of the outer end of the clavicle and division of the coracoacromial joint.[20] *Cuff tear arthropathy* has been described in which a massive capsule tear results in superior displacement of the humeral head, disuse atrophy and osteoporosis of the shoulder, and collapse of the proximal aspect of the humeral articular surface.[53] These findings must be correlated with the clinical features.

An arthrogram of the shoulder is indicated when physical findings suggest a shoulder cuff tear, or when further information is required. This may be deferred until a follow-up visit after conservative therapy has been attempted. However, if the Moseley test is positive, an arthrogram should be obtained immediately. Repair of a torn muscular cuff is difficult if the tear is not recognized promptly. In other musculotendinous cuff disorders, an arthrogram may be of some diagnostic help, but it is invasive and may not change the treatment program. Ultrasonography of the rotator cuff and biceps tendon may be a reliable, noninvasive method of investigation. Middleton et al.[53a] reported over 90% sensitivity and specificity of ultrasound in detecting a rotator cuff tear.

Differential Diagnosis. The differential diagnosis of shoulder pain includes referred pain from diaphragmatic irritation, neurovascular compression, systemic inflammatory diseases, and tumor. Patients with diffuse shoulder pain, without objective tenderness or limitation of movement, may have diaphragmatic irritation with referred pain. In such patients the pain may be reproduced by gentle but firm pressure over the epigastrium. When this is found, roentgenography of the upper gastrointestinal tract for hiatus hernia, reflux esophagitis, gastric ulcer, or peptic ulcer should be considered. An infraspinatus trigger point commonly refers pain to the shoulder, and should not be overlooked. A careful neurologic examination for cervical disc disease or studies to exclude hypothyroidism may be rewarding (see Table 4–3 and the Decision Chart, Table 4–4).

Management. Management begins with the recognition of one or more of the musculotendinous rotator cuff disturbances, and exclusion of systemic or referred pain conditions. The clinician should explain the problem to the patient, in order to have the patient and the physician together try to recognize and avoid aggravating factors. In the case of sport-induced injury, correction of improper shoulder use can often alleviate future recurrences.[23] Work habits, particularly overhead arm use,[52] may require evaluation by an occupational therapist. Conservative measures include prevention as stated above, and training. This should include adequate warmup before strenuous arm use, and strengthening exercises when needed. Sports activities that require repetitive use of shoulders may find isokinetic exercises helpful. Overuse must be avoided.

Local treatment includes ice applications for 10 minutes following workouts. If a paper cup or fruit juice can is filled with water and then frozen, the ice stick thus formed can be pushed up or peeled as it is used, then returned to the freezer. For acute lesions, ice prevents swelling and reduces pain. Ultrasound has been advocated for treatment of impingement disorders, but is not so helpful in subacromial bursitis.[54] Nonsteroidal antiinflammatory agents may be used.[24,31,55,56] Use of aspirin before weekend sports is helpful. DMSO (dimethyl sulfoxide) has received notoriety in the lay press for years as an effective

balm. A double blind study of 70% aqueous DMSO versus 5% aqueous DMSO in the treatment of rotator cuff tendinitis and tennis elbow revealed no statistical value in its use.[57]

Pain relief in tendon problems about the shoulder may be obtained in dramatic fashion if a corticosteroid-anesthetic mixture is injected into the correct tendon site (Figs. 4–12, 4–13). However, if the arm is to be used for any stressful job or sport, local use of corticosteroids is to be avoided. When used intralesionally in other patients, the arm should be exercised passively, and not stressed for at least 2 weeks. A prospective study of intralesional corticosteroid and local anesthetic treatment in patients with shoulder pain, reported by Roy and Oldham[58] demonstrated good results in 58 of 60 shoulders with painful arc syndrome which had a normal passive range of motion at the time of treatment. The injection sites in all patients were the subacromial bursa and the glenohumeral joint. In this study 20 mg of methylprednisolone was administered, while in another study, Kessel and Watson[20] reported good results with 40 mg of methylprednisolone and 5 ml of local anesthetic injection intralesionally in 66 of 68 patients with rotator cuff tendinitis involving the internal or external rotators. Surgical procedure was necessary in 10 of 12 patients with supraspinatus tendinitis and degenerative disease of the acromioclavicular arch.[20] Use of arthrography to assure that the steroid is placed into the shoulder joint cavity has been advocated.[59]

In another prospective study, Berry et al.[60] compared treatment with acupuncture, ultrasound, and tolmetin sodium with intralesional methylprednisolone (injected anteriorly only) or placebo therapy. The patients did have some limitation of motion in abduction. After 4 weeks, all groups showed significant pain relief, with no differences among the treatment groups. Range of motion also improved in all groups without significant differences among the treatment measures. The authors conclude that their study might have been flawed by having a charming and persuasive therapist administer treatment! Her

Table 4–4. Decision Chart, The Shoulder

Problem	Action	Other Actions
A. Not acute, unilateral myofascial shoulder pain: Diffuse dull, episodic Use-related Trigger points + + + Aggravates sleep No limitation of motion	CONSERVATIVE CARE Recognize aggravating factors Pain relief: NSAIDS; local injection; vapocoolant spray Prescribe exercises	
B. Unilateral tendinitis Motion impaired in one plane only		

C. Frozen shoulder
Diffuse dull, episodic pain
Use-related
Trigger points + + +
Aggravates sleep
Motion limited actively and passively in all planes
		Order roentgenograms
		Tests for inflammation
		If results uncertain:
		  do bone scan, +/– RA Latex
		  +/– Arthrogram
		Consult with physical therapist
		Reexamine patient

D. Acute bursitis Constant severe pain Marked guarding to passive motion	→ Oral or intralesional anti-inflammatory Rx first	→ CONSULTATION Rheumatologist Orthopedist Physiatrist
E. Symmetrical tendinitis or capsulitis Morning stiffness Little rest pain Palpable tendinitis or limited motion bilaterally.	→ Also begin workup for inflammatory rheumatic diseases	
F. DANGER LIST Swelling, warmth Fever, chills Numbness or tingling Aggravated by neck movement Referred from elsewhere Axillary pain	→ Take immediate appropriate action	

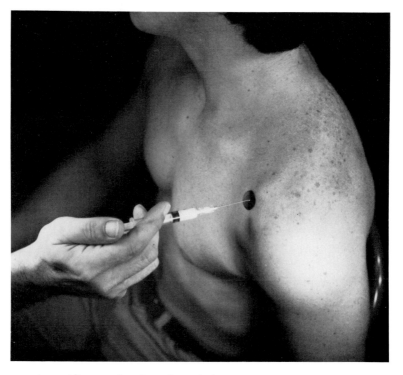

Fig. 4–12. Having located the site of tendinitis beneath the acromioclavicular joint, a short No. 23 needle is threaded into the supraspinatus tendon and a corticosteroid-anesthetic mixture administered.

personality and charm might have exerted a therapeutic influence upon the patients. Also, the site for the steroid injection determined by the protocol may have been too arbitrary; many injections may not have been placed into the site of the lesion.

The importance of accurate diagnostic assessment before injection was stressed in a prospective study reported by Hollingworth et al.[61] In this randomized and double blinded study in 77 patients with local shoulder pain that could be reproduced by examination, the authors localized the individual tendon involvement by selective tissue tension using resisted active arm movements. Patients were randomly allocated into two groups both of which received 80 mg of methylprednisolone acetate mixed with a local anesthetic. One group received the injection into a specific anatomic area (tendon sheath, bursa, or joint space). The other group had a trigger point injection, in which the most tender point which reproduced pain was identified

by deep palpation and then injected. After 1 week, 20% of the tender point injection group improved, whereas 60% of the anatomic injection site patients improved. A crossover was carried out for those still in pain. Overall, 12 of 63 tender point injections were successful, whereas 41 of 69 injections into more specific sites were successful.[62] A local anesthetic alone may be administered to test whether pain is relieved before adding the corticosteroid. Relief from the injection provides diagnostic value in bicipital tendinitis, supraspinatus tendinitis, subacromial and subcoracoid bursitis, and the impingement syndrome.[1,6,23,34] After the injection, the patient should be discouraged from participating in stressful shoulder activities for 2 to 3 weeks, although the pain has been relieved.

Every patient with a musculotendinous cuff problem should have a home exercise program directed toward the involved site. Exercise therapy for supraspinatus or bicipital tendinitis is important for the prevention

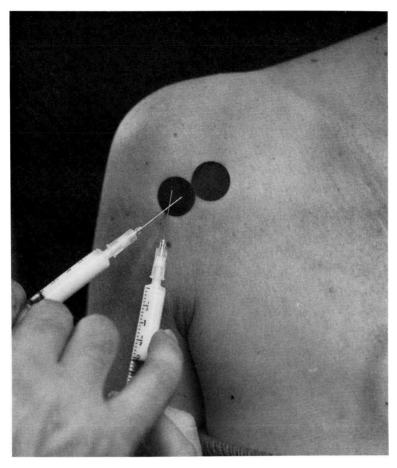

Fig. 4–13. In performing injection for biceps tendinitis, the needle should be directed parallel to the tendon after puncturing the skin.

of stiffness. Passive exercises are performed after application of heat by having the patient move the arm through motion within the limits of pain and with the assistance of the other arm. Pendulum exercises (Exercise 3, Table 4–5) should be performed with the arm relaxed while making small circles. This may be followed by light stroking massage for relaxation. Recalcitrant trigger point nodules in muscles may respond to ultrasound and local massage followed by whole limb massage. Rhythmic stabilization exercises performed by a therapist has been advocated.[40] These movements include active flexion followed by active extension, each against the therapist's resistance. Further mobilizing exercises may be used within the patient's tolerance (see

Exercises 1–4, Table 4–5). In the case of bursitis and supraspinatus tendon inflammation, pendulum exercises should be initiated as soon as acute symptoms are relieved, followed by gentle stretching of the shoulder capsule (Figs. 4–14, 4–15). Bicipital tendinitis in particular requires a gentle stretching out of the biceps tendon to release adhesions between the tendon and its sheath. This can be performed with a wand exercise (Fig. 4–16). See Wand Exercises 5 and 6, Table 4–5. In general, it is wise to perform the exercises twice daily, and continue them for several weeks after the pain has been relieved.

When calcific tendinitis is present and the deposit is greater than 1.5 cm in diameter,

Table 4–5.   Shoulder-Region Exercises

1. Back up to a wall with feet about 6 inches from the wall. Place hands behind head and push buttocks against the wall. The hands act as a cushion between the head and the wall; then push head and shoulders back against the wall; now begin a gradual forceful thrust of the head backward to the wall, keeping the chin tucked in like a military soldier at attention. As the head is thrust backward the arms are loose, just allowing the hands to act as a cushion behind the head. There should be a sensation of muscle tension in the back of the neck. This thrust is maintained for up to 30 seconds and then relaxed for a second; repeat exercises for 1 to 2 minutes (See Fig 2–7, p. 37).

2. Shoulder shrugging: Mobilize the neck and shoulder muscles with weights in each hand; gradually increasing weight from 2 to 10 pounds. These can be made from socks lined with a plastic freezer bag and then filled with gravel, sand, or dirt. The weights can be held at the sides of the body or draped over each shoulder. Arms are held down along the sides of the body while seated or standing. Then the shoulders are slowly drawn upward, then backward, then slowly let down. The shoulder blades are thus brought toward each other as the shoulders are raised. This movement is repeated slowly for a total of 1 to 2 minutes twice daily (See Fig. 3–5, p. 54).

3. Pendulum exercises: Stand or sit but lean slightly to the painful side. Then, while grasping a 2- to 5-pound weight, swing the arm in a small circle the size of the top of a pail. Proceed slowly in a smooth circular motion for a minute or two every few hours (See Fig. 4–14, p. 82).

4. Wall circles: If the shoulder is very painful and excercises are difficult, perform a warmup by reaching forward to a wall and drawing large circles on the wall. Then turn sideways to the wall and draw large circles with your hand on the wall.

5. Wand exercise to stretch biceps tendon: Grasp a yardstick or broom handle with hands wide apart. The good or better arm is always used to push the bad arm. The wand is held across the chest and then used to force the involved arm out and away and slightly back. Push gradually with increasing force to loosen scar tissue. After 1 minute, slowly draw the arm back down (See Fig 4–15, p. 82).

6. Additional wand exercises: Lift the wand upward and overhead. Keep the wand close to the head, bending the elbows to do so. Try to get the wand over and then behind the head. Hold position a moment and repeat 10 times. Next, put the wand behind the buttocks, with the elbows straight, raise the wand backward and upward. The movement is performed slowly and steadily for 1 minute (See Fig. 4–18, p. 87).

7. The wall-ladder exercise: Stand sideways to the wall, reaching out to the wall with the involved arm. Stand away from the wall so that just the fingertips reach the wall, then begin to walk up the wall but keep the body sideways. Don't turn the shoulders or chest toward the wall. The arm must be kept directly out to the side from the trunk. Begin climbing the fingers upward and slightly backward. When the arm can go no higher, note the location that was reached, stay at this extreme position for one minute, then slowly slide the hand back down the wall. DO NOT DROP the arm abruptly or the rotator cuff may be injured. If this cannot be performed sideways, then begin it frontward by facing the wall and reaching forward, walking the fingers straight up the wall. If there is improvement, the sideways technique should be tried (See Fig. 4–17, p. 86).

8. Supraspinatus muscle strengthening: The patient is seated, arms at shoulder height, palm down; raise and lower the arms adding small weights as the exercise is progressively better tolerated.

9. Infraspinatus and teres minor strengthening: This is performed in the side-lying position with the bad side up and the arm held close to the side and the elbow flexed 90 degrees; the forearm then is rotated palm forward while the elbow remains close to the body. Small weights are added subsequently (See Fig. 4–19, p. 88).

10. Subscapularis strengthening: Lie on back, affected arm held close to the side and the elbow bent 90 degrees. The arm is raised upward while the forearm is rotated across the front of the chest; the arm is then lowered slowly (See Fig. 4–23, p. 92).

Table 4–5. *Continued*

11. Pulley exercise: Using an eyescrew and pulley fastened to a doorway or beam, pass a thin rope of sashcord through the pulley. Tie a pillowcase with 6 to 20 pounds to one end. Tie a tea towel (opposite corners) to the other end to fashion a sleeve through which the involved forearm can be placed. Sit sideways to pulley, about 6 to 8 feet away. The pulley then passively pulls the affected arm outward, sideways and up. Apply ice to the shoulder while receiving the traction. The traction is used for 10 to 20 minutes twice daily.

12. Additional pulley exercise:
     With the loose ends of the rope, grasp one end with the good arm up, while seated with back to pulley. Then the good arm pulls downward, thus pulling the bad arm sideways and up. Repeat slowly. Then turn chair sideways and directly under pulley. Grasp rope with good arm in front and up, bad arm behind body and at level of hip. Now pull down with good arm, thus raising bad arm back and up. Repeat slowly. Lastly, reverse arms, so that bad arm is in front of body, at waist, and pulled upward. Spend 1 or 2 minutes in each position twice daily.

13. Shoulder capsule stretching:
    a. The patient sits on a well-padded high back chair, with a blanket on the back of the chair. The involved arm is draped over the back of the chair with the armpit firmly fixed over the back of the chair. The patient then grasps the arm just above the elbow, with the good arm grasping the involved one, then pulling downward and employing rhythmic oscillations. This is followed by using the same position but have the patient perform the pendulum exercise (See Fig 4–24, p. 93).
    b. With a pillow tucked up in the armpit, patient standing, the arm is first moved across and in front of the chest, then behind the chest, with the elbow bent. In each position the good arm is used, grasping the involved arm at the wrist and pulling across to the good side thus creating joint stretching.
    c. Seated beside a table with body at edge of chair, the involved arm is placed across the table, then the body weight is lowered, rhythmically. The arm may be directed forward, sideward, or backward to accomplish different capsular stretching.
    d. Seated sideways to a table, the involved upper arm is positioned so that it is entirely resting against the tabletop (the armpit is right at the edge). The elbow is bent to 90 degrees. The good arm grasps the ventral aspect of the wrist and then rotates the involved arm so that the arm is rotated upward.
    e. Stand facing a high ledge, shelf, mantle, or counter with the hand resting palm down on the edge of the counter with the elbow extended. Then the patient lowers his body. Changing the body's position in relation to the counter will provide additional passive shoulder exercise (See Fig. 4–25, p. 93).
    f. Using a door frame, passive motion can be accomplished by placing the back of the hand against the frame while holding the elbow at the side of the body. Then the patient walks forward as the arm rotates. Repeat the technique with the palm on the door frame (See Fig. 4–26, p. 94).

14. Shoulder-blade stretch: Sit in a chair, grasp a 2- to 5-pound weight with the hand of the painful side. First reach out straight in front, then slowly cross the arm until it is over the knee on the opposite side. Slowly bend the body straight forward and draw the weighted hand beyond and to the outside of the opposite foot. The body should end up bent forward, the head centered and looking down, the arm crossed to the other side, and the weighted hand about 6 inches from the floor, 12 inches in front and 12 inches to the outside of the opposite foot. For example, if the right shoulder blade is painful, the right hand holds the weight and crosses beyond and to the left side of the left foot. The position is held for 20 seconds and the exercise repeated three times in succession several times a day (See Fig. 4–21, p. 90).

15. Holding a towel behind the chest, the involved arm is held in extension, and the elbow is bent so that the hand is behind the head, the good arm is holding the lower end of the towel, and the lower arm pulls the upper one.

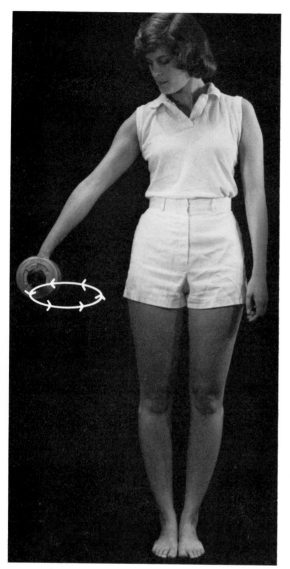

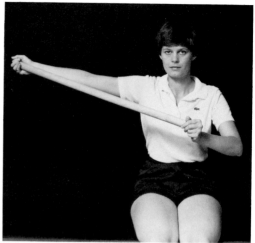

Fig. 4–15. Wand exercise in which the good arm gently forces the arm on the bad side out and away, thus stretching the shoulder capsule. After a minute or so, the good arm draws the bad arm back toward the midline.

Fig. 4–14. Pendulum or Codman's exercise for shoulder cuff mobilization: Using 5 or more pounds, the patient rotates the arm in a 12-in. diameter circle while leaning slightly to the side. This is performed for a minute in each direction.

aspiration and irrigation (with a large No. 16 to No. 18 bore needle) may be helpful if initial corticosteroid injection does not provide relief. Following corticosteroid injection, pain may be aggravated for the first 24 hours. Ice can be applied, particularly during the night following injection. Relief generally occurs within a few days. Rarely is more than one injection necessary. If a tendon requires two or more injections, orthopedic consultation should be considered.[1,63] On occasion, use of ultrasound to disperse the steroid crystals is helpful, and is performed immediately following injection of a steroid anesthetic mixture.

When calcific tendinitis occurs in a young adult, calcium apatite deposition disease should be suspected. The use of colchicine (0.6 mg, 2 to 4 times daily)[37] or nonsteroidal anti-inflammatory drugs may be prescribed for long-term use.

Strengthening exercises as outlined by Jobe and Moynes[41] can be started when tenderness and range of motion have improved. See Exercises 8–10, Table 4–5 and Figure 4–19.

Impingement within the coracoacromial arch, with associated tendinitis or coracoid bursitis, may respond to local injections with procaine and/or steroids. The subcoracoid region should be tender to palpation suggesting local inflammation. During injection, care must be taken to avoid adjacent nerves and vessels. If a spur is evident on roentgenographic examination, whether beneath the

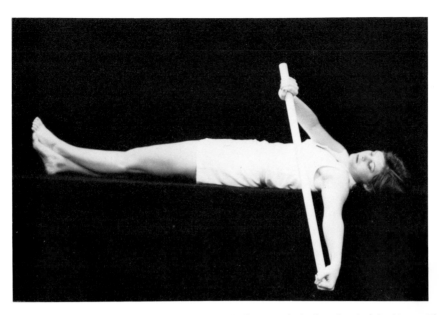

Fig. 4–16. Wand exercise: Performed off the side of the bed to stretch the long head of the biceps. The arm of the good side gently forces the shoulder into posterior extension, thus stretching the biceps tendon.

acromion or from the acromioclavicular joint, stretching exercises as in Figures 4–14 and 4–15 may still be of benefit. The presence of spurs are not predictive of outcome. In our experience, the presence of significant acromioclavicular joint osteoarthritis characterized by joint space narrowing, bony enlargement, or bony cysts, signifies a poor prognosis; spurs alone do not. Surgical consultation is advised in young and middle-aged persons with palpable joint enlargement. Resection of the coracoacromial ligament as well as any other site of impingement including the anterior acromion, acromial spurs, exuberant greater tuberosity, or osteoarthritic enlargement of the acromioclavicular joint is essential for good surgical result.[20,24,64] Surgical treatment of the spur should be considered only after 6 months of conservative measures including rest, exercise, local and oral anti-inflammatory measures have been used.

Outcome and Additional Suggestions. Richardson reported that prognosis of musculotendinous rotator cuff disorders correlated with passive range of movement. A good result was seen in nearly all patients following injection and exercise, if there was a good passive range of motion of the shoulder at the start of treatment.[65] Of patients with these disorders, 90% will obtain satisfactory recovery within 3 to 6 weeks.[1,23,34] Only 10% of patients with musculotendinous disorders require surgical consideration.[34] Patients who do not respond to conservative therapy, or young or middle-aged patients with a definite injury history and features of a rotator cuff tear, should have orthopedic consultation.[17,23]

Prolonged immobilization for a tear of the musculotendinous cuff may promote adhesive capsulitis (frozen shoulder). Early use of assisted passive range of movement exercise is the best preventive program. A trial of assisted passive exercises followed by active exercises should be undertaken (See Exercises 3–7, Table 4–5).

FROZEN SHOULDER (ADHESIVE CAPSULITIS)

The term "frozen shoulder" aptly describes a common disturbance of the shoulder with a *limitation of shoulder motion in all directions.* Described as periarthritis, adhesive capsulitis, frozen shoulder, adhesive bursitis, check rein disorder,[1] and DuPlay's disease,[34] this disorder may involve one or both shoulders. Frozen shoulder is a symptom complex that may result from diverse conditions.[18] Of these, "adhesive capsulitis" is the most common. The loss of motion is noted by examination with both active and passive motion restricted in all planes. The disorder is demonstrable by arthrography in which features of diminished capsular volume and loss of the capsular recesses can be detected.[66] Arthroscopy may not reveal intra-articular adhesions.[67,68] As will be noted later, neither inflammation nor adhesions are constant findings. Thus terminology remains difficult. The term adhesive capsulitis and frozen shoulder should be reserved for patients who lack other recognizable disorders affecting the shoulder joint. This disorder often occurs in women with cardiovascular disease,[17] but is frequently seen in men as well. It is rare in persons under the age of 40.

Onset usually begins on one side and is insidious. The usual presenting complaint is pain at night in a shoulder that has lost range of motion.[69] The earliest motion lost may be that which is necessary when reaching backward to fasten a brassiere or slip into a coat. Later, shoulder elevation is lost. The ache is described in the anterolateral aspect of the shoulder, the anterolateral arm, and the flexor portion of the forearm; occasionally the pain radiates to the chest wall. Throbbing discomfort or neuritic symptoms seldom occur. The condition may follow any underlying shoulder disorder. Untreated, adhesive capsulitis develops in three stages: "freezing," "frozen," and "thawing."[1] However, it is uncommon for an untreated frozen shoulder to dissipate completely and return to normal function.[19,70] More commonly, pain improves, but motion remains limited. The pain may fluctuate from day to day, depending upon physical activity.

Physical examination reveals a loss of active and passive shoulder movement in all directions. At first, only elevation and internal rotation are lost; later, all ranges of movement are lost, with the exception of forward extension. As the examiner puts the patient through passive movement, limitation of movement is noted even in the most relaxed patient. Tenderness is elicited regularly upon palpation of the tendons that form the musculotendinous rotator cuff.[17] Upon palpation, the humeral head may be felt higher in the shoulder joint, approximating the acromion, when compared to the uninvolved side. Patients with long-standing limitation of motion may have atrophy of the entire shoulder girdle musculature. Dystrophic changes in the remainder of the upper extremity are rare.

Etiology. Frozen shoulder has been considered the result of an extension of inflammation of adjacent tendon structures,[17] or of work in which the arm is kept abducted and motionless, as in typing. Conditions associated with adhesive capsulitis include trauma, myocardial infarction, pulmonary tuberculosis, diabetes, thyroid disease, cervical disc disease, cerebral hemorrhage and tumor, hemiplegia, cancer of the lung, and scleroderma.[71] Immobilization after trauma, or use of intravenous tubing for prolonged periods may lead to this entity.

Insulin-dependent diabetes has been linked to frozen shoulder. In one study of patients with frozen shoulder, 5 to 10% had diabetes.[9] No increased frequency of diabetic neuropathy was noted, and a third of the patients were insulin-dependent. Of patients with adhesive capsulitis and diabetes, 6% also had Dupuytren's contracture of the hand.[9] A relation to ischemic heart disease was also noted.[9,72,73]

Neviaser described the pathology of the shoulder capsule as thickened and contracted, with a chronic inflammatory infiltration.[74] The capsule appeared to suffer from a "glueing down," particularly in the region of the long head of the biceps. Synovial fluid is scant; synovial fluid studies have not been performed.[71] Lundberg compared surgical pathology with controls and reported no significant inflammation. The main finding was fibroplasia resembling that seen in Dupuytren's contracture. More fibroblasts were seen in adhesive capsulitis specimen.[75]

Immunologic abnormalities have recently been studied in patients with frozen shoulder. Initial reports of an association with HLA B27[76] have not been confirmed by others.[77] Also noted was a decreased immunoglobulin A level, and a decreased lymphocyte transformation.[78] Bulgen speculates that in the genetically susceptible host, an autoimmune inflammatory reaction follows supraspinatus tendon degeneration and leads to the frozen shoulder.[78] Drugs implicated in some patients include phenobarbital, iodides, and isoniazid.[79] The condition appears less common in blacks.[71]

Laboratory and Radiographic Examination. In the early stages of an adhesive capsulitis, the erythrocyte sedimentation rate may be elevated. Tests for diabetes should be performed. Roentgenography including an anterior posterior view of the shoulder with both internal and external rotation is useful to exclude fractures, degenerative arthritis, calcific tendinitis, chondrocalcinosis, malignancy, avascular necrosis, and dislocation.[71] Arthrography has been used to define the extent of the disorder. Reduced joint volume and diminution of the size of the subscapularis recess and the axillary recess are diagnostic of adhesive capsulitis.[66,80] Neither arthrography nor scintigraphy was of prognostic value but arthrography may demonstrate an associated capsule tear.[81,82] An arthrogram will seldom be necessary. Differential diagnosis from capsular tear is not difficult, and the presence of any remote underlying tear is unimportant clinically.

Differential Diagnosis. The causes of a painful stiff shoulder include degenerative, traumatic, and systemic inflammatory disorders. These include osteoarthritis, calcific tendinitis and bursitis, fractures and dislocations, rheumatoid arthritis and the spondyloarthropathies, polymyalgia rheumatica and temporal arteritis, and rarely gout, pseudogout, calcium apatite deposition disease, "Milwaukee Shoulder", tumors, Paget's disease, hyperthyroidism, myeloma, reflex dys-

trophy, psychogenic rheumatism, or malingering.[71,83] Frozen shoulder begins insidiously, is not associated with constitutional features, is not often a cause for severe pain. If the result of the erythrocyte sedimentation rate is greater than 70 mm/hr by the Westergren test, one must consider polymyalgia rheumatica and giant cell arthritis. Rheumatoid arthritis can produce a frozen shoulder. Careful evaluation during follow-up visits is necessary. A general examination of the patient with a frozen shoulder should be undertaken to observe for subtle features of systemic rheumatic disease.

Management. The importance of prescribed exercise for the relief of shoulder pain must be constantly stressed.[44] The patient can be informed that pain-free motion should occur but may take many months to achieve. Normal routine activity can be maintained during this time. However, until complete recovery occurs, active arm use should be limited so as not to precipitate severe pain. The exercise program for frozen shoulder must be progressive. Beginning with pendulum exercises, the patient should progress to wand manipulation,[3,85] and finally to overhead-pulley exercises.[17] Wall-ladder exercises can be used from the beginning if the patient has at least 60 degrees of abduction (Fig. 4–17). The duration of therapy depends on the patient pursuing an exercise program *despite pain*. Pain is the patient's worse enemy in trying to recover from frozen shoulder. As the patient attempts to perform an exercise program, the muscles comprising the musculotendinous cuff of the involved shoulder must be kept relaxed while stretching. This is accomplished by performing wand exercises (Fig. 4–18). The patient should be encouraged to gently, but persistently, stretch *beyond pain* to her tolerance (See Exercises 3–7, 11, 12, Table 4–5). Mobilization techniques should be performed by a therapist who has experience with joint mobilization techniques. In patients with acute pain and limitation of motion, such treatment is best begun with the arm held down at the side while the therapist begins with tech-

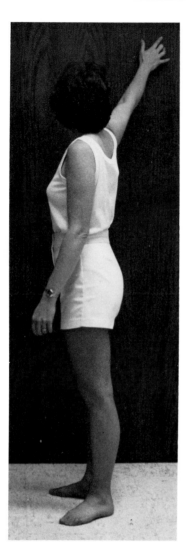

Fig. 4–17. Wall-ladder exercise for shoulder mobilization. The patient stands approximately 3 feet from a wall at a 90-degree angle. The fingers reaching for the wall "walk" in an upward and slightly posterior direction. Once the highest point possible has been reached, the hand is slowly lowered.

niques for elevation and relaxation. Later in the treatment, therapy can move on to progressive long axis "distraction," followed by an inferior gliding traction to the glenohumeral joint.[86] Similar motions can be performed by the patient alone.[86] (See Exercise 13, Table 4–5). Studies using physical therapy with exercise alone have revealed conflicting results.[58,87–89] Most agree, however, that ex-

ercise is an important adjunct to treatment.[87] Use of a TENS unit was of benefit in one series studied.[90]

Most authors currently recommend corticosteroid injections of the shoulder cuff, as well as intra-articular administration. A non-aqueous crystalline steroid suspension and local anesthetic mixture, injected into multiple locations about the shoulder capsule and into the joint, may be the best method of relieving pain. When steroids are used locally, a comprehensive program, in addition, is essential. When steroid injections were given with no other treatment, Hollingworth, Ellis, and Hattersley[61] reported a 26% success rate. Others compared manipulation and local steroid injection compared to steroid injection alone.[89] Thomas et al. reported 40% success with the combination of manipulation and injection versus 13% success with steroid injections alone.[91] We find that intralesional corticosteroid injections used in conjunction with exercises and joint protection advice is helpful in restoring nearly normal motion in the majority of our patients who have no concomitant shoulder disease. Equal aliquots of the mixture are injected into each site: the supraspinatus tendon insertion area, the subacromial bursa anterolaterally, the bicipital tendon sheath, the joint capsule posteriorly in the region of the teres minor muscle, and the glenohumeral joint[3] (Fig. 4–20). The injection may be repeated if night pain recurs and if the first injection did provide some relief.[92] Most patients will require only one shoulder injection session. Physical therapy instructions provided by the physician are usually satisfactory. We do not generally refer patients to a physical therapist unless instructions are difficult for the patient to comprehend, or improvement in range of motion is not satisfactory (about 33% improvement in the first month and 66% after 2 months). Because capsule tears may occur during manipulation under anesthesia, this procedure is never performed until all other therapeutic procedures have been tried.

Outcome and Additional Suggestions. Of patients who benefit, 60 to 95% return to

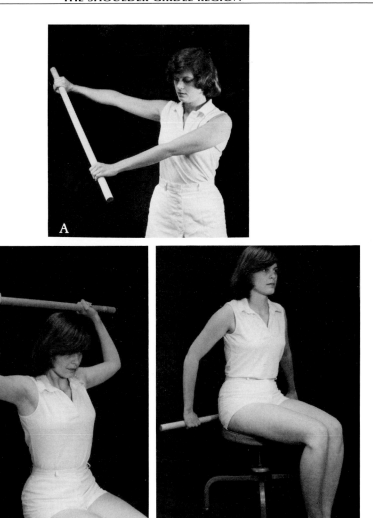

Fig. 4–18. Wand exercises to mobilize the frozen shoulder. The good arm is used to, *A,* force the arm on the involved side straight away, *B,* up and over head, and *C,* back and upward. Each position is performed as a single continuous movement or with short repetitions for 1 minute before going to the next movement.

normal, or at least near normal range of motion.[70,79,84,85] In our experience, the multiple shoulder injections, followed by immediate use of the wand exercises and wall-ladder exercises, provide relief from night pain in at least 90% of patients within 2 weeks. Once the patient has achieved 90 degrees of passive abduction (with the examiner assisting abduction), the shoulder motion nearly always returns to normal with home exercises alone. Some residual loss of motion can be seen in the elderly, but this may be "normal" for age.[19,70] The few who fail to respond can be referred to a physical therapist for stretching *manipulation,* and must continue to perform home exercises while under the therapist's care. In our experience, fewer than 1% of frozen shoulders need be manipulated under *anesthesia.* Of interest, insulin-dependent diabetic patients have the most intractable frozen shoulders, but the clinician cannot predict outcome just on this basis. If patients have failed to show progress following these maneuvers, infiltration brisement under

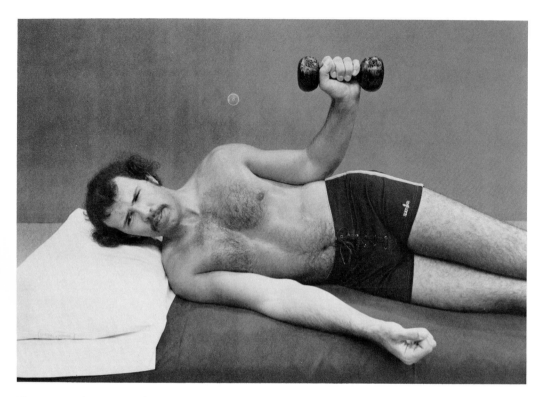

Fig. 4–19. Infraspinatus and teres minor strengthening. (From Jobe FW and Radovich Moynes D[41] with permission) (See Exercise 9, Table 4–5).

anesthesia (injecting an anesthetic and steroid suspension under pressure into the shoulder capsule), followed by manipulation under anesthesia, has been recommended.[34] Manipulation under anesthesia must be considered a last resort in the case of a frozen shoulder.[17] The addition of intra-articular corticosteroid injection following manipulation enhances results.[91]

SCAPULAR REGION DISORDERS

Normal scapular motion is an integral part of upper extremity movement. The "setting phase" of the scapula occurs during arm abduction or forward flexion. The scapulothoracic motion contributes significantly to shoulder motion.[17] The rhomboids, serratus anterior, levator scapulae, and pectoralis minor are important stabilizers of scapular movement, and may be the source of pain in and about the scapula. Three painful disorders of the scapula are described: snapping scapula, scapulocostal syndrome, and winging of the scapula.

Snapping Scapula

Audible and palpable sounds with discomfort may be due to alterations in the scapulothoracic articulations. Causes include anterior angulation of the superior scapular angle, rib deformities, the tubercle of Luschka (an enlarged bony nodule on the anterior aspect of the superior scapular angle), and scapular osteochondromatosis or tumors.[17] Scapular bursitis is an uncertain entity.[93] Oblique roentgenographic views of the scapula are necessary. The most common disturbance is an osteophyte on the superior medial border of the scapula.[94] Most cases are thought to arise from repetitive, forceful motion resulting in spur formation. A case in which a karate exercise resulted in injury to the insertion of the levator scapulae was re-

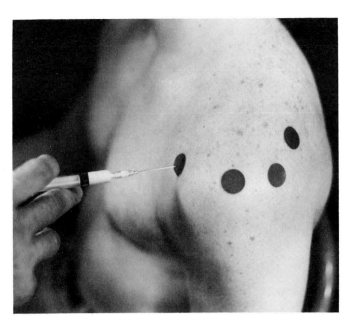

Fig. 4–20. The four points for injection of the frozen shoulder: Utilizing a suspension of a corticosteroid and local anesthetic, equal aliquots are injected into the supraspinatus tendon region, the subacromial bursa, the bicipital tendon sheath, and the joint capsule posteriorly in the region of the teres minor muscle. The latter site may be utilized also to inject the shoulder articulation.

ported.[95] The snapping scapula, which necessitates surgery, has been rare in our experience.

Scapulocostal Syndrome

The patient has insidious onset of pain in the superior and posterior aspects of the shoulder girdle radiating to the neck, upper triceps, deltoid insertion, and around the chest wall. Numbness and tingling of the hand occasionally accompany the scapulocostal syndrome.[17] Physical examination reveals diminished scapular motion on the involved side. Palpation reveals a trigger point located on the chest wall, medial and *beneath* the scapula. In order to locate the trigger point, the patient must draw the scapula laterally by reaching across her chest, placing her hand on the uninvolved shoulder, and rotating the involved shoulder forward. The trigger point is obviously tender, and palpation of the trigger point reproduces pain. Relief following infiltration of the lesion with an anesthetic and steroid injection confirms the diagnosis.

The cause may include friction between the scapula and the thoracic cage, myofascial strain from poor posture, scoliosis,[96,96A] disuse, trauma, or tumors about the scapula. Treatment includes posture exercises, scapular stretching (Fig. 4–21), and one or two sequential injections of a crystalline steroid-local anesthetic mixture.[17]

Other Myofascial Scapular Region Pain

Scapular region pain may result from postural strain when the trunk is forward flexed 30 to 50 degrees for long periods and the arm is held down and forward.[16] Triceps tendinitis at the site of attachment of the long head of the triceps to the infraglenoid tubercle of the scapula may result from vigorous throwing. It can be reproduced during examination by extending the shoulder and having the patient attempt to extend the flexed elbow against resistance. Exercises are the best treatment for such injuries. (See Exercises 14 and 15, Table 4–5).[97] The infraspinatus and teres minor muscles may be injured during

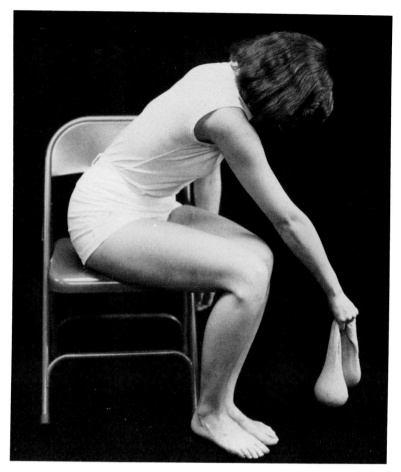

Fig. 4–21. Scapular stretching. Grasping a 2- to 5-pound weight, the patient slowly thrusts the arm forward; then leaning forward while keeping the trunk straight, she brings the arm on the involved side across the chest. The weight is allowed to approach the floor (but should not rest on the floor), in front and to the side of the foot, stretching the parascapular muscles. A pulling feeling in the area of pain will be noted. The position is held for 10 to 20 seconds and repeated 3 to 6 times twice daily.

racquet sports. Stretching and resistance exercises and physical therapy are helpful[97] (see Exercise 15, Table 4–5).

Trigger points under the scapula may be identified by having the patient rotate the scapula laterally by placing the ipsilateral hand across the chest and around the other shoulder, thus drawing the involved shoulder forward. After palpation and identification of a trigger point along the medial border of the scapula a local anesthetic injection can assist in both diagnosis and treatment.[96]

Travell reports the serratus posterior superior muscle medial to the superior pole of the scapula as the most frequent source of parascapular pain.[4] However, it seldom acts alone as the source of myofascial pain. The infraspinatus trigger point may cause local and referred pain to the outer and anterior upper arm. The supraspinatus and trapezius muscles commonly have trigger points located approximately ½-inch from each other in the center of the belly of the muscles. The trigger point is palpable as an indurated, elongated muscle band that rolls under the examiner's finger and is quite tender.[98] Treatment includes injecting the trigger point with a crystalline nonaqueous steroid anesthetic mixture (Fig. 4–22), stretching and postural correction exercises, and avoiding strain.

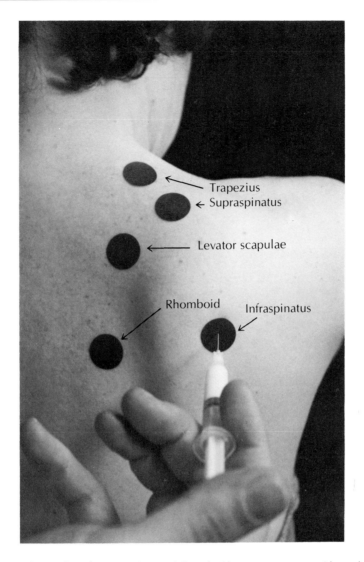

Fig. 4–22. The scapular myofascial trigger points are injected with a nonaqueous steroid-anesthetic mixture.

Physical therapy for myofascial scapular region pain includes wet heat followed by kneading massage of the tender points with or without skin rolling. This is followed by light stroking massage for relaxation. Recalcitrant trigger point nodules in muscles may respond to ultrasound using low wattage for a minute or so.[40] When tenderness is improved, conditioning exercises for the involved muscle should begin. The use of fluorimethane spray while the patient stretches has been helpful in our experience. The patient is seated leaning forward with arm crossed in front of the chest or hanging loosely between knees. The patient should arch or "hump" the spine and allow the arms to pull the scapula forward. The spray is swept from the trigger points across the scapula, laterally. The spray always is directed from the trigger point to the zone of pain referral. Two slow sweeps of the spray are used.[99] Joint protection advice (Table 4–2) is important to prevent recurrences. Reaching from the front seat of a car across to the back seat, and then

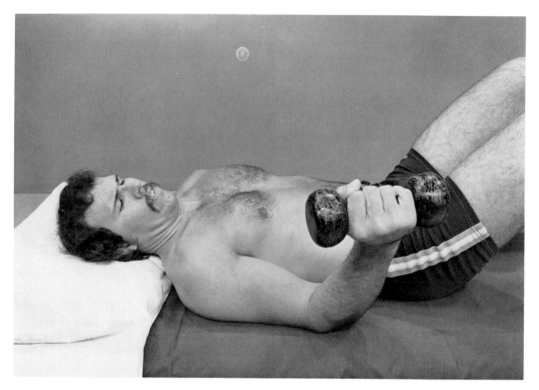

Fig. 4–23. Subscapularis strengthening. (From Jobe FW and Radovich Moynes D[41] with permission) (See Exercise 10, Table 4–5).

pulling a briefcase forward, is a common strain. Traveling salesmen are often seen with a myofascial scapular pain syndrome.

OTHER SHOULDER REGION DISORDERS

Winging of the Scapula

The patient with paresis or paralysis of the serratus anterior muscle may present with painless limitation of shoulder elevation, particularly the last 30 degrees of overhead-arm extension. There may be parascapular discomfort. As the physician observes the patient going through active shoulder motion, the scapula may be seen to draw away from the thoracic cage. While the patient presses his outstretched arms against a wall, the physician observes the involved scapula project from the thorax. This condition is the result of neurogenic paralysis of the serratus ante-

rior muscle. Paralysis may result from injury to the long thoracic nerve or brachial plexus from a direct blow to the suprascapular region, and has been described in army recruits carrying heavy packs with resultant nerve injury. Six cases of long thoracic nerve injury following first rib resection for thoracic outlet syndrome have been reported.[100] Tetanus antitoxin, typhoid, measles, or influenza vaccination may result in brachial plexitis and lead to winging of the scapula.[6] Bilateral suprascapular neuropathy resulting from weightlifting exercise with stretching injury to the suprascapular nerve was reported.[101] In patients with winging of the scapula, electrodiagnostic studies can demonstrate nerve injury as the cause, and may be useful in following the progress of the condition, which often requires a year or two for recovery. Treatment is expectant with exercises to preserve normal glenohumeral joint motion. Transcutaneous nerve stimulation may help alleviate discomfort.

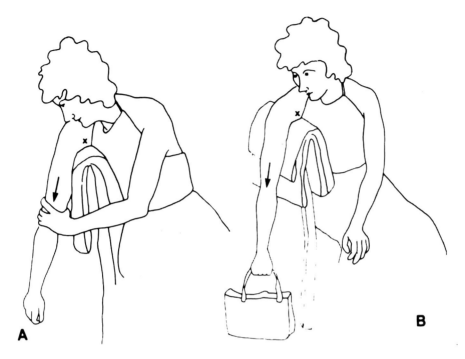

Fig. 4–24. Shoulder capsule stretch. (From Kessler RM, Hertling D[86] with permission) (see Exercise 13a., Table 4–5).

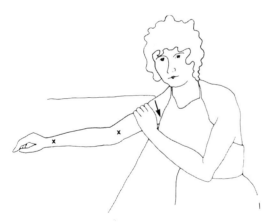

Fig. 4–25. Passive shoulder capsule stretch. (From Kessler RM, Hertling D[86] with permission) (See Exercise 13e., Table 4–5).

Acromioclavicular Joint Pain

Pain in the region of the acromioclavicular joint may result from trauma with subluxation or separation of the acromioclavicular joint, from a tear or strain of the coracoclavicular ligament,[28] or from tendinitis of the musculotendinous cuff of the shoulder. Osteoar-

thritis of the acromioclavicular joint may cause joint swelling and tenderness following excessive shoulder action. Synovitis of the acromioclavicular joint should alert the physician to the presence of a systemic inflammatory process, such as rheumatoid arthritis, spondyloarthritis, or giant cell arteritis.[102] Degenerative joint disease with bony enlargement is seldom the only cause of pain in the region of the acromioclavicular joint. A more likely cause is nearby tendinitis or bursitis. Careful palpation is essential. Frequently, acromioclavicular pain can be relieved by injecting a local anesthetic-corticosteroid mixture beneath the joint in the vicinity of the supraspinatus tendon (Fig. 4–12).

Soft Tissue Enlargement of the Shoulder

This unusual complaint is mentioned for completeness. Soft tissue thickening about the point of the shoulder may occur in amyloidosis (shoulder pad sign) or acromegaly, and from massive synovitis in patients with

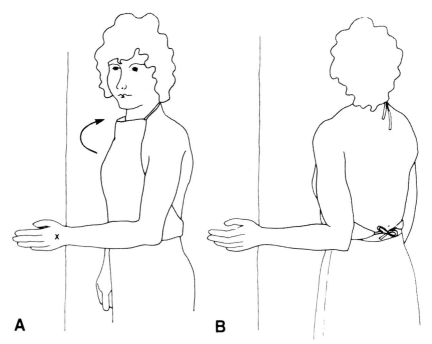

Fig. 4–26. Passive shoulder stretching in a doorway. (From Kessler RM, Hertling D[86] with permission) (See Exercise 13f, Table 4–5).

rheumatoid arthritis. Also, lipomas may occur about the shoulder. Amyloid infiltration has a rubbery feel upon examination. No fluctuance is noted. The enlargement is diffuse and does not follow any tendon-sheath pattern. The physician encountering such a disturbance should check the erythrocyte sedimentation rate, complete blood count, and serum protein electrophoresis. Features of acromegaly will be obvious, if it is kept in mind.

Abduction Contracture of the Shoulder

The inability to return the raised arm back down to the side of the body may result from repeated injections of any medication in large volume into the deltoid muscle. Two cases resulted from prolonged self administration of dimenhydrinate and pentazocine, and one case followed parenteral injections of lincomycin.[103] A band of dense scar tissue forms in the intermediate part of the deltoid and leads to contracture; permanent arm abduction follows. Surgical excision of the band may be required for relief.[103]

REFERENCES

1. Bland JH, Merrit JA, Boushey DR: The painful shoulder. Semin Arthritis Rheum 7:21–46, 1977.
2. Boyle AC: Joints and their diseases. Br Med J 3:283–285, 1969.
3. Kozin F: Painful shoulder and the reflex sympathetic dystrophy syndrome. *In* Arthritis and Allied Conditions. 10th Ed. Edited by DJ McCarty. Philadelphia, Lea & Febiger, 1985.
4. Travell J, Rinzler S, Herman M: Pain and disability of the shoulder and arm. JAMA *120*:417–422, 1942.
5. Kummel BM, Zazanis GA: Shoulder pain as the presenting complaint in carpal tunnel syndrome. Clin Orthop 92:227–230, 1973.
6. Duthie RB, Ferguson AB: Mercer's Orthopedic Surgery. 8th Ed. Baltimore, Williams & Wilkins, 1983.
7. Pinals RS: Traumatic arthritis and allied conditions. *In* Arthritis and Allied Conditions. 10th Ed. Edited by DJ McCarty. Philadelphia, Lea & Febiger, 1985.
8. Pinals RS, Short CL: Calcific periarthritis involving multiple sites. Arth Rheum 9:556–574, 1966.
9. Bridgman JF: Periarthritis of the shoulder and diabetes mellitus. Ann Rheum Dis *31*:69–71, 1972.
10. Wright V, Haq AM: Periarthritis of the shoulder. II. Radiological features. Ann Rheum Dis 35:220–226, 1976.
11. Cofield RH, Simonet WY: The shoulder in sports. Mayo Clin 59:157–164, 1984.
12. Bjelle A, Hagberg M, Michaelson G: Occupational and individual factors in acute shoulder-neck dis-

orders among industrial workers. Br J Ind Med 38:356–363, 1981.

13. Luopajarvi T, Kuorinka I, Virolainen M, et al: Prevalence of tenosynovitis and other injuries of the upper extremities in repetitive work. Scand J Work Environ & Health 5 [Suppl. 3]:48–55, 1979.

14. Myerson GE, Goldman J, Miller SB: Arcade arthritis-videogame violence. (Abstract #E83) Arth Rheum 25 (No. 4) [Supp], 1982.

15. Sheon RP: A joint protection guide for nonarticular rheumatic disorders. Postgrad Med 77 (5):329–338, 1985.

16. Hamilton PG: Chronic rhomboid strain: An illustration of an approach to fibrositis. Practitioner 222:841–843, 1979.

17. Turek SL: Orthopaedics: Principles and Their Application. 4th Ed. Philadelphia, JB Lippincott, 1984.

18. Matsen FA, Kirby RM: Office evaluation and management of shoulder pain. Ortho Clin N Am 13:453–475, 1982.

19. Clarke GR, Willis LA, Fish WW, Nichols PJR: Preliminary studies in measuring range of motion in normal and painful stiff shoulders. Rheumatol Rehab 14:39–46, 1975.

20. Kessel L, Watson M: The painful arc syndrome, clinical classification as a guide to management. J Bone Joint Surg 59-B:166–172, 1977.

21. Cyriax J: Textbook of Orthopaedic Medicine. I. Diagnosis of Soft Tissue Lesions. 7th Ed. London, Bailliere Tindall, 1978.

22. Hadler NM: Industrial rheumatology: Clinical investigations into the influence of the pattern of usage on the pattern of regional musculoskeletal disease. Arth Rheum 20:1019–1025, 1977.

23. Neer CS, Welch RP: The shoulder in sports. Orthop Clin N Am 8:583–591, 1977.

24. Penny JN, Welsh RP: Shoulder impingement syndromes in athletes and their surgical management. Am J Sports Med 9:11–15, 1981.

25. Laumann U: The so-called periarthritis humeroscapularis possibilities of an operative treatment. Arch Orthop Traumat Surg 97:27–37, 1980.

26. Kennedy JC, Hawkins RJ: Swimmer's shoulder. Physician Sports Med 2:25–35, 1974.

27. Ciullo JV, Guise ER: Coracoacromial arch impingement: Mechanical origin, clinical findings and treatment of so called subdeltoid bursitis. (Abstract #180) Arth Rheum 25 (No. 4) [Supp], 1982.

28. Nelson CL: The painful shoulder. Postgrad Med 29:71–78, 1970.

29. Cone III RO, Resnick D, Danzig L: Shoulder impingment syndrome: radiographic evaluation. Radiology 150:29–33, 1984.

30. Misamore GW, Hawkins RJ: Shoulder impingement syndrome: when to suspect, what to do. J Musculo Med (July):55–63, 1984.

31. Hawkins RJ, Kennedy JC: Impingement syndrome in athletes. Am J Sports Med 8:151–158, 1980.

32. McIntyre DI: Subcoracoid neurovascular entrapment. Clin Orthop 108:27–30, 1975.

33. Rathbun JB, Macnab I: The microvascular pattern of the rotator cuff. J Bone Joint Surg 52B:540–553, 1970.

34. Simon WH: Soft tissue disorders of the shoulder:

frozen shoulder, calcific tendinitis, and bicipital tendinitis. Ortho Clin N Am 6:521–535, 1975.

35. White RH, Hardy DC, Paull DM: Rotator cuff tendinitis: correlation of clinical features and radiographic findings with response to therapy. (Abstract #63) (No. 4) Arth Rheum [Supp], 1985.

36. Cannon RB, Schmid FR: Calcific periarthritis involving multiple sites in identical twins. Arth Rheum 16:393–396, 1973.

37. Thompson GR, Ting M, Riggs GA, et al: Calcific tendinitis and soft tissue calcification resembling gout. JAMA 203:464–472, 1968.

38. Codman EA: The Shoulder. Boston, Thomas Todd, 1934.

39. McKendry RJR, Uhthoff HK, Sarkar K, Hyslop P: Calcifying tendinitis of the shoulder: Prognostic value of clinical, histologic, and radiologic features in 57 surgically treated cases. J Rheum 9:75–80, 1982.

40. Zohn DA, Mennell J McM: Musculoskeletal Pain: Diagnosis and Physical Treatment. Boston, Little, Brown & Co., 1976.

41. Jobe FW, Radovich-Moynes D: Delineation of diagnostic criteria and a rehabilitation program for rotator cuff injuries. Am J Sports Med 10:336–339, 1982.

42. Andrews, JR, Carson WG: Shoulder Joint Arthroscopy. Orthopedics 6:1157–1162, 1983.

43. Cofield RH: Arthroscopy of the shoulder. Mayo Clin Proc 58:501–508, 1983.

44. McCarty DJ, Halverson PB, Carrera GF, et al.: "Milwaukee shoulder"—Association of microspheroids containing hydroxyapatite crystals, active collagenase, and neutral protease with rotator cuff defects. I: Clinical aspects. Arth Rheum 24:464–473, 1981.

45. Halverson PB, Cheung HS, McCarty DJ, et al.: "Milwaukee shoulder"—Association of microspheroids containing hydroxyapatite crystals, association with rotator cuff defects. II: Synovial fluid studies. Arth Rheum 24:474–483, 1981.

46. Petersson CJ: Ruptures of the supraspinatus tendon, cadaver dissection. Acta Orthop Scand 55:52–56, 1984.

47. Hagberg M, Kvarnstrom S: Muscular endurance and electromyographic fatigue in myofascial shoulder pain. Arch Phys Med Rehabil 65:522–525, 1984.

48. Schumacher HR, Smolyo AP, Tse RL, Maurer K: Arthritis associated with apatite crystals. Ann Intern Med 87:411–416, 1977.

49. McCarty DJ, Gatter RA: Recurrent acute inflammation associated with focal apatite crystal deposition. Arth Rheum 9:804–819, 1966.

50. Dieppe PA, Crocker P, Huskisson EC, Willoughby DA: Apatite deposition disease; A new arthropathy. Lancet 1:266–268, 1976.

51. Kvarnstrom S: Occurrence of musculoskeletal disorders in a manufacturing industry, with special attention to occupational shoulder disorders. Scand J Rehab Med 8:1–114, 1983.

52. Vigario GD, Keats TE: Localization of calcific deposits in the shoulder. Am J Roentgen Rad Therap Nuc Med 108:806–811, 1970.

53. Neer CS, Craig EV, Fukuda H: Cuff-tear arthropathy. J Bone Joint Surg 65A:1232–1244, 1983.

53a. Middleton WD, Reinus WR, Totty WG, et al.: Ultrasonographic evaluation of the rotator cuff and biceps tendon. J Bone Joint Surg 68A:440–450, 1986.

54. Downing D, Weistein A: Ultrasound Therapy of Subacromial Bursitis: A Double Blind Trial. Arth Rheum 26:37, 1983.

55. Cogan L: Medical Management of the Painful Shoulder. Bull Rheum Disease 32:54–58, 1982.

56. Guerin BK, Burnstein SL: Conservative Therapy of Acute Painful Shoulder. Ortho Review 11:29–37, 1982.

57. Percy EC, Carson JD: The use of DMSO in tennis elbow and rotator cuff tendonitis: a double-blind study. Med Sci in Sports Exer 13:215–219, 1981.

58. Roy S, Oldham R: Management of painful shoulder. Lancet 1:1322–1324, 1979.

59. Weiss JJ: Intra-articular steroids in the treatment of rotator cuff tear: reappraisal by arthrography. Arch Phys Med Rehabil 62:555–557, 1981.

60. Berry H, Fernandes L, Bloom B, et al.: Clinical study comparing acupuncture, physiotherapy, injection and oral anti-inflammatory therapy in shoulder-cuff lesions. Curr Med Res Opin 7:121–126, 1980.

61. Hollingworth GR, Ellis RM, Hattersley TM: Comparison of injection techniques for shoulder pain: results of a double blind, randomised study. Br Med J 287:1339–1341, 1983.

62. White RH, Paull DM, Fleming KW: Rotator cuff tendinitis: comparison of local corticosteroid injections versus nonsteroidal therapy. (Abstract #63) Arth Rheum 28 (No. 4) [Supp], 1985.

63. Crenshaw AH, Kilgore WE: Surgical treatment of bicipital tenosynovitis. J Bone Joint Surg 48A:1496–1502, 1966.

64. Ha'eri GB, et al: Shoulder Impingement Syndrome, results of operative release. Clin Orth 168:128–132, 1982.

65. Richardson AT: The painful shoulder. Proc Roy Soc Med 68:731–736, 1975.

66. Loyd JA, Loyd HM: Adhesive capsulitis of the shoulder: arthrographic diagnosis and treatment. Southern Med J 76:879–883, 1983.

67. Wiley AM, Older MWJ: Shoulder arthroscopy. Am J Sports Med 8:31–38, 1980.

68. Ha'eri GB, Maitland A: Arthroscopic findings in the frozen shoulder. J Rheum 8:149–152, 1981.

69. Hazleman BL: The painful stiff shoulder. Rheum Phys Med 11:413–421, 1972.

70. Reeves B: The natural history of the frozen shoulder syndrome. Scand J Rheum 4:193–196, 1975.

71. Rizk TE, Pinals RS: Frozen shoulder. Seminars Arth Rheum 11:440–452, 1982.

72. Sheldon PJH: A retrospective survey of 102 cases of shoulder pain. Rheum Phys Med 11:422–427, 1972.

73. Wright V, Haq AM: Periarthritis of the shoulder. I. Aetiological considerations with particular reference to personality factors. Ann Rheum Dis 35:213–219, 1976.

74. Neviaser JS: Adhesive capsulitis of the shoulder; A study of the pathological findings in periarthritis of the shoulder. J Bone Joint Surg 27:211–222, 1945.

75. Lundberg BJ: The frozen shoulder. Acta Orthop Scand Suppl 119, 1969.

76. Brewerton DA, Hart FD, Nicholls A, et al.: Ankylosing spondylitis and HL-A27. Lancet 1:904–907, 1973.

77. Stodell MA, Sturrock RD: Frozen Shoulder. The Lancet 1:527, 1981.

78. Bulgen D, Hazleman B, Ward M, McCallum M: Immunological studies in frozen shoulder. Ann Rheum Dis 37:135–138, 1978.

79. Steinbrocker O, Argyros TG: Frozen shoulder: Treatment by local injections of depot corticosteroids. Arch Phys Med Rehabil 55:209–213, 1974.

80. Reeves B: Arthrographic changes in frozen and post-traumatic stiff shoulders. Proc R Soc Med 59:827–830, 1966.

81. Binder AI, Bulgen DY, Hazleman BL, Tudor J, Wraight P: Frozen shoulder: an arthrographic and radionuclear scan assessment. Ann Rheum Dis 43:365–369, 1984.

82. Binder AI, Bulgen DY, Hazleman BL, Roberts S: Frozen shoulder: a long-term prospective study. Ann Rheum Dis 43:361–364, 1984.

83. Mens J, Van Der Korst JK: Calcifying supracoracoid bursitis as a cause of chronic shoulder pain. Ann Rheum Dis 43:758–759, 1984.

84. Russek AS: Role of physical medicine in relief of certain pain mechanisms of shoulder. JAMA 156:1575–1577, 1954.

85. Weiser HI: Painful primary frozen shoulder mobilization under local anesthesia. Arch Phys Med Rehabil 58:406–408, 1977.

86. Kessler RM, Hertling D: Management of Common Musculoskeletal Disorders. Philadelphia, Harper & Row, 1983.

87. Duncan BF: The Frozen Shoulder Syndrome—Rehabilitative Approach to Treatment. Contemp Ortho 6:69–72, 1983.

88. Binder AI, Bulgen DY, Hazleman BL, Roberts S: Frozen shoulder: a long-term prospective study. Ann Rheum Dis 43:361–364, 1984.

89. Bulgen DY, Binder AI, Hazleman BL, Dutton J, Roberts S: Frozen shoulder: prospective clinical study with an evaluation of three treatment regimens. Ann Rheum Dis 43:353–360, 1984.

90. Rizk TE, Christopher RP, Pinals RS, Higgins AC: Adhesive capsulitis (frozen shoulder): A new approach to its management. Arch Phys Med Rehabil 64:29–33, 1983.

91. Thomas D, Williams RA, Smith DS: The frozen shoulder: a review of manipulative treatment. Rheum Rehab 19:173–179, 1980.

92. Moskowitz RW: Clinical Rheumatology; A problem-oriented approach. 2nd Ed. Philadelphia, Lea & Febiger, 1982.

93. Coventry MB: Recurring scapular pain. JAMA 241:942, 1979.

94. Riggins RS: The shoulder. In Musculoskeletal Disorders. Edited by RD D'Ambrosia, Philadelphia, JB Lippincott, 1977.

95. Strizak AM, Cowen MH: The snapping scapula syndrome. J Bone Joint Surg 64A:941–942, 1982.

96. Cohen CA: Scapulocostal syndrome: Diagnosis and treatment. Southern Med J 73:433–437, 1980.

96A. Emans JB: Scoliosis: detecting the curves that mandate treatment. J Musculoskeletal Med (March):11–24, 1985.

97. Curwin S, Stanish WD: Tendinitis: Its Etiology and Treatment. Lexington, Mass, The Collamore Press, 1984.

98. Reynolds MD: Myofascial trigger points in persistent posttraumatic shoulder pain. Southern Med J 77:1277–1280, 1984.

99. Simons DG, Travell JG: Myofascial origins of low back pain—1. Principles of diagnosis and treatment. Post Grad Med 73:66–108, 1983.

100. Wood VE, Frykman GK: Winging of the scapula as a complication of first rib resection: a report of six cases. Clin Orth 149:160–163, 1980.

101. Saeed MA, Kraft GH: Bilateral suprascapular neuropathy. Orthopaedic Rev 11:135–137, 1982.

102. Miller LD, Stevens MD: Skeletal manifestations of polymyalgia rheumatica. JAMA 240:27–29, 1978.

103. Groves RJ, Goldner JL: Contracture of the deltoid muscle in the adult after intramuscular injections. J Bone Joint Surg 56A:817–820, 1974.

104. Goodman CE, Serebro LH: Sorting out the shoulder syndromes. J Musculoskeletal Med (June):37–45, 1984.

5

The Elbow

The elbow is a common site of involvement for many arthritides, including secondary osteoarthritis, rheumatoid arthritis, and gout. Elbow pain often occurs from disturbances of the regional soft tissue supporting structures. Furthermore, the clinician must keep in mind that elbow pain and dysfunction may be secondary to disorders arising in the neck, shoulder, wrist, or hand (Table 5–1). The three cardinal bony landmarks are the medial and lateral epicondyles and the olecranon.[1] An abnormal relationship suggests dislocation. Hyperextension greater than 10 degrees may indicate generalized joint laxity seen in the hypermobility syndrome.

The two major muscle components of the forearm serving the wrist and hand include the flexor pronator group (pronator teres, flexor carpi radialis, palmaris longus, flexor carpi ulnaris, flexor digitorum sublimis) and the extensor muscle group (extensor carpi radialis longus, extensor carpi radialis brevis, extensor digitorum communis, extensor indicis proprius, extensor carpi ulnaris). The flexor pronator group arises from the medial epicondyle region of the elbow. Conversely, the extensor group joins to form the extensor communis tendon, which inserts onto the lateral epicondyle of the humerus (See Anatomic Plates VI and VII). In addition to the well-known olecranon bursa, another bursa lies between the triceps and olecranon prominence. Also, a bursa may occur between the neck of the radius and the biceps tendon.[1]

The Examination. The history should include the quality, location, and duration of pain or disability. The physician must include in the history whether neck, shoulder, wrist, or hand position or movement aggravates the elbow problem. Numbness and tingling, in addition to pain, may suggest a local entrap-

Table 5–1. Danger Signs for the Elbow Region

1. Fever and chills
2. Peribursal erythema and edema
3. Lymphadenopathy
4. Malalignment of bony landmarks
5. Lateral instability during passive examination
6. Muscle atrophy
7. Night pain in the arm

ment syndrome, cervical nerve root impingement, or a carpal tunnel syndrome. Aggravating factors, such as occupational repetitive movement, hobbies, sports, or other possible injury-provoking work preceding the onset of pain, should be established. Improper sleep position, particularly with the involved arm in hyperabduction; use of the elbow as a prop when reading or driving; and use of the elbow to push up from bed are other possible aggravations to be elicited by history[3] (Table 5–2). Possible factors causing neuropathy (e.g., diabetes, alcoholism) should be elicited. A past history of tendinitis about the shoulder or other areas may suggest multifocal calcific tendinitis, although the elbow is an uncommon site for this.

Evaluation for evidence of generalized disorders, such as rheumatoid arthritis, osteoarthritis, neuropathy, gout, hyperlipidemia, and other medical conditions, should be carried out as indicated. Regional examination of the neck, shoulder, wrist, and hand may reveal disturbances at these locations, which can refer pain to the elbow.

Examination of the elbow includes muscle and neurologic examinations of the upper extremity. Palpation may demonstrate swelling of the tendon of the biceps anteriorly, swelling of the olecranon bursa, tophi, or rheumatoid nodules within the bursa. Points of tenderness at the epicondyles should be com-

Table 5–2. Joint Protection for the Elbow Region (From Sheon[3])

Harmful	Helpful
■ Using the elbow to push the body up when arising from bed or to prop it up when sitting can result in pressure injury to nerves at the elbow.	■ Use the abdominal muscles to help roll the body out of bed; when sitting, keep the elbows in space.
■ Repeatedly using tools that must be twisted and forced (e.g., screwdriver, pipe wrench) may injure tendons near the elbow. Improperly gripping golf clubs, rackets, or other pieces of sports equipment may be injurious to the elbow.	■ Grip tools less tightly; use foam-plastic pipe insulation (sold at hardware stores) on tool handles; take frequent short breaks. Learn the proper techniques for gripping various pieces of sports equipment.
■ Unconsciously clenching the hands while sleeping or driving may produce elbow pain.	■ Wear gloves (seams to the outside) to bed. Use a padded steering wheel. Learn to use relaxation techniques.

pared with the uninvolved elbow. The forearm muscles, approximately 1 to 2 inches distal to the elbow, should be palpated for cord-like induration. This may provide the examiner with evidence of a tear or adhesion within one or more of the forearm tendons. The painful elbow may be the presenting complaint in the fibrositis syndrome. Look for tender points in other locations such as the midpoint of the trapezei, the costochondral junctions, and perform a skin-rolling test above the midpoint of the trapezei. Tenderness is suggestive of the fibrositis syndrome.[4]

Usually the presentation of pain at the elbow area is found to be the result of only one predominant entity. However, on occasion more than one condition may be found, such as a tennis elbow and carpal tunnel syndrome, or olecranon bursitis and tendinitis of the biceps insertion of the elbow.[5] In Nirschl's series of 1213 patients with tennis elbow, a small number had associated musculoskeletal abnormalities including 13 cases with shoulder tendinitis, 8 cases with carpal tunnel syndrome, 4 cases with cervical disc or lumbar disc disease, and 2 patients with fibrositis.[6] Sometimes elbow pain may be the initial presentation of a systemic illness. Table 5–3 provides a decision chart for appropriate study. Furthermore, these soft tissue nonarticular rheumatic disorders may be superimposed upon other arthritic disorders. Relief from these soft tissue disturbances may provide the patient with satisfactory use of the elbow, despite persistence of other rheumatic disorders.

TENNIS ELBOW

In recent years the term "tennis elbow" has been applied to several soft tissue rheumatic disorders. Similar symptoms may also result from nerve root entrapment.[7,8] Tennis elbow most accurately includes disturbances that result in pain and tenderness in the lateral epicondyle region of the elbow.[9] "Golfer's elbow" has been used to describe similar disturbances in the medial epicondyle region. The term "tennis elbow" has gained preference over "epicondylitis" or "radiohumeral bursitis," perhaps because we know little about etiology, and neither inflammation of the epicondyle nor a radiohumeral bursitis has been described.[2]

The patient with tennis elbow may present with acute, intermittent, subacute, or chronic pain during grasping or supination of the wrist. The most common subjective symptom of tennis elbow is pain in the elbow during hand movement. In addition, rest pain, and pain during resisted movement of the wrist and fingers is common. Objective signs in-

Table 5–3. Decision Chart: The Elbow

Problem	Action	Further Action

A. Tennis Elbow
  No visible swelling
  Pain with use/grip
  No numbness/tingling
	CONSERVATIVE CARE
	Splint/rest
	Mobilizing exercise
	Local steroid injection
	  or NSAIDS
	ASA before play
		Examine for cervical disease
		Orthopedic consultation
		Surgery only after at least 6 months
		  of conservative treatment

B. Tendinitis
  No visible swelling
  Local tenderness
  Pain with finger motion
    against resistance		

C. Bursitis
  Visible swelling
  No joint limitation of movement
  With or without warmth/redness
  No skin penetration by injury
	Immediate aspiration
	Fluid examined for
	  gram stain/culture
	  sugar content
	  wbc and diff/crystals
		→ Orthopedic consultation

D. Nerve entrapment
  Pain on finger extension/or
    wrist supination
  Numbness/tingling
  Weakness of grip
	Inject site of entrapment
	  with steroid/local anesthetic
		→ Neurosurgery consultation

clude local tenderness at the epicondyle during palpation and a decrease in grip power.[10] It is an occupational hazard in carpenters, gardeners, dentists, and politicians.[11] It is seen often in patients previously afflicted with shoulder tendinitis or myofascial back pain.[1] This disorder is seldom bilateral; the lateral epicondylar site is more common than the medial epidondylar site.[5,12] Tennis elbow is seldom seen in persons under the age of 40 or over the age of 60.[5,13] The patient often points to a prominent point of the lateral epicondyle as the area of maximum pain and tenderness. Often, however, the clinician can detect a cord-like, firm scar within one of the extensor tendons leading to the epicondyle. This indurated tendon generally lies approximately 2 inches distal to the epicondyle; careful palpation is needed to locate it. Passive stretching of the extensor communis will be accompanied by a sensation of tautness or of a pulling on the involved side when compared to the uninvolved arm. The pain is reproduced by having the patient extend his wrist against the examiner's resistance. Elbow motion usually is not limited by uncomplicated tennis elbow.

Etiology. A controlled pathologic study carried out by Goldie,[14] and confirmed by Nirschl,[13] revealed no evidence of a bursa on the epicondyle; rather, a subtendinous space with granulation tissue, edema, and increased vascularity was found in these patients. Fibroblast proliferation of the extensor aponeurosis was also noted,[13] and no periostitis was found.[14] Nirschl[6] also reported the consistent finding of a lesion at the origin of the extensor carpi radialis brevis in 88 operated elbows. There was immature fibroblastic proliferation and vascular infiltration at this site. Sartar and Uhthoff described a tendinopathy of the common extensor tendon with ultrastructural features of mesenchymal cell proliferation and aggregates of newly formed vascular channels.[15] In another series, Bernhang noted a chronic synovitis with an inflamed synovial fringe in 11 of 21 operated elbows.[16] The presence of a sharp longitudinal linear ridge or spur on the lateral epicondyle

lying at 90 degrees to fibers of the conjoint extensor tendon may be detected in some patients during roentgenography.[17] The result is considered by most authors to be due to a strain or tear resulting from over-use of the forearm musculature.[2,5,9,12,18,19] More serious injury to elbow structures might present as tennis elbow, but examination for joint laxity should reveal these injuries (tear of the joint capsule or radial collateral ligament).[18] Tennis players, particularly novices, suffer tennis elbow often as a result of pressure-grip strain during backhand shots performed with a "leading elbow." The novice errs in performing a backhand shot with the elbow pointed toward the net. Also, tennis elbow is more common in loose-jointed tennis players.[19] Squash players with a "wristy backhand" or who play a lob from the front of the court are at risk for tennis elbow, as are badminton players.[20] Priest reported that 45% of 84 world class tennis players suffered from tennis elbow, though most continued to play.[21] In one large series most cases resulted from sport injuries or auto accidents and few were of occupational origin.[16] Another possible cause is unconscious hand clenching, which may occur during sleep, while driving, or when reading.

Laboratory and Radiographic Examination. Elbow joint roentgenographs in patients with tennis elbow rarely reveal an abnormality.[9] Unless tennis elbow is superimposed upon another inflammatory disease process, tests for inflammation are normal.

Differential Diagnosis. As mentioned, the term tennis elbow refers to pain resulting from myofascial injury, yet similar features can result from nerve entrapment, cervical nerve root impingement, or carpal tunnel syndrome. In addition, a trigger point in the anterior scalene muscle may give rise to pain in the lateral epicondyle area[22] (Table 5–3, Decision Chart). Failure to respond to local measures should raise the suspicion of these other disorders.

Management. The clinician and patient must recognize and alter aggravating activities that excessively contract the extensor

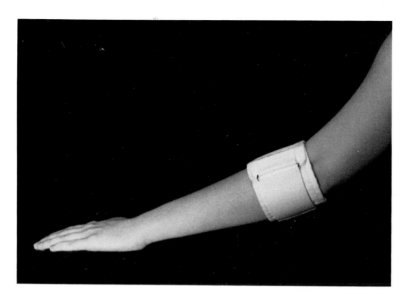

Fig. 5–1. The tennis elbow band: Although the rationale for use is uncertain, the protective influence of a tennis elbow band during arm use is helpful in most patients with tennis elbow. This is one of many available styles.

muscle group (Table 5–2). A "tennis elbow band" with velcro fastening may be helpful (Fig. 5–1). Generally, the band is 2 to 3 inches wide, and is applied across the epicondyles of the elbow just distal to the joint. It should be used during forearm work. Aggravating hand use should be avoided for at least 1 month after pain is relieved, in order to prevent recurrence.[9]

Exclude nerve entrapment syndromes, including carpal tunnel syndrome, thoracic outlet syndrome, or cervical radiculopathy.

Measures to relieve pain on the first visit depend on degree and location of tenderness elicited during the examination. If pain or tenderness is not disabling, and a well-localized point of tenderness is not found, then local corticosteroid injections should be withheld until a future visit. In such a patient, stretching exercises, protection from strain, and the use of local heat or ice may suffice. Nonsteroidal anti-inflammatory drugs, rub-ons, or simple analgesics may be useful. Splinting with a removable low temperature plastic resting splint may be valuable in acutely painful cases. As the pain subsides, gradual exercise is initiated beginning with active range of motion exercises. The patient is instructed to support the forearm on a table with the wrist suspended over the edge and to perform wrist extension with radial and ulnar deviation, pronation to supination, wrist flexion, and wrist circumduction.[23] Tendon stretching should follow (see Exercises 1 and 2, Table 5–4 and Figures 5–3 and 5–4). As the tendons lengthen, the patient is aware that the hand can be raised higher against the door or wall before the pulling sensation is detected in the forearm musculature. The exercises should be performed at least for 1 minute twice daily and until the elbow is pain free for 6 weeks.[5,9,11,13,19] For pain at the medial epicondyle, the exercise is reversed (See Exercise 3, Table 5–4). In one study, use of local therapy and exercise without injections resulted in complete relief of symptoms in 50% of athletes; a further 25% had marked relief of pain. Most required less than 5 weeks of exercise therapy.[20]

Use of ultrasound was considered of value in one double blind study.[24] Dimethyl sulfoxide (DMSO) was also studied in double blind fashion; no difference in benefit was noted between users of a 70% solution and those who used a 5% (placebo) solution. Side effects were noted in 66% of the treatment group.[25]

Friction massage from light to deep can be given to the affected fibers of the extensor carpi radialis brevis at the anterior aspect of the lateral humeral epicondyle. The massaging hand of the therapist is placed so that the thumb is over the affected fibers, and counterpressure is applied by the therapist's fingers lying against the medial proximal aspect of the forearm. The thumb is drawn across the site of the lesion in a direction perpendicular to the fibers by alternating supination and pronation of the therapist's arm.[26]

However, if a cord-like induration is elicited, or if symptoms are severe, local infiltration with a crystalline steroid-local anesthetic mixture with a No. 23 or No. 25 needle is usually helpful. In addition, the epicondylar region should be approached from one or more directions, so that the steroid mixture is injected into a region covering 2 cm[5] (Fig. 5–2). This is helpful in preventing local steroid atrophy. The patient should be forewarned that local pain may be worse the first day or two following injection, in which case cold applications are helpful. In a large series described by Nirschl, use of joint protection,

and an average of 5 steroid injections provided relief in the majority of patients; despite long duration of symptoms (21.6 months for men, 51 months for women); only 7% (88 of 1213 cases) required surgical procedure.[6] Similar results were noted by Bernhang who stressed the need to inject both the point of maximum tenderness and the area of the tendon and ligament insertion. Up to three injections were required and only 10% required surgery.[16] In a third study using these conservative measures, Nevalos noted recurrences in only 18% of patients after 6 months of followup.[27] Local injection and rest are also the procedure of choice for sport enthusiasts. O'Donoghue recommends up to four injections with avoidance of activities that caused the trouble, until symptoms and tenderness have improved.[28] Splinting is used only during acute pain; normal use is more helpful than was further splinting.[29]

Outcome. These conservative measures have provided relief in over 90% of patients.[5,6,19] Tennis elbow is generally a self-limiting disorder of several months' duration; in some patients, however, symptoms may last up to 12 months.[9,11,13]

In patients with continuing disability, care-

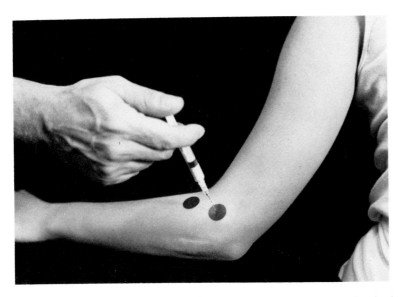

Fig. 5–2. Injection of the lateral epicondyle and the band-like trigger in the extensor tendon for the patient with tennis elbow.

Table 5–4. Elbow Exercises

1. Stretching exercise for tennis elbow: Stand facing a wall; place involved arm straight to a door, put back of hand to door, fingers toward floor. Start with wrist at about belt level, then slide wrist and hand slowly upward until a pulling sensation is felt near the elbow. Hold position 1 minute, perform one exercise and repeat twice daily (Fig. 5–3).

2. Mobilizing exercise for tennis elbow: Place arm on a table, grasp a 3-pound weight in hand, allow hand to hang over edge of table, first palm down, then palm up. In each position, let weight pull hand down below table then raise it back up. Repeat 30 times palm down, then palm up (for 1 to 2 minutes). Perform twice daily (Fig. 5–4).

3. Stretching exercise for golfer's elbow: Perform as above but place palm to door, point fingers to floor, slide upward until pulling sensation is felt near the elbow (Fig. 5–5).

4. Biceps stretch: Lie on back with the elbow at edge of bed and the arm extended beyond the bed. Grasp a 5-pound weight, with palm upward and allow the weight to pull the arm straight. Slowly bend and straighten the arm, allowing the weight to passively stretch the elbow with each movement. Repeat slowly for 1 minute. Repeat twice daily (Fig. 5–6).

5. Triceps strengthening exercise: Grasp 1- to 5-pound weight (begin with the most that is comfortable); hold elbow out at shoulder height, elbow bent 90 degrees, now raise arm to extend elbow to 180 degrees, in line with shoulder. Increase weight by 1 pound increments weekly (Fig. 5–7).

ful neurologic investigation should be performed. Gunn reported that 42 patients with symptoms of tennis elbow had accompanying cervical radiculopathy. Of these 42 patients, 39 had relief with conservative measures directed to the neck. Electrodiagnostic tests, carefully performed, proved useful in recognizing a cervical-nerve-root cause for tennis elbow.[7] This result requires confirmation. Other nerve entrapment lesions about the elbow should be considered. Tennis- or golf-related injuries may require a professional consultation for ascertaining an improper stroke.[14] An occupational therapist may be required for occupational reeducation. Local injections of corticosteroid-anesthetic mixture should generally not be required for more than a few times. Plaster immobilization is an additional therapeutic modality. Fewer than 5% of patients require surgery for chronic recurrent tennis elbow. A "lateral release" of the common origin of the radial extensors is one of the surgical procedures recommended.[30]

OLECRANON BURSITIS

The olecranon bursa occupies the posterior point of the elbow and has a synovial membrane. Inflammation or effusion of the bursa may result from gout, rheumatoid arthritis, sepsis, or trauma (Fig. 5–8). Traumatic bursitis occurs from pressure, either while seated with the elbow leaning on something, or as part of an occupational problem (e.g., carpet layers). Acute olecranon bursitis with warmth or erythema can occur in gout, pseudogout, rheumatoid arthritis, infection, or hemorrhage.[2,12] Peribursal edema and pain on motion were particular features of septic bursitis.[31] Whether bursitis appears acutely or subacutely in onset, septic bursitis must always be excluded. Septic bursitis may appear subacutely;[32–34] therefore, septic bursitis must be excluded by aspiration and the performance of appropriate diagnostic tests.

Laboratory and Radiographic Examination. If trauma with possible foreign body penetration is a consideration, roentgenographs with soft tissue techniques may be helpful to visualize the foreign body. Aspiration and evaluation of the bursal fluid are diagnostically helpful, and are essential if septic bursitis is even remotely suspected. Inspection of the fluid in most cases reveals a thin, watery, yellow- or brown-tinged fluid. The fluid should be examined for white blood cell count and differential, Gram stain, sugar content, and culture. A white blood cell count as low as 1400 cells/ml[3] does *not* exclude in-

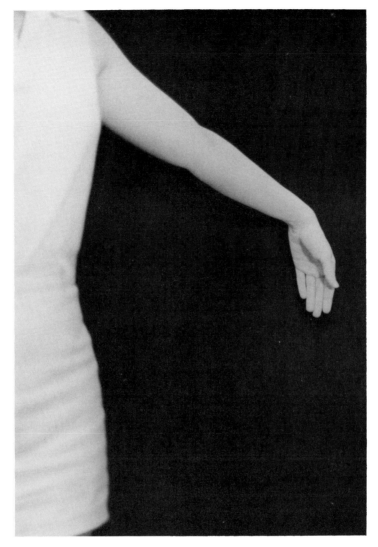

Fig. 5–3. Stretching exercise of the extensor forearm muscles for the patient with tennis elbow.

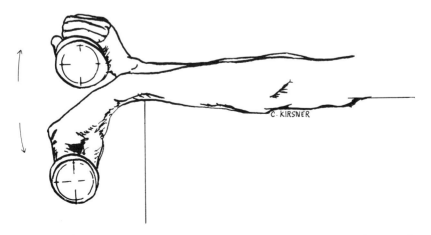

Fig. 5–4. Mobilizing and strengthening exercise for the forearm muscles in patients with tennis elbow.

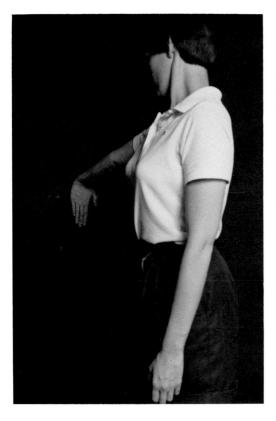

Fig. 5–5. A technique that stretches the forearm flexor muscles.

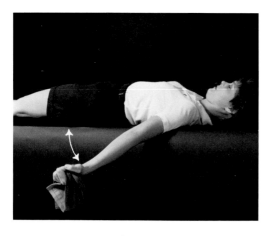

Fig. 5–6. Biceps stretching exercise.

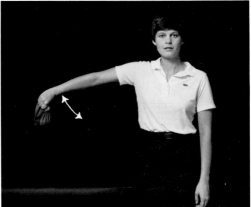

Fig. 5–7. Resistance exercise for strengthening the triceps muscle.

fection.[32,33] Comparison of bursal fluid sugar content to a simultaneously obtained serum sample may be helpful in cases of suspected sepsis. The majority of patients with septic bursitis have a low bursal fluid sugar level, but even this criterion is not absolute.[32] Septic bursitis may occur even in the absence of a penetrating injury. In general, the white blood cell count is less than 1000 cells/ml[3] in nonseptic bursitis fluid.[32] Crystal identification with polarizing microscopy should be performed in any patient with a history of gout, pseudogout, or recurrent olecranon bursitis.

Differential Diagnosis. Most patients with olecranon bursitis do not have a systemic disorder, yet careful palpation of the bursa for nodules can suggest the presence of rheumatoid arthritis, gout, or hyperlipidemia, before other typical features emerge. Our concern for low-grade sepsis as a cause for bursitis has been emphasized.

Management. Recognition and avoidance of aggravating pressure injury are necessary to prevent recurrence. Patients should be informed that their elbows should be kept away from the arms of chairs, or the arm rest of an automobile. In hospitalized patients, the provision of foam rubber protectors should be considered. Two studies of traumatic bursitis suggest that aspiration without local injection of steroidal agents is preferable to local in-

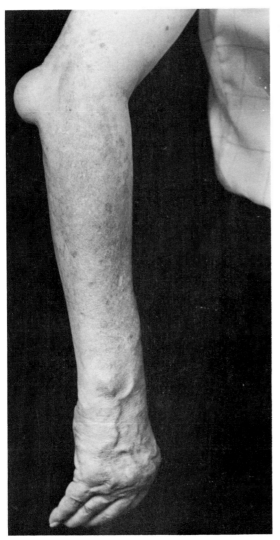

Fig. 5–8. Example of a patient with olecranon bursitis.

jection of corticosteroids. Weinstein et al. noted skin atrophy and persistent local pain in the steroid injected patients.[35] However, the patients treated with aspiration alone required 2 to 16 weeks for resolution compared to only 1 to 2 weeks for those injected with corticosteroids. Persistent swelling in 2 of 4 steroid injected patients was reported by Jaffe and Fetto.[36] This has not been our experience in traumatic bursitis. Iatrogenic infection is rare if the procedure is carefully done. We see recurrent swelling following steroid injection of traumatic bursitis.

Following aspiration of the bursal fluid, it is our practice to instill .5 ml of a crystalline steroid-local anesthetic mixture. Obviously, if there is a high index of suspicion for sepsis, the steroid should be withheld.

Outcome. Most patients who have suffered an olecranon bursitis recognize and avoid repeated local injury. Occasionally a patient with chronic bursitis and a thickened synovial membrane requires surgical excision of the bursa.

OTHER BURSAL AND CYSTIC SWELLINGS AT THE ELBOW

A diagnosis of bursitis between the biceps insertion and the head of the radius may be considered in patients with pain at the elbow during wrist rotation.[2] The discomfort is milder than that of tennis elbow, and tenderness is detected over the head of the radius and accentuated during wrist rotation. Relief from a local anesthetic injection into the region of the head of the radius assists diagnosis. Exercises to stretch the lower end of the biceps are helpful.

Tendinitis and bursitis at the insertion of the triceps on the olecranon process may also cause posterior elbow pain. In this instance, there is no palpable swelling. Local anesthetic injection into the point of tenderness, with protection of this region from pressure, is usually all that is required.

Patients may report swelling at the medial anterior border of the elbow or in the antecubital area due to antecubital cyst formation. These cysts are seen most commonly in rheumatoid arthritis and are readily demonstrated by arthrography.[37] We have seen such rheumatoid cysts dissect above the elbow into the triceps region as well.

TENDINITIS

Tendinitis of the distal insertion of the biceps muscle may cause pain in the antecubital fossa of the elbow with restriction of full elbow extension. Pain is dull and felt rather diffusely throughout the anterior elbow region. In all patients with elbow pain, palpation of the distal end of the biceps tendon in the antecubital space should be performed with the elbow in full extension. When biceps tendinitis is present, tenderness can be elicited along the lower ½-inch of the biceps tendon. This should be distinguished from bursitis in the area of the head of the radius. Injection of a steroid anesthetic mixture, *parallel to*, but not into the biceps tendon, provides prompt relief. Using a #23 one inch needle, 0.5 ml of methylprednisolone and 0.5 ml of procaine can be injected (see Table 15–4). Home physical therapy with gentle stretching of the biceps should be performed twice daily and continued for several weeks following relief from pain (See Exercise 4, Table 5–4).

Tendinitis slightly distal to the elbow can occur traumatically without giving rise to tennis elbow. Careful palpation of the individual tendons during finger movement and wrist movement should allow the examiner to discern which tendon is involved. Local corticosteroid anesthetic injection and avoidance of strain should provide benefit. *Myositis ossificans* may present with flexion contracture, a hard bony mass, and pain. Ten cases that resulted in elbow contractures following football injuries have been reported.[38] All patients had eventual resolution of the elbow contractures regardless of activity restriction or surgical procedure. Only 3 cases with prolonged symptoms were operated upon; recurrence of the bony mass occurred in 2 of 3 patients.

NERVE ENTRAPMENT SYNDROMES

Ill-defined, diffuse, upper-forearm pain, aggravated by particular movement, should alert the clinician to the possibility of a nerve entrapment syndrome. Nerve entrapment is characterized by a positive *tourniquet test*, in which a tourniquet applied above the painful area accentuates the pain. Paresthesia may result.[8] Electrodiagnostic tests may delineate the level of entrapment (Fig. 5–9).

Radial Tunnel Syndrome

The radial nerve courses from medial to lateral around the posterior surface of the humerus, then pierces the lateral muscular septum. Compression by a contracted muscle or band may give rise to symptoms of pain and tenderness in the area of the lateral epicondyle. Of particular diagnostic value, the pain is reproduced with passive stretching or resisted extension of the middle finger. In a study of 15 patients, reported by Moss and Switzer, a variety of symptoms involving the lateral epicondylar area were observed. These included sensations of popping, paresthesias and paresis. Long finger extension tests were positive in all. Steroid injections and physical therapy were of no benefit. Two anomalies were found at surgery: one case demonstrated a completely tendinous proximal border of the extensor carpi radialis brevis and the other a bifid origin of the extensor carpi radialis.[39] Temporary relief following anesthetic injection is diagnostically helpful. Paresthesia may or may not be present in the distribution of the superficial radial nerve. A Tinel test (tapping over the nerve), performed over the radial head, may produce tingling along the course of the nerve. Finger-extension weakness may be noted; limitation of full extension of the elbow may also be observed.

Causes include adhesions to tissue overlying the radial head, constriction by the extensor carpi radialis brevis, or compression by the supinator muscle.[40] Direct trauma of a minor nature to the elbow is a common etiology. A "double crush" syndrome of the nerve, in which compression of the nerve occurred both at the arcade of Frohse and at the distal border of the supinator was reported by Sponseller and Engber.[41] In this patient, radial sensory and motor function were clinically normal as were nerve conduction velocities and electromyography showed polyphasic motor units in radially innervated muscles. Three surgical explorations were required before complete diagnosis was made and recovery occurred.

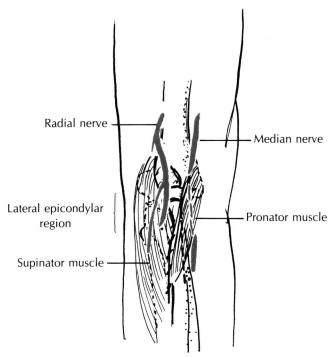

Fig. 5–9. Nerve entrapment of the elbow region: The *radial tunnel syndrome* may result from radial nerve compression in the region of the lateral epicondyle. The *pronator syndrome* results from median nerve entrapment by the pronator muscle.

Compression of the posterior interosseus nerve, the deep branch of the radial nerve, within the supinator muscle may result from forceful supination-pronation tasks such as hammering, carrying objects with the elbow fully extended, and from use of a heavy purse. An early sign is the inability to extend the little finger. Pain over the extensor muscles and lateral epicondyle may present as a tennis elbow.[42] Nerve conduction tests may reveal slowing of impulses from the spiral groove to the medial portion of the extensor digitorum communis. In patients suspected of having radial nerve entrapment, surgical exploration and release from the overlying muscle often provide good relief.[43] The radial tunnel syndrome, as a cause for *chronic* epicondylar (tennis elbow) pain, has been refuted.[44]

Compression of the musculocutaneous nerve at the elbow by the biceps aponeurosis and tendon against the fascia of the brachialis muscle may result from trauma or may occur as a chronic condition; pain is located at the anterolateral elbow. Only acute lesions were associated with paresthesias. Direct tenderness over the area where the musculocutaneous nerve exits from beneath the biceps tendon, and decreased sensation distally along the radial aspect of the volar part of the forearm are noted. Of 11 patients reported in one series, 4 responded to local rest and intralesional steroid injections. Surgical exploration and decompression relieved symptoms in the remainder.[45]

Pronator Syndrome

Median nerve entrapment by the pronator muscle may result in diffuse pain in the arm and weakness of wrist pronation.[46,47] The pain is reproduced by resistance to pronation of the forearm and flexion of the wrist.[8] Other features include paresthesias along the median nerve distribution, paresis of thumb muscles, and sometimes a positive Tinel's sign over the pronator teres. In 1 patient with bilateral involvement, an intralesional steroid injection was not helpful.[48] Surgical consultation for consideration of nerve release should be obtained.

Ulnar Nerve Entrapment (Cubital Tunnel Syndrome; External Compression Syndrome)

Ulnar nerve palsy may result from pressure injury to the ulnar nerve. The ulnar nerve lying behind the medial epicondyle may be palpably thickened, secondary to repeated minor trauma from pressure.[8,49,50] Paresthesia, with weakness and intrinsic atrophy in an ulnar nerve distribution, is noted. Similar symptoms may result from subluxation of the nerve, or by compression from a congenital supracondylar process of the humerus. If weakness or other motor nerve signs are absent, local corticosteroid injection along the ulnar groove may be effective. Use a #25 ¾ inch needle, inject a mixture of procaine and steroid cautiously into the groove, *parallel* with the nerve. Use a Tinel test to locate the nerve. When the needle is inserted ask the patient if there are any sensations distributed along the ulnar nerve area, so that nerve penetration by the needle can be avoided.

Carpal Tunnel Syndrome

Retrograde paresthesia into the forearm and arm may be caused by carpal tunnel syndrome. Symptoms may be reproduced by tapping over the median nerve at the wrist. (See Chapt. 6, "Carpal Tunnel Syndrome.")

REFERENCES

1. Conwell HE: Injuries to the elbow. Clin Symp (CIBA) 21:35–62, 1969.
2. Turek SL: Orthopaedics: Principles and Their Application. 4th Ed. Philadelphia, JB Lippincott, 1984.
3. Sheon RP: A joint protection guide for nonarticular rheumatic disorders. Postgrad Med 77(5): 329–338, 1985.
4. Wolfe F, Sheon, RP: When aching is generalized, consider fibrositis. *Diagnosis* (July) 1984.
5. Boyd HB, McLeod AC Jr: Tennis elbow. J Bone Joint Surg 55A:1183–1187, 1973.
6. Nirschl RP, Pettrone FA: Tennis elbow: The surgical treatment of lateral epicondylitis. J Bone Joint Surg 61A:832–839, 1979.
7. Gunn CC, Milbrandt WE: Tennis elbow and the cervical spine. Can Med Assoc J 114:803–806, 1976.
8. Dan NG: Entrapment syndromes. Med J Aust 1:528–531, 1978.
9. Swezey RL: Arthritis: Rational Therapy and Rehabilitation. Philadelphia, WB Saunders, 1978.
10. Waris P, Kuorinka I, et al.: Epidemiologic screening of occupational neck and upper limb disorders. Scand J Work Environ and Health 5:25–36, 1979.
11. Medical Letter: Management of tennis elbow. Medical Letter 19:33–36, 1977.
12. Pinals RA: Traumatic arthritis and allied conditions. *In* Arthritis and Allied Conditions. 10th Ed. Edited by DJ McCarty. Philadelphia, Lea & Febiger, 1985.
13. Nirschl RP: Tennis elbow. Primary Care 4:367–382, 1977.
14. Goldie I: Epicondylitis Lateralis Humeri. (Epicondylalgia or tennis elbow): A pathologic study. Acta Chir Scand (Suppl) 339:110–112, 1964.
15. Sartar K, Uhthoff HK: Ultrastructure of the common extensor tendon in tennis elbow. Virchows Arch A Path 386:317–318, 1980.
16. Bernhang AM: The many causes of tennis elbow. NY State J Med. (Aug):1363–1366, 1979.
17. Begg RE: Epicondylitis or Tennis Elbow: Frequent finding of gunsight type spur in lateral epicondyle of distal humerus. Orthop Rev 9:33–42, 1980.
18. Gardner RC: What to do about 'tennis elbow'. Consultant 11:61–62, 1971.
19. Bernhang AM, Dehner W, Fogarty C: A scientific approach to tennis elbow. Ortho Rev 4:35–41, 1975.
20. Curwin S, Stanish WD: Tendinitis: Its Etiology and Treatment. Lexington, Mass., The Collamore Press, 1984.
21. Priest JD, Jones HH, Tichenor CJC, Nagel DA: Arm and elbow changes in expert tennis players. Minn Med 60:399–404, 1977.
22. Zohn DA, Mennell J McM: Musculoskeletal Pain: Diagnosis and Physical Treatment. Boston, Little, Brown & Co., 1976.
23. Duncan BF: Rehabilitation of the tennis elbow syndrome. Contemp Ortho 7:61–65, 1983.
24. Binder A, Parr G, Hazleman B: Ultrasound in tennis elbow. Ann Rheum Dis 42:309, 1983.
25. Percy EC, Carson JD: The use of DMSO in tennis elbow and rotator cuff tendonitis: a double-blind study. Med Sci in Sports Exer 13:215–219, 1981.
26. Kessler RM, Hertling D: Management of Common Musculoskeletal Disorders. Philadelphia, Harper & Row, 1983.
27. Nevelos AB: The treatment of tennis elbow with triamcinolone acetonide. Curr Med Res Opin 6:507–509, 1980.
28. O'Donoghue Don H: Treatment of Injuries to Athletes. 4th Ed. Philadelphia, WB Saunders, 1984.
29. Little TS: Tennis elbow—to rest or not to rest? The Practitioner 228:457, 1984.
30. Rosen MJ, Duffy FP, Miller EH, et al: Tennis elbow syndrome: Results of the "lateral release" procedure. Ohio State Med J 76:103–109, 1980.
31. Canoso JJ, McGinnis G: Physical findings in olecranon bursitis (OB), A clue to its etiology. (Abstract #E41). Arth Rheum 25 (No. 4) [Supp], 1982.
32. Thompson GR, Manshady BM, Weiss JJ: Septic bursitis. JAMA 240:2280–2281, 1978.
33. Ho G Jr, Tice AD, Kaplan SR: Septic bursitis in the

prepatellar and olecranon bursae. Ann Intern Med 89:21–27, 1978.

34. Ho G Jr, Tice AD: Comparison of nonseptic and septic bursitis: Further observations on the treatment of septic bursitis. Arch Intern Med 139:1269–1273, 1979.

35. Weinstein PS, Canoso JJ, Wohlgethan JR: Longterm follow-up of corticosteroid injection for traumatic olecranon bursitis. Ann Rheum Dis 43:44–46, 1984.

36. Jaffe L, Fetto JF: Olecranon bursitis. Contemp Ortho 8:51–54, 1984.

37. Ehrlich GE: Antecubital cysts in rheumatoid arthritis. A corollary to popliteal (Baker's) cysts. J Bone Joint Surg 54A:165–169, 1972.

38. Huss CD, Puhl JJ: Myositis ossificans of the upper arm. Am J Sports Med 8:419–424, 1980.

39. Moss SH, Switzer HE: Radial tunnel syndrome: A spectrum of clinical presentations. J Hand Surg 8:414–420, 1983.

40. Kopell HP, Thompson WAL: Peripheral Entrapment Neuropathies. Huntington, NY, RE Krieger Publishing, 1976.

41. Sponseller PD, Engber WD: Double-entrapment radial tunnel syndrome. J Hand Surg 8:420–423, 1983.

42. Feldman RG, Goldman R, Keyserling WM: Peripheral nerve entrapment syndromes and ergonomic factors. Am J Indus Med 4:661–681, 1983.

43. Roles NC, Maudsley RH: Radial tunnel syndrome. J Bone Joint Surg 54B:499–508, 1972.

44. Rossum JV, Buruma OJS, Kamphuisen HAC, et al: Tennis elbow—A radial tunnel syndrome? J Bone Joint Surg 60B:197–198, 1978.

45. Bassett FH, Nunley JA: Compression of the musculocutaneous nerve at the elbow. J Bone Joint Surg 64A:1050–1052, 1982.

46. Brown, PW: Peripheral nerve lesions. In Musculoskeletal Disorders. Edited by RD D'Ambrosia. Philadelphia, JB Lippincott, 1977.

47. Nigst H, Dick W: Syndromes of compression of the median nerve in the proximal forearm (pronator teres syndrome: anterior interosseous nerve syndrome). Arch Orthop Traum Surg 93:307–312, 1979.

48. Wiggins CE: Pronator syndrome. Southern Med J 75:240–241, 1982.

49. Wadsworth TG, Williams JR: Cubital tunnel external compression syndrome. Br Med J 1:662–666, 1973.

50. Clark CB: Cubital tunnel syndrome. JAMA 241:801–802, 1979.

6

The Wrist and Hand

Pain and disability of the hand and wrist may result from local factors, or may result from systemic diseases with onset in the wrist or hand, in which case presenting features may be manifest as changes in skin color or texture, nodular lesions, or tendon and ligament problems before other systemic features are evident.

Physical Examination. The normal wrist can flex and extend approximately 80 degrees respectively from the horizontal. Ulnar wrist deviation is approximately twice the capability of radial wrist deviation (40 degrees versus approximately 20 degrees, respectively). Finger flexion should be tested by having the patient bend the distal phalanx to approximate the proximal phalanx. Flexor tendon sheath swelling, or true joint arthritis, may cause limitation of flexion of proximal interphalangeal (PIP) or distal interphalangeal (DIP) finger joints. Thumb abduction should approximate 80 to 90 degrees from a line drawn proximally along the long finger.

Camptodactyly, flexion contracture of the proximal interphalangeal joint, is a genetic disorder. When present, it may be a clue to a recently described syndrome consisting of camptodactyly, scoliosis, torticollis with fusion of cervical vertebrae, and limitation of motion of other upper extremity joints.[1] Another syndrome consists of congenital camptodactyly, chronic persistent synovitis, and a tendopathy of hands and feet with marked thickening of synovial sheaths, adhesions between tendons and their sheaths, and tendon degeneration. A significant portion of the finger tendons is replaced with fibrous tissue.[2] Similar contractures seen in insulin dependent (Type II) diabetes with *cheiroarthropathy* may be superficially confused with Dupuytren's contracture. Inspection for skin and nail color and texture may provide clues of systemic disease. Palpate the skin of the dorsal surface of the digits for texture and looseness (see Anatomic Plates VI–VIII).

Thumb adduction should reach to the base of the little finger. Flattening or atrophy of the thenar eminence should be noted (suggesting carpal tunnel syndrome with median nerve compression). Wasting of the interossei with "valleys" between the extensor tendons on the back of the hand may suggest ulnar nerve dysfunction. The metacarpophalangeal (MCP) collateral ligaments are tested for stability with the finger flexed to 90 degrees at the MCP joint. This tightens the collateral ligaments and allows little passive lateral finger motion (Fig. 6–1). Dorsal-volar motion of the wrist should be tested. The examiner attempts to move the patient's hand up and down within the horizontal plane of the patient's wrist. Wrist and PIP hypermobility may suggest *hypermobility syndrome* with its multiple presentations. Note the texture of the skin, presence of telangiectasia, pitting, or smoothness of the distal fingertips.

DISORDERS OF THE LOWER ARM AND WRIST

Whether from sport injury or from falling on the outstretched wrist, injury may involve tendons, ligaments, or the articular disc, or may result in joint laxity.[3,4] Acute tenosynovitis, resulting from injury or unaccustomed movement, generally involves the tendons of the lower dorsal forearm. Swelling and painful crepitus during hand extension may be detected;[4] tenderness can be elicited and internal joint derangement may be suspected.[5] In the acute stage, swelling and pain over the dorsal aspect of the wrist or over the distal radioulnar joint may occur. Clicking during

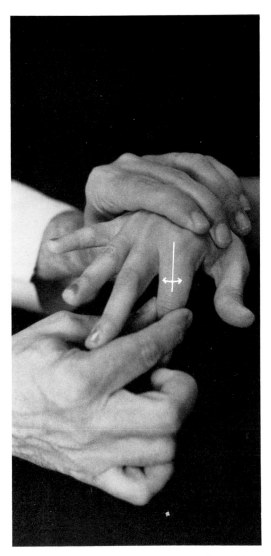

Fig. 6–1. Metacarpophalangeal (MCP) collateral ligament stability test: The finger is flexed to 90 degrees at the MCP joint in order to tighten the collateral ligament. Normally, lateral finger motion is minimal in this position.

hand activity may be noted. Locking does not occur. Grip strength is weakened by these injuries, and treatment requires orthopedic consultation when carpal instability is suspected.

A *compartment syndrome* may occur following trauma to the wrist and hand, particularly after a crush injury. Each of the interosseous muscles is surrounded by a tough investing fascial envelope; following trauma, swelling within this compartment may cause neurovascular compression particularly involving the more radially situated muscles. Paresis, pain on passive motion of the metacarpophalangeal joint, and an elevated tissue pressure measurement are usual findings. A case of a compartment syndrome of the hand that followed heroin injection into the region of the anatomic snuffbox was recently described.[6]

Microwave ovens are in wide use and injuries are rare. Repeated exposure can, however, induce soft tissue injury with superficial and deep second degree burn.[7]

Prominence of the distal ulna with hypermobility ("piano key" motion) may occur spontaneously, or as a result of injury or rheumatoid arthritis (Fig. 6–2). It is more prevalent in adolescents, but may follow a Colles' fracture of the wrist in others. Often, no treatment is required.[8]

If trapezium-first metacarpal joint sprain results in subluxation with limitation of pinch grasping, the region at the base of the thumb may be injected with a steroid-local anesthetic mixture, and a thumb splint provided that allows pinch grasping, yet stabilizes the carpometacarpal joint.[4] Persistent symptoms may indicate a need to consider arthroplasty.

Lastly, the pisiform-triquetral joint may be sprained, resulting in the pisiform being displaced distally. This results in pain with wrist flexion or ulnar deviation motions. The pisiform is tender to palpation in the hypothenar aspect of the palm. Reconstructive surgery may be indicated.[9]

Patients who have suffered wrist sprain and have persistent symptoms should have repeat roentgenograms, including oblique views and special scaphoid roentgenograms to detect a fracture of the scaphoid. Also, flexion and extension wrist views help to determine instability.

SYSTEMIC DISEASES AFFECTING THE WRIST AND HAND

Systemic Rheumatic Diseases

The presenting symptom of rheumatoid arthritis is swelling of the joints of the digits,

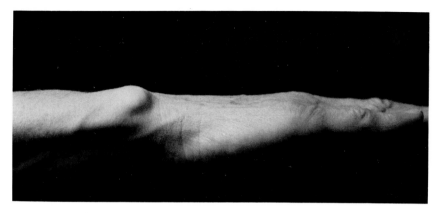

Fig. 6–2. Post-traumatic laxity of the distal ulna. Examination with downward pressure results in "piano key" movement of the distal ulna.

or sometimes of the flexor tendon sheaths (tenosynovitis). The patient may complain only of slight morning stiffness in the fingers and inability to fully flex the finger joints. Any patient with this complaint should have careful palpation of the flexor portion of the proximal phalanges. Swelling of the flexor tendons can be discerned as a rubbery, firm swelling when compared to the practitioner's own normal finger. Similarly, rheumatoid disease may cause flexor or extensor tendon sheath swelling in the forearm musculature, giving rise to carpal tunnel syndrome or loss of grip strength. Associated swelling of MCP and PIP joints is common. Tenosynovitis may also result from calcific tendinitis, tophaceous gout, psoriatic arthritis, Reiter's syndrome, mixed connective tissue disease, and occasionally dermatomyositis. Finger joints or tendon swelling may result from pseudogout or giant cell arteritis. The hands may be diffusely swollen in the early stage of progressive systemic sclerosis; telangiectasias, fingertip ulcers, or binding of the dorsal finger skin should suggest the diagnosis.

Clubbing of distal fingers, with or without associated periostitis or synovitis, may alert the physician to the presence of hypertrophic pulmonary osteoarthropathy and intrathoracic disease, or clubbing may be a benign inherited characteristic. The hand examination can provide clues to many systemic diseases, ranging from subacute bacterial endocarditis

to hyperlipidemia; the clinician should look carefully (see Danger Signs, Table 6–1, and the Decision Chart, Table 6–4).

Diabetic Cheiroarthropathy

As described earlier, the appearance of camptodactyly, palmar scarring, and associated tendon and nerve entrapment in insulin dependent diabetics has been well described.[10–12] Diabetic cheiroarthropathy results in nerve entrapments, trigger fingers, tenosynovitis, and carpal tunnel syndrome. The skin may have a waxy appearance over the dorsal surface of the fingers.[10,11] Similar findings have now been reported in adult non-insulin dependent diabetics.[12] These patients may be at greater risk for microvasculature disease. The skin and tendon changes may precede overt vascular complications.[11] Inspection of nailfold capillaries for changes in morphology, distribution and den-

Table 6–1. Danger Signs for the Wrist and Hand

1. Fever and chills
2. Lymphadenopathy
3. Dusky cyanosis of finger tips
4. Nailfold infarcts (at nail edges)
5. Diminished pulse at wrist
6. Associated arm claudication
7. Diffuse swelling of a hand with warmth and erythema
8. Numbness and weakness of sudden onset

sity can discriminate cheiroarthropathy from early scleroderma.[13] Local treatment with splinting, stretching, joint protection measures, and judicious use of intralesional local corticosteroid injection of the individual soft tissue components does result in local relief, sometimes for 6 to 12 months. We have treated several adults with repeated local intralesional crystalline corticosteroid injections and joint protection measures for over 10 years with good results and no complications. We do outline a sliding scale of insulin dose after a steroid injection as follows: On the evening of the day of injection, if the urine glucose dipstick registers 3 or 4 plus, then the insulin dose, next morning, is raised 2 to 6 units depending on the patient's usual dosage. Similarly, the next evening the urine is checked with the following day's insulin similarly raised. Only once in our experience did a diabetic get into serious trouble following local corticosteroid treatment. For others, tenolysis may be performed in order to provide full range of motion.[14] Use of sorbinil, an aldose reductase inhibiting agent, in a dose of 250 mg per day has been reported to be of benefit in a small series of patients. Range of motion and strength of digital flexion improved.[15]

Calcific Tendinitis

Calcific tendinitis may be part of recurrent multifocal attacks of tendinitis that involve the shoulder, wrist, and ankle regions. In the wrist, it may involve the lateral region with an attack of redness and swelling. Similar involvement of the palm, or dorsum of the hand, with systemic fever, intense pain, and local swelling without adenopathy may occur. Fluffy calcification is evident on roentgenography.[16] In another report, swelling of the thumb following gardening was the initial presentation of calcific tendinitis.[17] Radiographic detection of periarticular calcification should alert the clinician to the disorder[18,19] (see "Calcific Tendinitis," Chapt. 4). The soft tissue calcifications associated with dermatomyositis and scleroderma do not usually present as an acute lesion; rather they

may be associated with low-grade swelling and inflammation when calcific deposits are near the surface.

JOINT LAXITY AND THE HYPERMOBILITY SYNDROME

Minor structural skeletal disorders are common and important causes for regional rheumatic pain and disability. Joint laxity (hypermobility) is the most common.[20,21] Joint laxity is practically never mentioned by the patient. Most patients, even physicians, when presented with their own features of joint laxity did not realize that this was abnormal! The diagnosis of the hypermobility syndrome is based upon finding 3 or more areas of joint laxity[22–24] (Table 6–2).

The diagnosis is difficult in children, who have greater joint laxity than adults.[25] For older children, a goniometric quantitative measurement technique has been devised to assist in measurement and diagnosis.[26]

CASE REPORT: N.T., a 26-year-old secretary, presented with the chief complaint of hand pain and swelling. She could no longer complete her typing and secre-

Table 6–2. Features of the Benign Hypermobility Syndrome

A. History
  1. Symmetrical joint pain and stiffness
  2. Sensation of joint swelling of brief duration
  3. Onset of joint symptoms after prolonged inactivity
  4. Joint laxity in other family members
  5. No other contributing illness or disease
B. Presence of three or more areas with joint laxity:
   Passive apposition of thumb to forearm (Fig. 6–3A)
   Passive hyperextension of fingers
   Active hyperextension of elbow >10 degrees (Fig. 6–3B)
   Active hyperextension of knee >10 degrees (Fig. 6–3C)
   Ability to flex spine and place palms on the floor without bending knees

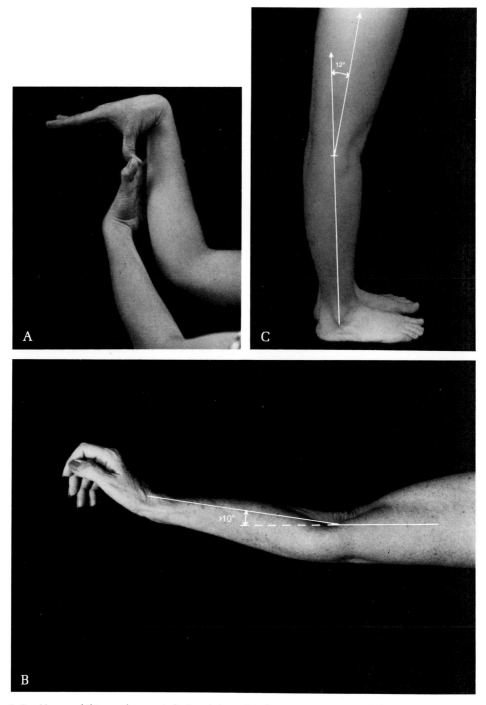

Fig. 6–3. Hypermobility syndrome: *A,* laxity of the wrist allows approximation of the thumb to the patient's ipsilateral forearm; *B,* laxity of the elbow with greater than 10 degrees of joint extension; *C,* laxity of the knee with greater than 10 degrees of joint extension.

tarial tasks because of pain and weakness when typing or writing for any length of time. The swelling was limited to her fingers and was characterized by a sensation, not visible swelling. It was present upon arising from sleep. She noted stiffness as well, and this lasted about an hour. She did not have numbness or tingling. Her rings felt tight, the fingers were stiff. The sensation occurred after any handwork such as typing, writing, or peeling vegetables, and it lasted 3 to 4 hours. The problem began shortly after she returned to work having been on medical leave to care for her new child. There was no family history of rheumatic disease. She had been athletic and participated in gymnastics in school, then joined an aerobics group until she became pregnant. Now she wanted to know if arthritis would prevent her from returning to aerobics.

Physical examination revealed normal features on inspection. No skin hyperelasticity or striae were noted. A high arched palate was not present. General examination revealed no abnormalities. Joint palpation revealed no synovitis but the proximal interphalangeal joints (PIP joints) were definitely tender. She did have flat feet. Joint range of motion revealed excessive mobility at the shoulder, elbow, wrist, thumb, and PIP joints. The latter revealed excessive side to side mobility. Laxity was also present at the hip, spine, and ankles. Roentgenographs of the hands and wrists, and appropriate laboratory studies for inflammation were within normal limits.

The patient in summary, had a history of joint "swelling" that lasted for too brief a duration for inflammation, joint laxity in 3 or more joints, and no other features of underlying disease. These features constitute a syndrome known as the benign hypermobility syndrome.

The first known reference to joint laxity is attributed to Hippocrates who, in the 4th Century BC, described the Scythians as being "so-loose-limbed that they were unable to

draw a bow-string or hurl a javelin."[28] Joint laxity may result from more serious diseases of the connective tissues such as Marfan's syndrome, hyperlysinemia, osteogenesis imperfecta, pseudoxanthoma elasticum, homocystinuria, and Ehlers-Danlos syndrome as well as rheumatic fever, rheumatoid arthritis, acromegaly, and neurologic disease (Table 6–3). Joint hypermobility as an inherited cause for congenital joint dislocation has been reported many times in the past century.[28A] These are rare when compared to the much more common benign hypermobility syndrome, described by Kirk, Ansell, and Bywaters.[29] They defined the hypermobility syndrome as generalized joint laxity with musculoskeletal complaints in an otherwise normal person. Recently, Biro et al. emphasized similar features in children having juvenile arthritis.[30] They and others[30-34] found that 5.7% of children seen for a diagnosis of juvenile arthritis actually had the benign hypermobility syndrome. Only 3 patients with inflammatory juvenile arthritis had coexisting joint laxity.

Thompson and colleagues noted joint laxity in 1.3% of high school athletes.[20] Raskin and Lawless[21] reported results of a careful musculoskeletal examination of healthy medical students and 85 structural disorders were noted among the 123 students. Of these, 22 had at least one lax joint and 14 others had three or more lax joints. Limited joint motion was detected in 33 students. Other studies suggest that 5% of children and 1% of adults have joint laxity. Joint laxity is more common in the right limb, in females, in blacks, and in children from families with higher socioeconomic status. Thus, joint laxity is common, and usually not symptomatic. As pointed out earlier, joint laxity may occur as a result of other diseases of connective tissues, or it may result from metabolic, rheumatic, or neurologic causes. Furthermore, as an inherited disorder, joint laxity may occur in association with clubfoot, recurrent dislocations of hips, shoulders, or patellae. Toe deformities are commonly associated as well.[27]

In an orthopedic practice, Finsterbush and

Table 6–3. Disorders Associated with Joint Laxity*

Ehlers-Danlos syndrome	Acute rheumatic fever
Marfan's syndrome	Rheumatoid arthritis
Pseudoxanthoma elasticum	Poliomyelitis
Osteogenesis imperfecta	Tabes dorsalis
Myotonia congenita	Familial joint deformities
Homocystinuria	Clubfoot
Hyperlysinemia	Dislocation of shoulder, hip, patellae
Acromegaly	Toe deformities

*Source: Sheon, Kirsner, Farber, Finkel[27]

Pogrund noted that among 100 consecutive patients with joint laxity in 3 or more joint regions and without other discernible disease, 44% had generalized pain that was of long duration with acute exacerbations. In the remaining patients, pain in the knees or feet were common presenting complaints. They also noted 65% of first degree relatives (mostly mothers) had joint laxity.[22]

Our experience suggests that in a private rheumatology practice, benign hypermobility syndrome is as common as rheumatoid arthritis. But because joint laxity is so common in the general population, careful examination to exclude other more serious disease is essential.[34] The "marfanoid syndrome", with added features of Marfan's syndrome and Ehlers-Danlos syndrome including joint laxity, cardiac valvular lesions, symmetrical striae and a high arched palate is occasionally seen.[23,35,36] In our patients with joint laxity, a high arched palate, and striae, we have not seen any serious cardiac abnormalities. However, Grahame[24] and colleagues noted an increased frequency of mitral valve prolapse among their patients; this is not the experience of others.[37]

As pointed out, these patients may have generalized or regional complaints. Many patients with hypermobility syndrome have additional features of sleep disturbance and trigger points that provide an additional diagnosis of fibrositis.[38] The patients with both disorders may have axial pain of fibrositis and peripheral joint complaints of the hypermobility syndrome. The significance of joint laxity to back pain also requires emphasis. Howes and Isdale reported the 'loose back' as a common

and often unrecognized cause for backache among women. They reported that of 102 consecutive cases of "problem" back patients, musculoskeletal examination with careful attention for joint laxity revealed no cases of generalized joint laxity among the 59 men; all but 17 of the 59 men had disc or other skeletal lesions. Among the 17 males without a specific organic back disorder, 3 had one or more lax joints. Of the 43 women, 23 had local back derangements, but 20 females remained without cause for backache. Whereas 2 women with a definable back condition also had joint laxity, 17 of the 20 without another cause for backache had joint laxity. This possible association of joint laxity with backache in women has also been recognized in several industrial centers in Europe.[39] The importance of proper body mechanics and the value of joint protection for this condition is speculative but recognition and trial of protection measures is certainly safe and may be cost effective (see Joint Protection, Table 6–5).

Two sequelae to joint laxity are chondrocalcinosis and precocious osteoarthritis.[33,40] Our patients had no more frequent osteoarthritis than that seen in the general population. Nevertheless, these patients should be warned to respect pain during repetitive activities. Those who say "I'm going to finish this even if it kills me!" may cause cartilage injury due to joint laxity and overuse.

Laboratory and Radiologic Examination. Tests for inflammation and rheumatoid factor are normal. Roentgenograms are usually normal, although in the older patient with hypermobility syndrome, they may reveal chondrocalcinosis or degenerative changes beyond that expected for age.[33]

Management. Treatment consists of explanation, extensor muscle strengthening, joint protection (Table 6–5), and symptomatic treatment medication.[22,27,30] Upon reassuring the patient that serious crippling is not a consequence, and that sedentary activity leads to decreased muscle tone and support for lax joints, most patients are receptive to a conditioning program. The use of individualized resistance exercise to forearm extensors, quadriceps, and abdominal muscles has been helpful[22] (Table 6–6).

Finger extension exercises can be performed using a 2- to 3-inch wide stiff elastic band. The eight fingers are slipped into the band, sewn to fit snug. The band covers the distal ends of the fingers (Fig. 6–4). The patient repetitively extends the fingers against the elastic band, keeping the palms together.

Wrist extensor strengthening is performed against weight progressing from 1 to 7 pounds; the weight is draped across the extended fingers. The arm may rest upon a table top, and the hand is raised about an inch, then returned to a horizontal position. These exercises are perfomed twice daily. Exercises to strengthen extensor muscles across the knee may also be required.

Patients should be taught to avoid arm hyperextension during sleep. Since these patients can assume unusual sitting, lying, and resting body positions, the physician should review each of these positions with the patient. In particular, these patients should not sit with knees tucked under or Indian style. Proper shoes should be recommended if pes planus is present. Bracing is sometimes necessary for the knees.

Outcome. Joint protection principles for hand use, lower limb joints, and the back are essential.[41] Because the exercises may require several months until optimal strength is achieved, the patient should be told at the outset that exercise may seem to aggravate or not seem helpful for a month or longer. Use of nonsteroidal agents for joint pain is therefore recommended.[27,30,42] Once exercises

have provided improved strength, a lifelong sport or conditioning program should be strongly encouraged in order to maintain good muscle tone. Intralesional soft tissue corticosteroid injections are often helpful.[41] In our experience, most patients, even older patients with premature osteoarthritis, respond reasonably well to a resistance-exercise program. The younger the patient, the more complete has been the response to therapy. Probably these patients should be told to avoid occupations that require prolonged repetitive hand tasks as they grow older, in the hope of preventing premature osteoarthritis.[40]

PSYCHOPHYSIOLOGIC DISORDERS OF THE HAND

Hand clenching may be voluntary or involuntary and lead to hand fatigue, carpal tunnel syndrome, or tendinitis. Persons with hand symptoms that are worse after arising from sleep should be asked about hand clenching or jaw clenching, as many hand clenchers are also nocturnal jaw clenchers. Such persons also hand clench when driving or reading. They may describe themselves as "heavy handed" persons. Sometimes they are driven by caffeine sensitivity. The nocturnal hand clencher can sometimes break the habit by sleeping with nylon stretch gloves worn inside out (so that the seams do not constrict).[43] The less common clenched fist syndrome (see following) must also be considered.

The Clenched Fist Syndrome

This disorder, considered a conversion syndrome by Simmons and Vasile,[44] often follows a minor inciting incident. The patient has swelling, pain, and paradoxical stiffness in which the patient maintains the same degree of finger flexion despite changing the position of the wrist. Hand clenching is usually not noted on the first visit. Attempts to passively extend the fingers result in pain. The examiner can detect active use of the finger flexors. Secondary infection and maceration from the

Table 6–4. Decision Chart, The Wrist and Hand

Problem	Action	Other Actions

1. Pain and dysfunction: Thumb
    Trigger thumb
    DeQuervain's disease
    Writer's cramp
	CONSERVATIVE MEASURES
	General examination
	—Joint protection advice
	—Splinting
	—Stretching and mobilizing
	   exercises
	—Tendon sheath injection with
	   corticosteroid, judiciously
	—Electrodiagnostic studies
	   in *selected* cases
		Occupational therapist consultation
		Roentgenographic examination
		Tests for systemic rheumatic disease
		Orthopedic or hand surgery consultation
		Rheumatology consultation
		Other appropriate consultation

2. Pain and dysfunction: Finger
    Collateral ligament callus
    Trigger finger		

3. Pain, paresthesia, dysfunction
    Thoracic outlet syndrome
    Carpal tunnel syndrome
    Reflex dystrophy		

4. Hypermobility syndrome; Dupuytren's contracture		
6. Raynaud's phenomenon	Protection from cold exposure Therapeutic trials with reserpine, nifedipine, beta blockers Obtain screening ANA, thyroid tests.	

7. Danger Signs:
    Fever, swelling, lymphadenopathy
    Erythema, cyanosis
    Nailfold infarcts
    Sudden onset numbness, weakness
	→ General examination and
	   urgent consultation	

Table 6–5.   Joint Protection for the Hand (from Sheon RP[174])

Harmful	Helpful
■ Repetitively moving the fingers excessively, such as occurs in typing, peeling vegetables, knitting, needlepointing, playing cards, and some types of assembly-line work, is the most common cause of carpal tunnel syndrome (numbness, tingling combined with a sensation of swelling, and weak finger grip), tendinitis, trigger finger, and trigger thumb.	■ Restrict repetitive tasks to 20-minute periods separated by a short break. Keep the hands flat and open rather than making tight fists. Pad the handles on utensils and tools and the steering wheel with pipe insulation. Use stronger, larger joints for assistance. Use the palms and forearms to carry heavy objects. Push, slide, or roll objects instead of lifting them. Use both hands as much as possible when lifting heavy objects.
■ Writing, stapling, or using scissors for long periods can cause hand injuries.	■ Use pencil holders and pad the stapler; take frequent breaks.
■ Pushing off from chairs, clenching the hands, writing for prolonged periods, or doing work that requires repetitious wrist or hand motion can result in carpal tunnel syndrome.	■ Keep the hands off chairs when arising; be aware of hand clenching and wear gloves to bed if necessary; interrupt lengthy writing sessions. Consult an occupational therapist about work-induced problems.

prolonged flexed position may be noted. No organic disease can be detected, and the fingers can be extended under general anesthesia. Psychiatrically the patient manifests severe anger and has poor defenses to stress. The prognosis is poor. Similar occupational cramp disorders such as violinist's cramp and trumpeter's lip, or factitious lymphedema of the hand, and the syndrome of delicate self cutting, are additional psychologically motivated disorders.[44]

Writer's cramp may also occur as a psychologicaly motivated disorder, but may respond to operant conditioning techniques.[45] Sheehy and Marsden examined 29 patients with writer's cramp, 4 with typists' cramp, and 1 with pianists' cramp. They divided the features into two groups, simple, and dystonic. All had muscular spasm and apparent incoordination when attempting to write, play or type. Features of dystonic motion observed when writing included difficulty in picking up the pen, gripping it with a closed fist, or the patient would adopt a typical dystonic posture or jerky motion. When walking, some patients had loss of arm swing on the affected side; no other features of Parkinson's disease were noted. Increased limb tone was

noted in others. These features were variable from time to time so that patients might be considered as having simple writer's cramp on one visit, then dystonic disease at another time. Psychologic examination failed to demonstrate abnormality.[46]

DISORDERS OF THE THUMB

DeQuervain's Tenosynovitis[47a]

Stenosing tenosynovitis of the abductor pollicis longus or the extensor pollicis brevis may result from repetitive activity or direct injury. These tendons traverse a thick fibrous sheath at the radial-styloid process. Thickening of the tendon sheath results in stenosis and inflammation. The patient notes pain during pinch grasping or thumb and wrist movement. Palpation of the tendons in the anatomic "snuff box" area may reveal swelling when compared to the uninvolved side. Tenderness to palpation over the radial styloid is common. A triad of tenderness to palpation over the radial styloid, the presence of localized swelling in the vicinity of the radial styloid, and a positive Finkelstein sign are diagnostic for stenosing tenosynovitis of DeQuervain's disease.[47]

Table 6–6. Hand and Wrist Exercises

1. Thumb stretching: Grasp involved thumb with other hand and pull involved thumb straight away from forearm.
2. Finger flexor tendon stretch: Grasp involved finger and gently pull it backward until pulling sensation is noted in palm.
3. Finger strengthening exercise: Obtain foundation elastic, at least 2 inches wide. Sew a band large enough for the eight fingers to be inserted. Sew at an angle to keep band right at the little finger side. The fingertips should be within the top of the band. Then keep palms together and pull fingers apart against the band. The band should be snug so that the fingers cannot be drawn farther than 1 inch apart. Repeat for 1 minute twice daily, holding only a second or so for each motion (see Fig. 6–4).
4. Palm Flexor Stretching: Place the fingers on a table, palm down and while pressing the finger pads into the table, slowly draw the palms up thus stretching the ball of the hand. Do this slowly and to maximum tolerance. Hold 10 seconds, repeat 5 times.
5. Exercise for DeQuervain's disease: Have a 1 or 2 pound object placed in the toe of a woman's stocking: tie a loop knot above the heel of the stocking, this can slip over the interphalangeal joint. Then with the forearm held vertically, and the thumb pointed downward, the back of the hand directed forward, the thumb, tendon, and forearm should all be aligned with the weight tugging on the tendon downward. Then the thumb is slowly twirled for a minute clockwise and then counterclockwise, twice daily (see Fig. 6–17).
6. Conditioning exercise for tendinitis: Using a weight ranging from 7 to 10 pounds; the weight is grasped; the arm is rested upon a table, with the wrist hanging over the edge, palm down; the weight is raised as high as possible without lifting the arm from the table. This is performed for 7 to 15 repetitions with increases in the weight and the repetitions each week. Each hand is exercised with 7 pounds until able to do 15 repetitions, then the weight is increased to 8 pounds and 7 repetitions, etc. A second exercise is performed similarly but with the palm up, and raised as high as possible with the forearm maintained on a table.[82]
7. Exercise for carpal tunnel syndrome: Beginning with the hand and fingers aligned straight, the patient is asked to press the distal phalanges of the second to fifth fingers against the radial aspect of the opposite distal forearm, with maximum force, while slowly flexing only the involved wrist to at least 45 degrees and holding that position for about 5 seconds. Return to starting position, relax, and repeat 3 times in succession, every hour throughout the day, as feasible[129] (Fig. 6–13).

The Finkelstein sign to extend the tendon and reproduce symptoms is performed by having the patient fold the thumb into her palm with the fingers of the involved hand folded over the thumb. The examiner then grasps the patient's folded hand and rotates the wrist ulnarly, gently stretching the involved tendons (Fig. 6–5). Pain is exacerbated if DeQuervain's tenosynovitis is present. In some cases, the tenosynovitis has occurred bilaterally or has been recurrent. Differential diagnosis is important. In one study an incorrect diagnosis was made in 7 of 19 operated patients.[48] Correct diagnoses included an underlying osteoarthritis of the carpometacarpal joint (2 cases), peritendinitis of wrist extensors (2 cases), infectious tenosynovitis (1 case), a volar ganglion (1 case), and a flexor pollicis longus tenosynovitis (1 case). Attention to the site of maximum symptoms is important. Crepitus of tendons that lie more proximal and dorsal to the radial head can be detected in cases of long wrist extensor peritendinitis. Peritendinitis with crepitation

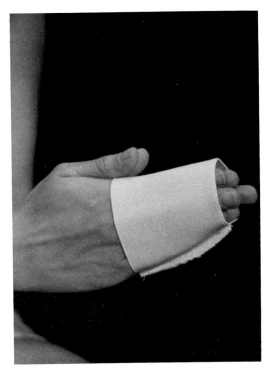

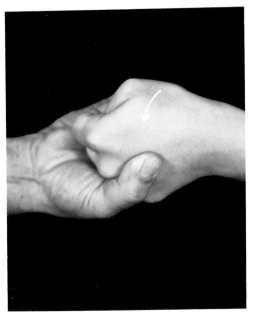

Fig. 6–5. The Finkelstein test: The examiner gently rotates the patient's wrist ulnarly (arrow) while the patient's fingers are folded over the thumb. DeQuervain's tenosynovitis can usually be distinguished from pain arising in the first carpometacarpal joint.

Fig. 6–4. Finger extension exercises are performed using a band made from foundation elastic. The band is sewn to fit snugly. The patient inserts eight fingers into the band and allows the band to cover the distal end of the fingers; the patient repetitively extends the fingers against the elastic band while keeping the palms together.

over the radial extensors of the wrist is a common manifestation of overuse and in particular, can be seen in oarsmen and canoeists.[49] Grinding maneuvers in which the thumb is rotated under pressure will usually result in pain when osteoarthritis is present.[48]

Treatment includes wrist protection with a splint, and one or two injections of a steroid-local anesthetic mixture into the tendon sheath, which is effective for acute relief (Fig. 6–6). Using a total of 1 ml of local steroid/anesthetic mixture (see Table 15–4) a ¾ inch #25 needle is inserted parallel to the tendon.[50–52] The clinician should observe or palpate the proximal tendon sheath as the injection proceeds and note that the sheath distends during the injection. This assures proper placement of the needle. Often an adhesion can obstruct the flow of fluid. Be

certain the needle is fixed tightly to the syringe, and inject with increasing pressure if an adhesion is apparent. Often, the adhesion will "pop". Ultrasound treatment may be beneficial[53] as well as friction massage.[54] All patients should try a simple exercise program that stretches the tendon (Table 6–6, Exercises 1 and 5). Joint protection measures must be provided in order to prevent recurrences (Table 6–5). Repetitive movement of the wrist as in wringing out clothes, canning, rapid writing, and knitting frequently predispose to a variety of regional hand disorders in addition to DeQuervain's disease. Tasks that require repetitive thumb movement or pinch grasping should be avoided.[55] About 75% of patients will have a good response to this conservative treatment.[56,57]

Trigger Thumb

Stenosing tenosynovitis of the flexor pollicis longus often results in a snapping or triggering movement of the thumb. The tendon

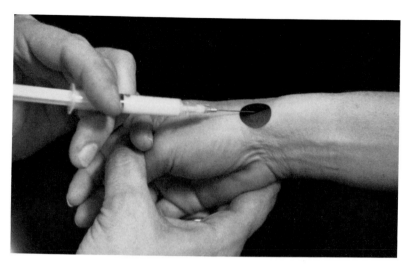

Fig. 6–6. Injection of the tendon sheath in a patient with DeQuervain's tenosynovitis.

becomes compressed against a prominence of the head of the first metacarpal bone or sesamoid. Thickening of the tendon sheath is often due to repetitive movement or pressure. Trigger thumb also occurs in infants.[58] Tenderness is noted at the base of the thumb in the palmar aspect. Often, a nodule on the tendon can be palpated as it moves during thumb flexion and extension. Detection and differentiation of a nodule from the normal sesamoids at the base of the thumb can be accomplished by having the patient flex and extend the PIP joint of the thumb while the examiner palpates and holds the metacarpophalangeal (MCP) joint straight. With the examiner's index finger palpating the flexor aspect of the MCP joint, the nodule can be felt to move with the tendon. Trigger thumb and trigger finger are frequently seen as industrial injuries.[9,59,60]

Treatment includes avoiding pressure at the base of the thumb during hand use, and injecting a steroid-local anesthetic mixture into the tendon region with a No. 25 to No. 27 gauge needle (Fig. 6–7). The tendon should then be stretched by having the patient grasp the involved thumb, and gently pull it away and back from the palm repetitively for 1 minute twice daily. If there is a recurrence, the tendon may be injected a second time, and a thumb splint provided for

use during work. Failure to provide benefit after two injections should lead to consideration for surgery. Rupture of the tendon is a rare complication of repeated tendon injections.

Bowler's thumb is a common stress syndrome that may present with a soft tissue mass at the base of the thumb web, with pain and stiffness of the digits that are used during bowling. For such problems, the bowling ball holes may be bevelled to reduce friction.[61]

Tenosynovitis of the flexor carpi radialis tendon sheath causes local swelling and pain just proximal to the wrist crease radial to the carpal tunnel. Pain is increased by dorsiflexion.[62] Splinting the thumb with a 2-inch elastic bandage and, if necessary, local intralesional steroid injection with 0.25 ml (10 mg) methylprednisolone mixed with procaine is usually helpful.

DISORDERS OF THE PALM AND FINGERS

Trigger Finger

Fusiform swelling of the flexor sublimus tendon over a metacarpal head, accompanied by constriction of the tendon sheath, results in the locking of a finger in flexion. Often, the patient first notices locking upon arising

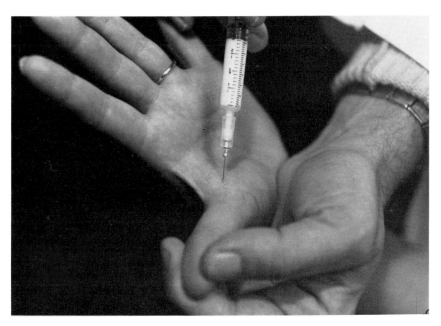

Fig. 6–7. Site for injection of a trigger thumb. Use a #25 or 27 needle, 0.25 ml (10 mg) crystalline corticosteroid with 0.25 ml local anesthetic without epinephrine. Inject parallel to tendon.

in the morning. The bent PIP joint should be passively returned to extension; a popping sensation is perceived sometimes as the finger is straightened.

Trigger finger is of increasing concern because it can economically impact upon health costs to industry.[59,60] Central to its etiology is overuse by performing repetitive tasks. The number of movements the tendon performs per unit of time and the degree of clenching during use is important.[57,59,60,63-73] In others, hand clenching can result from stress, from overuse by a compulsive homemaker, or from performing tasks with the attitude "I'm going to finish this if it kills me!" Hand clenching, any repetitive handwork, sport, or recreational activity can result in recurrences of trigger finger. Card playing, prolonged reading with rapid turning of pages, prolonged horseback riding with a tight grip on the reins, are examples to be searched for. "Arcade arthritis" includes digital callosities, arthralgia, and tendinitis following use of videogames played with rapid repetition of action[74] (see Joint Protection, Table 6–5). Direct trauma is a rare cause.[75]

Trigger finger may also result from rheumatoid arthritis, degenerative arthritis, Dupuytren's contracture, and ochronosis.[76-78] A hyperextension injury with partial flexor tendon rupture as a cause of trigger finger has been described.[79] Causes of similar symptoms include: slipping of an extensor tendon, particularly in rheumatoid arthritis, a collateral ligament catching on a bony prominence on the side of a metacarpal head, traumatic splitting of the joint capsule, and an abnormal sesamoid catching on a metacarpal head. Persistent symptoms despite treatment should raise suspicion for a tendon fibroma[80] or a systemic inflammatory rheumatic disease such as rheumatoid arthritis.

Treatment begins with avoiding repetitive activities, hand clenching, and tasks that require a tightly clenched fist. Wrapping the PIP joint with one inch "Kling" gauze may help remind the patient to protect the hand.[81] Prevention can be offered to workers by use of exercise as recommended by Peterson.[82] (see Exercise 6, Table 6–6).

Physical therapy may be helpful and includes joint mobilization techniques, glide and joint distraction maneuvers, ice massage,[54] ultrasound,[53] and passive stretching.

By far, the quickest relief can be obtained by intralesional injection with a local anesthetic and corticosteroid agent (see Table 15–4). Whereas the average industrial patient is off work for 3 to 6 weeks,[83] we see results in 7 to 10 days or less in most patients. A #25 or #27 needle should be kept parallel to the tendon and 0.5 ml of steroid injected slowly while the clinician palpates proximal to the nodule for distension of the sheath by the steroid (Fig. 6–8). Injection into the sheath is optimal, but good results can usually also be expected by delivery of the steroid to the region of maximum tenderness. Others also report success in up to 80% of cases.[55–57,75] We and others have performed thousands of injections safely.[50–52]

Infectious Tenosynovitis

Tuberculous tenosynovitis should be an immediate consideration if massive swelling of a single flexor tendon from the palm all the way out to the distal finger is noted. The cold swelling, with relatively little pain, should immediately be considered tuberculous until proved otherwise. Acute septic tenosynovitis

may result from gonococcal, staphylococcal, and syphilitic (rare) infections.[9,84]

Another presentation of tuberculous tenosynovitis of the wrist and hand is "compound palmar ganglion" in which gradually enlarging rubbery masses are noted. They are slightly tender but without evidence of inflammation. A case in which such masses developed over 3 years[85] emphasizes the mildness of presentation. Destruction of the enclosed tendons may occur.

Dupuytren's Contracture

Dupuytren's contracture, which is usually painless, represents a nodular fibrosing lesion within the palmar fascia that progresses to fibrous bands, and usually radiates distally to the fourth and fifth fingers (Fig. 6–9). Ultimately the fingers are contracted by the taut bands. The flexor tendons are not intrinsically involved. Soft tissue pads over the proximal interphalangeal joints on the extensor surface (knuckle pads) may be associated findings. Nodular lesions within the plantar fascia of the feet may also develop concurrently. Dupuytren's contracture occurs in 1 to 3% of Caucasian males. Sex ratio is predominately male (10:1). The condition is probably of genetic origin (by late age, 68% of male relatives

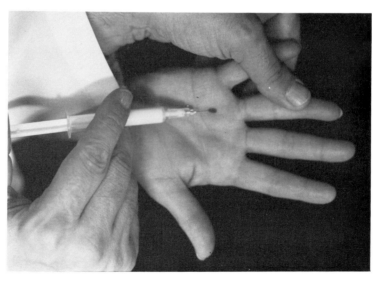

Fig. 6–8. Site for injection of a trigger finger. Use a #25 or 27 needle, 0.25 ml (10 mg) crystalline corticosteroid with 0.25 ml local anesthetic without epinephrine. Inject parallel to tendon.

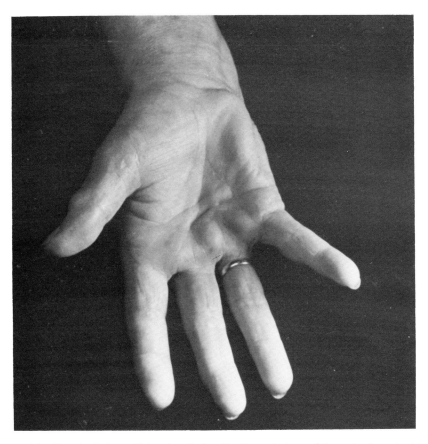

Fig. 6–9. Nodular fibrosing lesion with bands radiating distally are features of Dupuytren's contracture.

are reportedly affected), and no definite relation to occupation has been accepted by various investigators.[34,86,87] However, Bennett examined workers who performed bagging and packing tasks versus those who did no manual work and detected Dupuytren's contracture in 16/216 baggers, but in only 1/84 others.[88] Knuckle pads are benign thickened skin over the PIP joints. They occur in otherwise normal persons but are 4 times more common in patients with Dupuytren's contracture. They can spontaneously improve. Sometimes they can result in tethering of the extensor tendons, and in one reported case, caused loss of finger flexion.[89] Knuckle pads may occur without palmar lesions in relatives of patients.[87] An association with diabetes was not found to be statistically significant.[90] The fasciitis histologically demonstrates fibro-blastic proliferation with giant cells and vascular hyperplasia.[91]

Differential diagnoses include congenital flexion deformity of the fourth and fifth digits (camptodactyly), diabetic cheiroarthropathy, traumatic scars, Volkmann's ischemic contracture, or intrinsic joint disease.[86]

Treatment of patients with minimal Dupuytren's contracture includes passively stretching the involved digits (hyperextending the digits), avoiding a tight grip by means of built-up handles (pipe insulation, cushion tape),[92] and perhaps using a glove with padding across the palm during heavy grasping tasks. Surgery should be considered if functional impairment occurs, or if progressive deformity develops.[93] Unfortunately, the recurrence rate is considerable. Most patients who learn the benign nature of the contracture adapt to the disorder.

DORSAL EDEMA OF SECRETAN

Rarely, following injury to the dorsum of the hand, a peritendinous fibrosis may occur. This brawny, edematous swelling may gradually harden, and often becomes painlessly persistent. Early, consistent elevation of the affected hand may be beneficial in preventing edema.[92] Repeated injections of a corticosteroid or excision of the fibrotic tendinous tissue have been advocated.[57] Failure of surgical excision to shorten disability suggests that surgical procedure should be prescribed rarely if at all for this entity.[94]

NERVE ENTRAPMENT DISORDERS OF THE WRIST AND HAND

Carpal Tunnel Syndrome

Compression of the median nerve at the wrist may give rise to variable signs and symptoms. The most common and easily recognized symptoms are early morning numbness, tingling, or burning in the distribution of the median nerve of the hand. The patient awakes in the early morning hours, and shakes her hand, elevates it, or otherwise tries to restore sensation. At times the distress is exquisite. Symptoms may consist of sensory nerve complaints only, motor incoordination, or both. Altered motor function may predominate, in which case the patient has difficulty performing pinch grasping, writing, or holding small utensils. The symptoms generally are worse in the early morning or after prolonged use, such as knitting, working on needlepoint, or driving. Because of variable innervation, numbness, tingling, and sensory deficits may involve the entire palmar aspect of the hand, in contrast to the more typical median nerve distribution of the thumb, index, middle, and radial half of the ring fingers. Thenar flattening or atrophy are late manifestations. Raynaud's phenomenon may be seen.

Tests for nerve compression at the wrist include the Hoffman-Tinel test (Fig. 6–10) and the Phalen maneuver (Fig. 6–11). The Hoffman-Tinel test consists of a tingling sen-

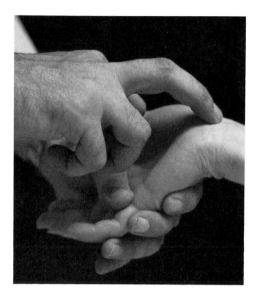

Fig. 6–10. The Hoffman-Tinel test: Tapping over a compressed nerve at the wrist reproduces pain and paresthesia, proximal or distal to the site of compression.

sation without pain, following tapping over the median nerve at the flexor surface of the wrist.[95] The Phalen maneuver is performed by having the patient approximate the back of both hands, one to the other, with fingers pointed downward, and wrists flexed maximally; this position is held for 60 seconds. A positive test reproduces numbness and tingling along the median nerve distribution.[69,96,97] Direct compression of the median nerve may give the same findings. Electrodiagnostic testing with abnormal nerve conduction velocity is supportive of the diagnosis.[98,99] Use of multiple sites for stimulation may improve localization of the entrapment.[100] The findings include slowed conduction velocity and increased latency of evoked response potential (terminal latency of the motor impulse > 4 to 5 msec). Of patients with carpal tunnel syndrome, 10% may have normal test results. Roentgenographic studies are rarely of value. Osteoarthritis of adjacent joints are palpably enlarged, and need not be confirmed by roentgenography. Thermography can provide evidence of thenar hypothermia before and after the Phalen maneuver; this finding correlated well

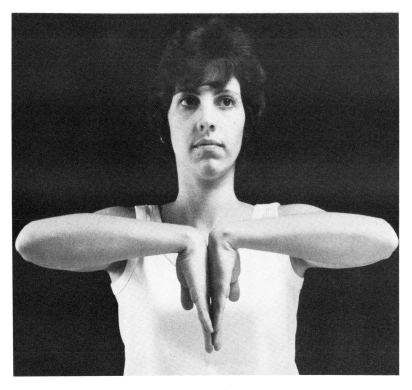

Fig. 6–11. The Phalen maneuver: Acute wrist flexion maintained for 30 to 60 seconds reproduces symptoms in patients with nerve compression in the carpal canal (the carpal tunnel syndrome).

with nocturnal symptoms and electrodiagnostic findings.[101]

Carpal tunnel syndrome may occur from occupations or activities that require repetitive flexor handwork such as typing or knitting,[102] or it may follow sleeping with the wrist in flexion, resting the wrists over a steering wheel, work that requires thumb rolling or kneading motion, or trauma with resulting tenosynovitis.[103] Only 3 of 658 patients with this disorder were performing heavy labor.[102] Occupations with pronounced repetitive hand use include typists, boot and shoe manufacturing and repairing, cashiers, machinists, cleaners, assemblers and packers, retail clerks when ticketing merchandise, exposure to vibrations and vibratory hand tools, rope coiling (fishermen), and prolonged writing or driving.[104–108] The carpal tunnel syndrome may occur secondarily to other conditions or diseases, including inflammatory connective tissue disease, chondrocalcinosis of the wrist,[109] secondary osteoarthritis, pregnancy, diabetes, myxedema, acromegaly, amyloid, hepatic disease,[110] peripheral neuropathy, fibrositis,[111] pyridoxine deficiency,[112,113] polymyalgia rheumatica,[114] or benign local tumors.[69,96,102,103,109,115] Pyridoxine deficiency was investigated in 4 series of patients whose diagnosis was based on electrodiagnostic studies: carpal tunnel syndrome, peripheral neuropathy, carpal tunnel syndrome and peripheral neuropathy, or those with normal findings. Erythrocyte glutamic oxaloacetic acid transaminase activity was measured before and after pyridoxal phosphate was added. This was used to assess pyridoxine status. Pyridoxine deficiency was associated only with peripheral neuropathy, not with carpal tunnel syndrome.[116] Others who reported pyridoxine deficiency in carpal tunnel syndrome[112,113] based the diagnosis on clinical findings only, and did not confirm the diagnosis with electrodiagnostic findings. Others found no evidence for pyridoxine deficiency in patients with carpal tunnel syndrome diagnosed by electrodiagnostic studies.[117]

Space occupying lesions as causes have also been described and include ulnar bursitis[118] and tuberculous "compound palmar ganglion".[85] Rheumatoid arthritis with tenosynovitis often occurs with a carpal tunnel syndrome, as can systemic lupus erythematosus.[115] The majority of patients with carpal tunnel syndrome do not have an underlying disease process. Rather, the disturbance results from repetitive finger motion or from forced wrist extension, such as pushing from the sides of a chair upon arising, or from development of a dense fibrotic volar-carpal ligament compressing the nerve. Pathologic findings suggest that obstruction of venous return results in increased pressure, fibrous tissue formation, and anoxia of the nerve trunk.[119] Direct measurement of the pressure between the median nerve and the carpal ligament preoperatively was carried out by Werner et al. At rest, pressure ranged from 18 to 64 mm Hg in 16 patients. Passive volar and dorsal wrist flexion increased the pressure about 3 times. Maximal muscle contraction increased the pressure 3 to 6 times more than the resting value.[120] Data concerning structural disorders such as hand and wrist size or carpal stenosis are conflicting. Thus Armstrong and Chaffin found no difference in wrist and hand size between workers with and those without symptoms of carpal tunnel syndrome.[121] Dekel et al. on the other hand, noted a significantly smaller cross-sectional carpal tunnel area in patients than in controls when studied by computed tomography of the wrist.[122]

If carpal tunnel syndrome has not resulted in atrophy of the thenar eminence, conservative treatment may suffice. These measures include 30-degree cockup wrist splinting, particularly at night,[125] avoiding aggravating activity, and injecting a steroid-local anesthetic mixture into the carpal canal (Fig. 6–12). The injection should be placed radially to the palmaris longus tendon.[123,124] Before injection, the patient should notify the phy-

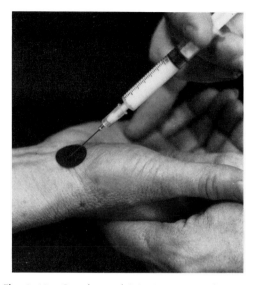

Fig. 6–12. Carpal tunnel injection: Many clinicians consider carpal tunnel injection to be diagnostic and therapeutic. The site for injection should be to the radial side of the palmaris longus tendon. The needle may be directed proximally and then distally, with aliquots of the corticosteroid-anesthetic injected in each direction. A ¾ inch, No. 25 gauge needle to inject 20 mg of methylprednisolone and 0.5 ml of procaine may be used.

sician if the needle accentuates the numbness and tingling, since this indicates penetration of the nerve, and must be avoided. In one prospective study of 160 wrists in 105 patients with this syndrome, conservative measures provided relief without progression (by electrodiagnostic measurement) in 65% of cases followed for an average of 37 months. Chronicity and severity of electrodiagnostic findings did not correlate with outcome.[125] These results are similar to ours and others.[56] They differ from other studies[126,127] but the differences may relate to the importance we place on joint protection principles (see Joint Protection, Table 6–5). Gelberman et al. analyzed results of conservative care and noted that patients who responded were those with mild symptoms, short duration, and no muscle atrophy.[127] Pyridoxine treatment has been reported of value in the treatment of carpal tunnel syndrome. In a double blind study, post-treatment electrodiagnostic studies were used, as well as clinical assessment. Significant improvement was reported in the pyridoxine treated patients. As mentioned, the diagnosis before treatment was not supported by electrodiagnostic studies.[112,113] Others report inconsistent benefit with pyridoxine treatment (100 mg per day for 9 to 26 weeks).[117,128]

Wiley recommends an exercise to loosen the flexor retinaculum[129] (see Exercise 7, Table 6–6 and Figure 6–13). The exercise utilizes bowstringing of the flexor tendons to stretch the flexor retinaculum; benefit was reported to occur within 6 weeks.[129] If conservative measures fail, or atrophy of the thenar eminence is detected, surgical release should be carried out. About 10% of postoperative patients unfortunately have recurrences and on occasion require repeat surgical intervention.[99] Patients under worker's compensation had 2.5 times higher failure rate in one study.[130] Surgical failures were analyzed retrospectively by Graham. Age of the patient and duration of symptoms were important but the choice of surgical incision seemed to have little bearing on complication rate.[131] Nevertheless, criticism of "microsurgery" in which a small incision is made and a blind section of the volar carpal ligament carried out is to be noted.[132] Incomplete sec-

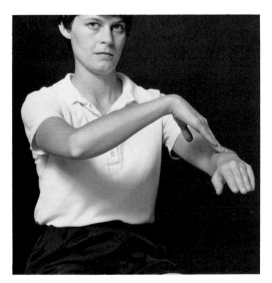

Fig. 6–13. Wiley's exercise to stretch the volar carpal ligament for carpal tunnel syndrome[129] (see Exercise 7, Table 6–6).

tioning may result in increased failures. Furthermore careful inspection is necessary to detect tumors, fibromas, ganglions, lipomas, or bony spurs.[132] After surgery, repetitive hand use at work may still not be tolerated. Surgery does not greatly improve motor function loss, but usually aids in relieving nocturnal discomfort and in preventing further motor dysfunction.[99]

Anterior Interosseous Nerve Syndrome

Sudden loss of distal interphalangeal flexion of the thumb and distal interphalangeal flexion of the index finger may result from injury to the anterior interosseous nerve. The injury occurs during lifting, which results in strain and compression of the anterior interosseous nerve by the flexor pollicis longus and flexor carpi radialis at the neck of the radius. Occasionally, a fibrous band is found on the underside of the flexor digitorum sublimus. Electrodiagnostic tests with nerve conduction measurement assist in diagnosis. Treatment includes use of a sling, galvanic stimulation, or surgical exploration.[9]

Ulnar Nerve Entrapment at the Wrist

This disorder may result from compression through Guyon's canal, where the nerve passes deeply into the muscles of the hypothenar eminence on the ulnar side of the wrist. Such compression results in typical ulnar nerve atrophy of the interosseous muscles, and paresthesia of ulnar nerve distribution. Nerve conduction determination will assist in diagnosis. Surgical intervention for release of the nerve is usually required.[69] Ganglia and anomalous musculature may be noted at the time of intervention.[133]

NEUROVASCULAR DISORDERS OF THE WRIST AND HAND

Raynaud's Disease and Phenomenon

Sequential discoloration of the digits, progressing from pallor to cyanosis to rubor, upon exposure to cold or emotional upset may occur as a secondary *phenomenon*. Raynaud's phenomenon accompanies, or may precede, other manifestations of systemic connective tissue disease, such as progressive systemic sclerosis, systemic lupus erythematosus, rheumatoid arthritis, or mixed connective tissue disease. Raynaud's phenomenon may also result from hypothyroidism,[134] trauma or frostbite, proximal large vessel obstruction, compression within the thoracic outlet, or use of vasoconstrictive drugs. In addition it has been described in association with use of vinblastine, bleomycin, and beta adrenergic blocking agents. Arterial disease, cryoprotein dyscrasias, vibratory tool use, neoplasms, primary pulmonary hypertension, and pheochromocytoma are additional associated disorders.[134,135]

The term Raynaud's *disease* is reserved for patients who demonstrate these manifestations, but in whom no primary underlying cause can be demonstrated after a prolonged period of time (Fig. 6–14). The diagnosis is often made only with great uncertainty, since a systemic disorder such as progressive systemic sclerosis may not appear for many years after onset of Raynaud's phenomenon. Antinuclear antibody studies are helpful in diagnosis.[136,137] Antinuclear antibodies are frequently present in patients with progressive systemic sclerosis (PSS). Antibody to Scl-70 antigen is almost specific for PSS; anticentromere antibody is seen in PSS, but is more consistently observed in patients with CREST syndrome (calcinosis, Raynaud's phenomenon, esophageal dysfunction, sclerodactyly, and telangiectasia). In vivo capillary microscopy of the periungual skin can be particularly helpful. Scleroderma is characterized by capillary dilatation and areas of capillary drop-out.[138,139] The magnifying glass of an otoscope can be used for this examination. Yet 90% of patients with Raynaud's phenomenon have no apparent underlying disorder at the time of Raynaud's onset.[140] The best that the clinician can do is to examine the patient carefully for subtle features of various associated disorders. The presence of distal fingertip pitting, skin telangiectasias or thickening raises concern for progressive systemic sclerosis. Physical examination of the pulses, thoracic outlet maneuvers, neurologic examination, and a general physical examination are essential.

The clinician should order rheumatoid factor test determination, antinuclear-antibody determination, serologic test for syphilis, complete blood counts, tests for sedimentation rate and cryoproteins, protein electrophoresis, urinalysis, a thyroid function test, and a chest roentgenogram.

The etiology and pathogenesis of Raynaud's phenomenon and disease involves the sympathetic nervous system. Indirect evidence suggests that norepinephrine release and sympathetic nervous system activity are increased in both primary and secondary cases.[141]

Treatment for Raynaud's disease and phenomenon includes total body protection from cold. Cold exposure of any body part can set off the disturbance. Patients with mild symptoms need only reassurance, environmental protection from cold, and perhaps abstinence from tobacco (not of proved value). Moderate symptoms often respond to use of oral (0.25 to 0.5 mg/day) or intra-arterial (0.5 mg) reserpine. Recently, there has been concern that reserpine may induce local gangrene or breast cancer. This relationship to breast cancer has been refuted.[142] We recommend that it be used only during the colder months. Calcium antagonist drugs that inhibit the contraction of smooth muscle cells have received much attention for symptomatic control of Raynaud's phenomenon. These include verapamil,[143] and nifedipine.[144-147] However, in one study of primary Raynaud's disease, the benefit was shortlived (30 to 60 mg/day), lasting only 5 weeks.[148] Verapamil has proved less effective than nifedipine in other studies.[149] Relief with sublingual nifedipine was also reported.[147] In one study, treatment with nifedipine for patients with Raynaud's phenomenon and scleroderma resulted in decreased peripheral blood flow and increased resistance when compared to control patients.[150] Other drugs that may be tried include prazosin (1 mg bid),[151,152] alpha-methyldopa (1 or

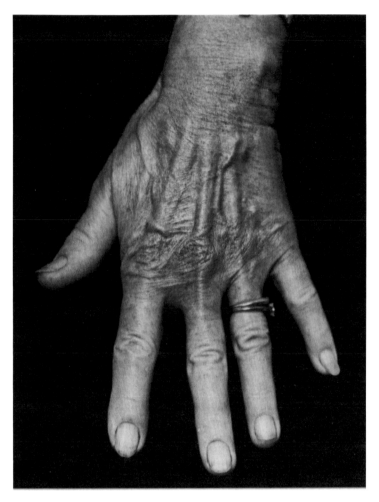

Fig. 6–14. Raynaud's disease: Despite blanching of the digits from the metacarpophalangeal joints to the fingertips for many years, this patient's hands failed to show evidence of atrophy or other features of connective tissue disease.

2 g/day), guanethidine (30 to 50 mg/day), phenoxybenzamine (20 to 60 mg/day), estrogen replacement,[140,142,151,153–155] and nitroglycerin ointment. Intravenous dextran or plasmapheresis have been used in intractable cases associated with scleroderma.[154] Stanozolol, a fibrinolytic anabolic steroid (5 mg bid) has recently been reported useful in severe cases secondary to progressive systemic sclerosis.[155] Hepatotoxicity is a limiting factor. Several new drugs are under study. Ketanserin, a selective antagonist of 5-HT$_2$ serotonin, provided symptomatic relief and improved digital circulation in 15 of 18 patients.[156] A Prostaglandin E$_2$ analogue, ad-ministered transdermally, reduced the frequency and severity of attacks in one recent study.[157] Dazoxiben, an inhibitor of thromboxane synthetase (thromboxane A2, produced by platelets, is a potent vasoconstrictor) was not helpful.[158] Sympathectomy has provided relief in some patients,[151] and long-term benefit has ranged from 20 to 80% in various reports. In our experience most patients benefit with reserpine or nifedipine,[151] often used only in the colder seasons.

We have had some rewarding experience with the use of biofeedback training in patients with either Raynaud's disease or phenomenon. Some patients have raised their skin temperatures by 8 to 10 degrees for sustained periods of time.[159-161]

Erythermalgia

Redness, burning sensation, and swelling of the hands and feet after exposure to heat or after exercise suggests erythermalgia. The disorder may be primary, or secondary to a hematologic disease, diabetes, or a connective tissue disease, including vasculitis with peripheral neuropathy. Similar features resulted from a carpal tunnel syndrome; later, digital gangrene occurred in one case report.[162]

The autonomic nervous system and platelet-mediated arteriolar inflammation have been implicated in the pathogenesis of erythermalgia. In one patient, autonomic nerve plexuses from four skin biopsies revealed a marked reduction in the density of both acetylcholinesterase-positive and catecholamine-containing nerve terminals in the periarterial and sweat glandular plexuses. Terminal axons containing either agranular or small dense-cored vesicles were present but much reduced in frequency in involved skin compared to uninvolved skin. A mecholyl skin test resulted in less sweating than would normally occur.[163] In 26 of 40 patents with thrombocythemia and hand complaints of erythermalgia, the symptoms were alleviated during busulfan-induced remission of the thrombocythemia; symptoms recurred during relapse.[164] The attack appears to be triggered by increased skin temperature (range from 32 to 36 degrees C). Therapy includes trials of aspirin, phenoxybenzamine hydrochloride (Dibenzyline), methysergide, or sympathectomy if a treatable underlying disorder is not found.[69,153,165]

Acrocyanosis

Painless cyanosis, coolness, and hypoesthesia of the extremities may occur in persons with vasomotor instability, or from causes listed for Raynaud's phenomenon. When underlying disease is not found, reassurance usually suffices for therapy.[69,153]

Other Vascular Syndromes

Other vascular disturbances to be considered include a *syndrome of acute blue fingers in women*.[166] This syndrome consists of acute onset of pain and discoloration of the volar aspect of the digit, then the entire digit, lasting for 2 or 3 days. Attacks recur one or more times per year. Some cases are familial. No other abnormal findings are detected on physical or laboratory examination. *The hypothenar hammer syndrome* consists of digital ischemia that involves the fourth and fifth fingers, and is a result of repetitive use of the hypothenar eminence as a hammer. Compression of the ulnar artery against the hook of the hamate can lead to segmental thrombosis.[167] Similarly, ulnar artery entrapment and occlusion within and distal to the canal of Guyon may follow a solitary blow to the region.[168]

NODULES

Pseudorheumatoid nodules (firm, rubbery, subcutaneous nodular lesions) may occur in multiple sites, particularly in the pretibial area and extensor finger regions, without the presence of rheumatoid arthritis. They may last for months or years, occur in both males and females but predominantly occur in children and young adults[169,169a] (Fig. 6–15).

Giant cell tumors of tendon sheaths or pigmented villonodular tenosynovitis usually occur in women between the third and fourth decade, and are the second most common noninflammatory lesions of a tendon sheath.[170] These growths generally occur on the flexor or extensor tendons, adjacent to a proximal interphalangeal joint. A review of 81 cases of solitary nodular, multiple nodular, and diffuse lesions suggests a common histogenesis characterized by proliferation of fibroblastic and histiocytic mesenchymal cells beneath synovium or tenosynovial lining cells.[171] Giant cell tumors of tendon sheaths also occur in the Achilles tendon, and are generally bilateral. Clinically, similar nodules are associated with hyperlipidemia or sarcoi-

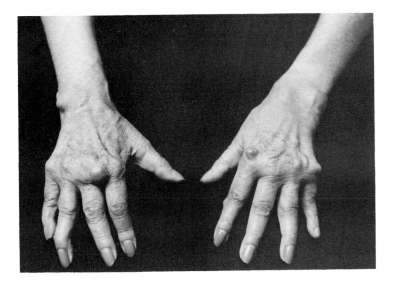

Fig. 6–15. Rheumatoid nodulosis: In patients with rheumatoid arthritis, firm nodules may erupt and persist adjacent to joints, or in the finger pulp. Similar lesions (pseudorheumatoid nodules) may occur on the extremities in the absence of rheumatoid arthritis.

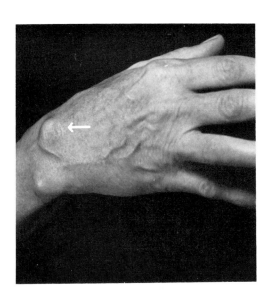

Fig. 6–16. Ganglion (arrow) on the dorsum of the wrist. Aspiration reveals a clear gelatinous fluid.

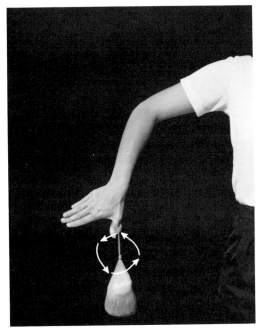

Fig. 6–17. Stretching exercise for first carpometacarpal joint and adjacent tendons (see Exercise 5, Table 6–6).

dosis; thse may be pea-size, yellowish, and lobulated, and in them giant cells with lipoid foamy cytoplasm are noted microscopically.

Presenting symptoms of hemochromatosis may be nodules at the elbow and over the extensor digitorum tendons.[172] Glomus tumors occur as painful, slow-growing neurovascular tumors of an extremity; 30% arise beneath a fingernail. Pain is described as excruciating, burning, or shooting. Local contact exacerbates the pain and suggests the presence of the lesion. Surgery is necessary. An occasional patient presents with acute painful swelling in the pulp of a distal finger pad, which may be due to an infection, known as a *felon.*

Epidermoid cysts or pearls are small, hard, pearl-like cysts several millimeters in diameter. These occur in the volar aspects of the palm, or in the web adjacent to the metacarpophalangeal joints, and generally are painless. These cysts are thought to arise from injury, when a small piece of epidermis becomes implanted in the subcutaneous tissue.[71] In most cases they disappear spontaneously.

GANGLIA

A ganglion is a cystic swelling overlying a joint or tendon sheath. It probably results as a herniation of synovial tissue from joint capsule or tendon sheath. Ganglia may be unilocular or multilocular. Inflammatory cells are not present. A soft jelly-like fluid can be aspirated from the lesion. Ganglia rarely occur after age 50, and may spontaneously regress or recur. Most commonly, a ganglion occurs at the dorsal aspects of the wrist (Fig. 6–16). Anomalies appearing as ganglia include anomalous extensor muscle bellies, lipomas, neuromas of the posterior interosseous nerve, synovial cysts of rheumatoid arthritis, radial artery aneurysm, dorsal exostoses, partial tendon rupture, periarticular calcareous deposits, plexiform neuroma, sarcomas, and giant cell tumor.[173] Ganglia transilluminate in most instances whereas solid tumors will not. Management may be one of the following:

leave it alone; aspirate and inject a crystalline steroid; or surgically remove the ganglion after tracing its connection to the tendon sheath or capsule, and repair the defect.

REFERENCES

1. Baraitser M: A new camptodactyly syndrome. J Med Genetics 19:40–43, 1982.
2. Ochi T, Iwase R, Okabe N, Fink CW, Ono K: The pathology of the involved tendons in patients with familial arthropathy and congenital camptodactyly. (Abstract #A10) Arth Rheum 26 (No. 4) [Supp], 1983.
3. Linscheid RL, Dobyns JH, Beaubout JW, et al: Traumatic instability of the wrist. J Bone Joint Surg 54A:1612–1632, 1972.
4. Maudsley RH: The painful wrist. Practit 215:42–45, 1975.
5. Posner MA: Injuries to the hand and wrist in athletes. Orthop Clin N Am 8:593–618, 1977.
6. Halperin JL, Coffman JD: Pathophysiology of Raynaud's disease. Arch Intern Med 139:89–92, 1979.
7. Zambrano J, Boswick JA: Microwave injury to the upper extremity: a case report. Contemp Ortho 9:91–93, 1984.
8. Adams JC: Outline of Orthopaedics. 9th Ed. London, Churchill, Livingstone, 1981.
9. Turek SL: Orthopaedics; Principles and Their Application. 4th Ed. Philadelphia, JB Lippincott, 1984.
10. Rosenbloom AL, Silverstein JH, Lezotte DC, et al: Limited joint mobility in childhood diabetes mellitus indicates increased risk for microvascular disease. N Engl J Med 305:191–194, 1981.
11. Knowles HB Jr: Joint contractures, waxy skin, and control of diabetes. N Engl J Med 305:217–218, 1981.
12. Fitzcharles MA, Duby S, Waddell RW, Banks E, Karsh J: Limitation of joint mobility (cheiroarthropathy) in adult noninsulin-dependent diabetic patients. Ann Rheum Dis 43:251–257, 1984.
13. Trapp RG, Springfield IL, Spencer-Green G, Soler NG: Nailfold capillary findings in type 1 diabetes: relation to musculoskeletal abnormalities and retinopathy. (Abstract #D63) Arth Rheum 27 (No.4) [Supp], 1984.
14. Robertson JR, Earnshaw PM, Campbell IW: Tenolysis in juvenile diabetic cheiroarthropathy. Br Med J 2:971–972, 1979.
15. Eaton RP, Sibbitt WL, Harsh A: The effect of an aldose reductase inhibiting agent on limited joint mobility in diabetic patients. JAMA 253:1437–1440, 1985.
16. Watson FM, Purvis JM: Acute calcareous deposits of the hand and wrist. South Med J 73:150–151, 1980.
17. Selby CL: Acute calcific tendinitis of the hand: an infrequently recognized and frequently misdiagnosed form of periarthritis. Arth Rheum 27:337–340, 1984.
18. Paty JG Jr: Flexor carpi ulnaris tendinitis. Arth Rheum 22:97–98, 1979.

19. Dieppe P: Crystal deposition disease and the soft tissues. Clinics in Rheumatic Disease 5:807–822, 1979.

20. Thompson TR, Andrish JT, Bergfeld JA: A prospective study of preparticipation sports examinations of 2670 young athletes: method and results. Cleve Clin Quart 49:225–233, 1982.

21. Raskin RJ, Lawless OJ: Articular and soft tissue abnormalities in a "normal" population. J Rheumatol 9:284–288, 1982.

22. Finsterbush A, Pogrund H: The hypermobility syndrome: musculoskeletal complaints in 100 consecutive cases of generalized joint hypermobility. Clin Ortho Research 168:124–127, 1982.

23. Walker BA, Beighton PH, Murdoch LJ: The Marfanoid hypermobility syndrome. Ann Intern Med 71:349–352, 1969.

24. Grahame R, Edwards JC, Pitcher D, Gabel A, Harvey W: A clinical and echocardiographic study of patients with hypermobility syndrome. Ann Rheum Dis 40:541–546, 1981.

25. Gedalia A, Person DA, Giannini EH, Brewer EJ: Joint hypermobility in juvenile episodic arthritis/arthralgia. Paper presented to the Central Region Interim Meeting, Chicago, American Rheumatism Association, 1984.

26. Fairbank JCT, Pynsent PB, Phillips H: Quantitative measurements of joint mobility in adolescents. Ann Rheum Dis 43:288–294, 1984.

27. Sheon RP, Kirsner AB, Farber SJ, Finkel RI: The hypermobility syndrome. PostGrad Med 71: 199–209, 1982.

28. Grahame, R: Joint hypermobility—Clinical aspects. Proc Roy Soc Med 64:32–34, 1971.

28a. Finkelstein H: Joint hypotonia. With congenital and familial manifestations. New York Med J 104:942–944, 1916.

29. Kirk JA, Ansell BM, Bywaters EGL: The hypermobility syndrome: musculoskeletal complaints associated with generalized joint hypermobility. Ann Rheum Dis 26:419–425, 1967.

30. Biro F, Gewanter HL, Baum J: The benign hypermobility syndrome in pediatrics. (Abstract #E33) Arth Rheum 25 (No. 4) [Supp], 1982.

31. Beighton PH, Horan ET: Dominant inheritance in familial generalized articular hypermobility. J Bone Joint Surg 52B:145–147, 1970.

32. Key JA: Hypermobility of joints as a sex linked hereditary characteristic. JAMA 88:1710–1712, 1927.

33. Bird HA, Tribe CR, Bacon PA: Joint hypermobility leading to osteoarthrosis and chondrocalcinosis. Ann Rheum Dis 37:203–211, 1978.

34. James JIP, Wynne-Davies R: Genetic factors in orthopaedics. In Recent Advances in Orthopaedics. Edited by AG Apley. London, J & A Churchill, 1969.

35. Goodman RM, Wooley CF, Frazier RL, Covault L: Ehlers-Danlos syndrome occurring together with the marfan syndrome. N Engl J Med 273:514–519, 1963.

36. Cotton DJ, Brandt KD: Cardiovascular abnormalities in the marfanoid hypermobility syndrome. Arth Rheum 19:763–768, 1976.

37. Jessee EF, Owen DJ Jr, Sagar KB: The benign hypermobile joint syndrome. Arth Rheum 23:1053–1056, 1980.

38. Goldman JA: Hypermobility—the missing link to fibrositis (Abstract #E64) Arth Rheum 28 (No. 4) [Supp], 1985.

39. Howes RG, Isdale IC: The loose back: An unrecognized syndrome. Rheum Phys Med 11:72–77, 1971.

40. Rowatt-Brown A, Rose BS: Familial precocious polyarticular osteoarthrosis of chondrodysplastic type. NZ Med J 65:449–461, 1966.

41. Peter Beighton, Rodney Grahame, Howard Bird: Hypermobility of Joints. Berlin, Springer-Verlag, 1983.

42. Sheon RP: Joint laxity and the hypermobility syndrome. Arthron (Fall):3–16, 1984.

43. Hess E.: Personal communication.

44. Simmons BP, Vasile RG: The clenched fist syndrome. J Hand Surg 5:420–427, 1980.

45. Sanavio E: An operant approach to the treatment of writer's cramp. J Behav Ther Exp Psychiat 13:69–72, 1982.

46. Sheehy MP, Marsden CD: Writer's cramp—a focal dystonia. Brain 105:461–480, 1982.

47. Pick RY: DeQuervain's disease: A clinical triad. Clin Orthop 143:165–166, 1979.

47a. de Quervain, Fritz: Uber eine Form von chronischer Tendovaginitis. Correspondenz-Blatt fur Schweizer Arzte 25:389–394, 1895.

48. Belsole RJ: DeQuervain's tenosynovitis diagnostic and operative complications. Orthopedics 4:899–903, 1981.

49. Williams JGP: Surgical management of traumatic non-infective tenosynovitis of the wrist extensors. J Bone Joint Surg 59B:408–410, 1977.

50. Carlson CS, Curtis RM: Steroid injection for flexor tenosynovitis. J Hand Surg 9A:286–287, 1984.

51. Cooney WP III: Bursitis and tendinitis in the hand, wrist, and elbow. Minnesota Medicine 66:491–494, 1983.

52. Wilson DH: Tenosynovitis, tendovaginitis and trigger finger. Physiotherapy 69:350–352, 1983.

53. Curwin S, Stanish WD: Tendinitis: Its Etiology and Treatment. Lexington, Mass., The Collamore Press, 1984.

54. Kessler RM, Hergling D: Management of Common Musculoskeletal Disorders. Philadelphia, Harper & Row, 1983.

55. Clark DD, Ricker JH, MacCollum MS: The efficacy of local steroid injection in the treatment of stenosing tenovaginitis. Plast Reconstr Surg 51:179–180, 1973.

56. Janecki CJ: Extra-articular steroid injection for hand and wrist disorders. Postgrad Med 68:173–181, 1980.

57. Wolin I: The management of tenosynovitis. Surg Clin N Am 37:53–62, 1957.

58. Swezey RL: Arthritis: Rational Therapy and Rehabilitation. Philadelphia, WB Saunders, 1978.

59. Hartwell SW Jr, Larsen RD, Posch JL: Tenosynovitis in women in industry. Cleve Clin Q 31:115–118, 1964.

60. Reed JV, Harcourt AK: Tenosynovitis: An industrial disability. Am J Surg 62:392–396, 1943.

61. Moidel RA: Bowler's thumb. Arth Rheum 24:972–973, 1981.
62. Green SM: Tenosynovitis of the hand. Ortho Review 6:55–64, 1985.
63. Hadler NM: The influence of repetitive tasks on hand structure. Occ Health & Safety 50:57–64, 1981.
64. Hadler NM: Industrial Rheumatology: Clinical investigations into the influence of pattern of usage on the pattern of regional musuloskeletal disease. Arth Rheum 20:1019–1025, 1977.
65. Greenberg L, Chaffin DB: Workers and their tools: A Guide to The Ergonomic Design of Hand Tools and Small Presses. Midland, Mich., Pendell Publishing Co., 1978.
66. Kuorinka I, Koskinen P: Occupational rheumatic diseases and upper limb strain in manual jobs in a light mechanical industry. Scand J Work Environ & Health 5:Suppl 3:39–47, 1979.
67. Luopajarvi T, Kuorinka I, Virolainen M, et al: Prevalence of tenosynovitis and other injuries of the upper extremities in repetitive work. Scand J Work Environ & Health 5 [Supp]:48–55, 1979.
68. Maeda K, Hunting W, Grandjean E: Localized fatigue in accounting machine operators. J Occup Med 22:810—816, 1980.
69. Duthie RB, Ferguson AB: Mercer's Orthopedic Surgery. 8th Ed. Baltimore, Williams & Wilkins, 1983.
70. Fahey JJ, Bollinger JA: Trigger-finger in adults and children. J Bone Joint Surg 36A:1200–1218, 1954.
71. Chuinard RG: The upper extremity: Elbow, forearm, wrist and hand. Musculoskeletal Disorders. Edited by RD D'Ambrosia. Philadelphia: JB Lippincott, 1977.
72. Burton RI: The jammed finger or thumb. Contemp Orthop 1:56–81, 1979.
73. McCue FC III, Baugher H, Burland WL, et al: The 'jammed finger': How to prevent permanent disability. Consultant 19:29–38, 1979.
74. Myerson GE, Goldman J, Miller SB: Arcade arthritis-videogame violence. (Abstract #E83). Arth Rheum 25 (No. 4) [Supp], 1982.
75. Quinnill RC: Conservative management of trigger finger. Practitioner 224:187–190, 1980.
76. Stewart GJ, Williams EA: Locking of the metacarpophalangeal joints in degenerative disease. The Hand 13:147–151, 1981.
77. Parker HG: Dupuytren's Contracture as a cause of stenosing tenosynovitis. J Maine Med Assoc 70:147–148, 1979.
78. Seradge H: Ochronotic stenosing flexor tenosynovitis—case report. J Hand Surg 6:359–360, 1981.
79. Rayan GM, Elias L: "Trigger finger" secondary to partial rupture of the superficial flexor tendon. Orthopedics 3:1090–1092, 1980.
80. Sammarco GJ, Sabogal J: Fibroma of the flexor tendon presenting as carpal tunnel syndrome and trigger finger. Orthopedics 4:299–300, 1981.
81. Swezey RL, Spiegel TM: Evaluation and treatment of local musculoskeletal disorders in elderly patients. Geriatrics 34:56–75, 1979.
82. Peterson RR: Prevention! A new approach to tendinitis. Occup Health Nursing 27:19–23, 1979.
83. Johns AM: Time off work after hand injury. Br J Accident Surg 12:417–424, 1980–81.
84. Bush DC, Schneider LH: Tuberculosis of the hand and wrist. J Hand Surg 9A:391–398, 1984.
85. Borgsmiller WK, Whiteside LA: Tuberculous tenosynovitis of the hand ("Compound palmar ganglion"): Literature review and case report. Orthopaedics 3:1093–1096, 1980.
86. Vilijanto JA: Dupuytren's contracture: a review. Sem Arth Rheum 3:155–176, 1973.
87. Ling RSM: The genetic factor in Dupuytren's disease. J Bone Joint Surg 45B:709–718, 1963.
88. Bennett B: Dupuytren's contracture in manual workers. Br J Ind Med 39:98–100, 1982.
89. Addison A: Knuckle pads causing extensor tendon tethering. J Bone Joint Surg 66B:128–130, 1984.
90. Bridgman JF: Periarthritis of the shoulder and diabetes mellitus. Ann Rheum Dis 31:69–71, 1972.
91. Gelberman RH, Amiel D, Rudolph RM, et al: Dupuytren's contracture. J Bone Joint Surg 62A:425–432, 1980.
92. Goodwin C, OTC: Personal communication.
93. Rodrigo JJ, Niebauer JJ, Brown RL, et al: Treatment of Dupuytren's contracture. J Bone Joint Surg 58A:380–387, 1976.
94. Redfern AB, Curtis RM, Wilgis EFS: Experience with peritendinous fibrosis of the dorsum of the hand. J Hand Surg 7:380–382, 1982.
95. Sonntag VKH: Tinel's sign. N Engl J Med 291::263, 1974.
96. Pinals RS: Traumatic arthritis and allied conditions. In Arthritis and Allied Conditions. 10th Ed. Edited by DJ McCarty. Philadelphia, Lea & Febiger, 1985.
97. Phalen GS: The carpal tunnel syndrome. J Bone Joint Surg 48A:211–228, 1966.
98. Bendler, EM, Greenspun B, Yu J, Erdman WJ: The bilaterality of carpal tunnel syndrome. Arch Phys Med Rehabil 58:362–364, 1977.
99. Harris CM, Tanner E, Goldstein MN, Pettee DS: The surgical treatment of the carpal tunnel syndrome correlated with preoperative nerve conduction studies. J Bone Joint Surg 61A:93–98, 1979.
100. Kimura J: The carpal tunnel syndrome: Localization of conduction abnormalities within the distal segment of the median nerve. Brain 102:619–635, 1979.
101. Rothschild BM, Fisherowitz J, Reiss J, et al: Pathophysiology of carpal tunnel syndrome: Electrothermographic assessment. (Abstract C2) Arth Rheum 28 (No. 4) [Supp], 1985.
102. Birkbeck MQ, Beer TC: Occupation in relation to the carpal tunnel syndrome. Rheumatol Rehabil 14:218–221, 1975.
103. Kopell HP, Thompson WA: Peripheral Entrapment Neuropathies. Huntington NY, RE Krieger, 1976.
104. Kaplan PE: Carpel Tunnel Syndrome in Typists. JAMA 205:821–822, 1983.
105. Cannon LJ, Bernacki EJ, Walter SD: Personal and Occupational Factors Associated with Carpal Tunnel Syndrome. J Occup Med 23:255–258, 1981.
106. Emlen W, Dugowsen C: A New Occupational Association with carpal tunnel syndrome. (Abstract #107) Arth Rheum 26 (No. 4) [Supp], 1983.
107. Feldman RG, Goldman R, Keyserling WM: Pe-

ripheral nerve entrapment syndromes and ergonomic factors. Am J Indus Med 4:661–681, 1983.

108. Wick WJ: Carpal tunnel syndrome: retailing. J Occup Med 23:524–525, 1981.

109. Gerster JC, Lagier R, Boivin G, Schneider C: Carpal tunnel syndrome in chondrocalcinosis of the wrist. Arth Rheum 23:926–931, 1980.

110. Massey EW, Folger WN, Holohan T, et al: Carpal tunnel syndrome in hepatic disease. Southern Med J 72:1030, 1979.

111. Richards AJ: Carpal tunnel syndrome and subsequent rheumatoid arthritis in the 'fibrositis' syndrome. Ann Rheum Ds 43:232–234, 1984.

112. Ellis J, et al.: Clinical results of a cross-over treatment with pyridoxine and placebo of the carpal tunnel syndrome. Am J Clin Nutrition 32: 2040–2046, 1979.

113. Ellis: Pyridoxine and carpal tunnel syndrome. Proc Natl Acad Sci (USA) 79:7494–7498, 1982.

114. Richards AJ: Carpal tunnel syndrome in polymyalgia rheumatica. Rheumat Rehab 19:100–102, 1980.

115. Sidiq MBBS, Kirsner AB, Sheon RP: Carpal tunnel syndrome as the first manifestations of systemic lupus erythematosus. JAMA 222:1416–1417, 1972.

116. Byers CM, DeLisa JA, Frankel DL: Pyridoxine metabolism in carpal tunnel syndrome with and without peripheral neuropathy. Arch Phys Med Rehab 65:712–716, 1984.

117. Smith GP, Rudge PJ, Peters TJ: Biochemical studies of Pyridoxal and Pyridoxal Phosphate status and therapeutic trial of Pyridoxine in patients with carpal tunnel syndrome. Ann Neurology 15:104–107, 1984.

118. Linscheid RL: Carpal tunnel syndrome secondary to ulnar bursa distention from the intercarpal joint: Report of a case. J Hand Surg 4:191–192, 1979.

119. Sunderland S: The nerve lesion in the carpal tunnel syndrome. J Neurology, Neurosurg, Psych 39:615–626, 1976.

120. Werner CO, Elmqvist D, Ohlin P: Pressure and nerve lesion in the carpal tunnel. Acta Ortho Scand 54:312–314, 1983.

121. Armstrong TJ, Chaffin DB: Carpal tunnel syndrome and selected personal attributes. J Occup Med 21:481–486, 1979.

122. Dekel S, Papaioannou T, Rushworth G, Coates R: Idiopathic carpal tunnel syndrome caused by carpal stenosis. Br Med J 120:1297–1303, 1980.

123. Crane RF, Hay EL: What to do when pain signals carpal tunnel syndrome. Consultant 19:81–86, 1979.

124. Moskowitz RM: Clinical Rheumatology. 2nd Ed. Philadelphia, Lea & Febiger, 1982.

125. Moore L, Bernat J, Taylor T: Carpal tunnel syndrome: A conservative management program. (Abstract #143) Arth Rheum 26 (No. 4) [Supp], 1983.

126. Wood MR: Hydrocortisone injections for carpal tunnel syndrome. The Hand 12:62–64, 1980.

127. Gelberman RH, Aronson D, Weisman MH: Carpal-tunnel syndrome. J Bone Joint Surg 62A:1181–1184, 1980.

128. Amadio PC: Pyridoxine as an adjunct in the treatment of carpal tunnel syndrome. J Hand Surg 10A:237–241, 1985.

129. Wiley BC: Exercise therapy for carpal tunnel syndrome. Aches Pains (Feb): 41–42, 1984.

130. Tountas CP, Macdonald CJ, Meyerhoff JD, Bihrle DM: Carpal tunnel syndrome a review of 507 patients. Minnesota Med 66:479–483, 1983.

131. Graham RA: Carpal Tunnel Syndrome, a statistical analysis of 214 cases. Ortho 6:1283–1288, 1983.

132. Editorial: Surgical treatment of carpel-tunnel syndrome. Lancet 1:1125, 1979.

133. McLean MV, Mir DJ: Resident Review #26: Case of an unusual forearm muscle creating an ulnar tunnel syndrome. Orthop Rev 10:103–105, 1981.

134. Shagan BP, Friedman SA: Raynaud's phenomenon and thyroid deficiency. Arch Intern Med 140:832–833, 1980.

135. Spencer-Green G: Raynaud Phenomenon. Bull Rheum Dis 33:1–8, 1983.

136. Kallenberg CGM, Wouda AA, The TH: Systemic involvement and immunologic findings in patients presenting with Raynaud's phenomenon. Am J Med 69:675–680, 1980.

137. Kallenberg CGM, Pastoor GW, Wouda AA, The TH:Antinuclear antibodies in patients with Raynaud's phenomenon: clinical significance of anticentromere antibodies. Ann Rheum Dis 41:382–387, 1982.

138. Harper FE, Maricq HR, Turner RE, Lidman RW, Leroy EC: A prospective study of Raynaud phenomenon and early connective tissue disease. Am J Med 72:883–888, 1982.

139. Maricq HR, Weinberger AB, Leroy EC: Early detection of scleroderma-spectrum disorders by in vivo capillary microscopy: a prospective study of patients with Raynaud's phenomenon. J Rheum 9:289–299, 1982.

140. Halperin HL, Coffman JD: Pathophysiology of Raynaud's disease. Arch Intern Med 139:89–92, 1979.

141. Hooper M, Condemi JJ, Izzo JL: Increased norepinephine turnover in Raynaud's syndrome. (Abstract #25) Arth Rheum 28 (No. 4) [Supp], 1985.

142. Labarthe DR, O'Fallon WM: Reserpine and breast cancer: A community-based longitudinal study of 2,000 hypertensive women. JAMA 243:2304–2310, 1980.

143. Kinney EL, Nicholas GG, Gallo J, Pontoriero C, Zelis R: The treatment of severe Raynaud's phenomenon with verapamil. J Clin Pharm 22:74–76, 1982.

144. Kahan A, Weber S, Amor B, Saporta L, Hodara M: Nifedipine and Raynaud's Phenomenon. Ann Intern Med 94:546, 1981.

145. Rodeheffer RJ, Rommer JA, Wigley F, Smith CR: Controlled double-blind trial of nifedipine in the treatment of Raynaud's phenomenon. N Engl J Med 308:880–883, 1983.

146. Smith CD, Mckendry RJR: Controlled trial of nifedipine in the treatment of Raynaud's phenomenon. Lancet 2:1299–1301, 1982.

147. Winston EL, Pariser KM, Miller KB, Salem DN, Creager MA: Nifedipine as a therapeutic modality for Raynaud's phenomenon. Arth Rheum 26:1177–1180, 1983.

148. Sarkozi J, Bookman AAM, Mahon W, Ramsay C, Keystone EC: Nifedipine in the treatment of idi-

opathic Raynaud's syndrome (IRS). (Abstract #71) Arth Rheum 27 (No. 4) [Supp], 1984.

149. Smith CR, Rodeheffer RJ: Treatment of Raynaud's phenomenon with calcium channel blockers. Am J Med 78:39–42, 1985.

150. Lindsey G, McCullough RGJ: Nifedipine may be harmful in the treatment of Raynaud's phenomenon secondary to systemic sclerosis—results of a double blind study. (Abstract #27) Arth Rheum 28 (No. 4) [Supp], 1985.

151. Waldo R: Prazosin relieves Raynaud's vasospasm. JAMA 241:1037, 1979.

152. Russell IJ, Lessard JA: Prazosin treatment of Raynaud's phenomenon: a double blind single cross-over study. J Rheum 12:94–98, 1985.

153. Spittell JA Jr: Raynaud's phenomenon and allied vasospastic conditions. Peripheral Vascular Diseases. Ed. by Juergens JL, Spittell JA Jr, Fairbairn JF II. 5th Ed. Philadelphia, WB Saunders, 1980.

154. Wong WH, Freedman RI, Rabens SF, et al: Low molecular weight dextran therapy for scleroderma: effects of dextran 40 on blood flow and capillary filtration coefficient in scleroderma. Arch Dermatol 110:419–422, 1974.

155. Jarrett PEM, Morland M, Browse NL: Treatment of Raynaud's phenomenon by fibrinolytic enhancement. Br Med J 2:523–525, 1978.

156. Seibold JR, Jageneau AHM: Treatment of Raynaud's phenomenon with Ketanserin, a selective antagonist of the serotonin 2 (5-HT2) receptor. Arth Rheum 27:139–146, 1984.

157. Kassam YB, Grace EM, Kean WF, Buchanan WW, Tugwell P, Norman G, Beattie WS: Transdermally administered prostaglandin E2 analogue for Raynaud's phenomenon. (Abstract #18) Arth Rheum 28 (No. 4) [Supp], 1985.

158. Ettinger WH, Wise RA, Schaffhauser D, Wigley F: Controlled double-blind trial of Dazoxiben and Nifedipine in the treatment of Raynaud's phenomenon. Am J Med 77:451–456, 1984.

159. Emery H, Schaller JG: Biofeedback in the management of primary and secondary Raynaud's. Abstract presented to Fortieth Annual Meeting Am Rheum Assoc, Chicago, 1976.

160. Editorial from the NIH: Biofeedback for patients with Raynaud's phenomenon. JAMA 242:509–510, 1979.

161. Blanchard EB, Haynes MR: Biofeedback treatment of a case of Raynaud's disease. H Behav Ther Exp Psych 6:230–234, 1975.

162. Aratari E, Regesta G, Rebora A: Carpal tunnel syndrome appearing with prominent skin symptoms. Arch Dermatol 120:517–519, 1984.

163. Uno H, Parker F: Autonomic Innervation of the skin in primary erythermalgia. Arch Dermatol 119:65–71, 1983.

164. Michiels JJ, Abels J, Steketee J, et al: Erythromelalgia caused by platelet-mediated arteriolar inflammation and thrombosis in thrombocythemia. Ann Intern Med 102:466–471, 1985.

165. Paulson GS: Erythromelalgia: a case report and a review of the literature. Intern Med 4:112–126, 1983.

166. Deliss LJ, Wilson JN: Acute Blue Fingers in Women. J Bone Joint Surg 64B:458–459, 1982.

167. Ettein JT, Allen JT, Vargas C: Hypothenar Hammer Syndrome. Southern Med J 74:491–493, 1981.

168. Cho KO: Entrapment occlusion of the ulnar artery in the hand. J Bone Joint Surg 60A:841–843, 1978.

169. Williams HJ, Biddulph EC, Coleman SS, Ward JR: Isolated subcutaneous nodules (pseudorheumatoid). J Bone Joint Surg 59A:73–76, 1977.

169a. Rush PJ, Bernstein BH, Smith CR, et al.: Chronic arthritis following benign rheumatoid nodules of childhood. Arth Rheum 28:1175–1179, 1985.

170. Stern RE, Gauger DW: Pigmented villonodular tenosynovitis. J Bone Jt Surg 59:560–561, 1977.

171. Rao S, Vigorita VJ: Pigmented villonodular synovitis (giant cell tumor of the tendon sheath and synovial membrane) 81 cases. J Bone Joint Surg 66:76–94, 1984.

172. Bensen WG, Laskin CA, Little HA, Fam AG: Hemochromatotic arthropathy mimicking rheumatoid arthritis. Arth Rheum 21:844–848, 1978.

173. Fogel GR, Younge DA, Dobyns JH: Pitfalls in the diagnosis of the simple wrist ganglion. Ortho 6:990–992, 1983.

174. Sheon RP: A joint protection guide for nonarticular rheumatic disorders. Postgrad Med 77(5):329–338, 1985.

7

The Thoracic Cage and
Dorsal Spine Region

Myofascial and other chest wall pain syndromes may occur as entities in and of themselves, may be secondary manifestations of other systemic disorders, or may coexist with other serious underlying diseases. Thus, a careful history and physical examination are essential. The physician may categorize the various causes for chest pain according to whether they arise from structures superior to the chest, within the chest (intrathoracic), inferior to the chest, posterior to the chest, or from structures involving the chest wall. Multiple etiologies are often operative, and consideration for more than one disorder is important to good diagnosis and management. A hands-on examination must not end with the use of a stethoscope! Careful palpation for myofascial tender points should also be performed. Important danger signs and symptoms must be delineated (Table 7–1). In addition, a Decision Chart, Table 7–2, may be helpful.

Table 7–1. Danger Signs for the Thoracic Cage

1. Fever and chills.
2. Effort pain radiating to neck, or to left or both arms.
3. Numbness and weakness in an upper limb.
4. Pain that radiates to the mid thoracic spine.
5. Pain that refers to the shoulder blade area.
6. Thoracic spine pain that awakens the patient.
7. Hemoptysis.
8. Pleuritic pain.
9. Lymphadenopathy.
10. Pain that refers to the axilla.

Chest Pain Arising from Structures Superior to the Chest. Disturbances arising in the head, neck, or thoracic outlet, such as cervical disc disease or thoracic outlet syndrome, may give rise to referred pain that involves the chest region.[1,2,3] When chest pain results from thoracic outlet syndrome, the site of origin of the symptoms can usually be detected by characteristic manifestations involving the upper extremity (see "Thoracic Outlet Syndrome," Chapt. 3). Chest wall tenderness may also result from irritation of the cervical or vagus nerves.[1] The history should include the presence or absence of numbness and tingling in the upper limbs. Precordial chest pain and features of angina may be caused by cervical nerve root irritation.[4] In addition to chest wall tenderness and pain, these patients may have a positive Spurling test (see Chapt. 2) and cervical myofascial trigger points.[5] These patients improve after treatment to the neck including cervical traction.

Chest Pain of Intrathoracic Origin. A brief list of the intrathoracic origin of chest pain is seen in Table 7–3.[6]

To distinguish intrathoracic diseases causing chest pain, a careful history of the quality, duration, radiation, and precipitating causes of the pain must be undertaken. The pain of classic angina occurs in the retrosternal region and may radiate into the neck, left arm, and occasionally into the medial aspect of both upper arms. Angina is usually distinguishable from pain of chest wall origin by its brief duration, its aggravation by cold and exertion, and its relief with rest. Chest wall pain by contrast lasts for hours or days, occurs at rest, and may improve with general activ-

Table 7–2. Decision Chart, Chest Pain

Problem	Action	Other Actions

1. Chest pain, unilateral, nonacute.
  Duration for hours
  Not only effort induced
  Trigger points present
	CONSERVATIVE CARE
	Correct aggravating factors
	Prescribe exercises
	Antidepressants, relaxants
	General examination
		Bone scan
		NSAID trial
		GI workup
		Antidepressants

2. Chest pain, bilateral, nonacute
  tender costochondral joints,
  symmetric
  Chest expanse limited (<4 cm.)
	+ Bone scan, tests for
	  inflammation
		Trial NSAIDS

3. Chest pain, bilateral, nonacute
  Numbness of upper limbs present
	+ Examine for thoracic
	  outlet syndrome	

4. DANGER LIST
  Fever, chills
  Effort pain
  Pain radiation to mid thorax,
  shoulder
  Numbness and weakness,
  upper limb
  Hemoptysis
  Pleural pain
  Axillary pain
	Chest roentgenogram
	⟶ Workup as appropriate
	Urgent consultation
		GI workup
		Cardiac workup
		⟶ Roentgenographs of
		chest and neck

Table 7–3. Sources of Chest Pain of Intrathoracic Origin

1. Classic Heberden's angina (arteriosclerotic heart disease)
2. Angina of pulmonary hypertension or aortic stenosis
3. Prinzmetal's angina (arteriosclerotic heart disease)
4. Acute myocardial infarction
5. Dressler's syndrome
6. Postcardiotomy syndrome
7. Pericarditis
8. Mitral prolapse
9. Dissection of the aorta
10. Diseases of the pleura
11. Pulmonary embolism
12. Pneumothorax
13. Disease of the esophagus
14. Mediastinal or pulmonary neoplasms
15. Diaphragmatic irritation

ity. Pericardial pain, which is retrosternal, is often worse while recumbent and improves by sitting up or forward, and may be accentuated by deep breathing. Complaints of chest discomfort, fatigue, dyspnea, palpitations, tachycardia, anxiety, and neurotic behavior have been described in the past under various labels, including "neurocirculatory asthenia," Da Costa's syndrome, or "effort syndrome."[7] It has been suggested that similar symptoms may be related to mitral valve prolapse (systolic click) syndrome. Although an interesting speculation, no data are available that definitively relate such symptoms to this syndrome.[13]

Mitral valve prolapse is often asymptomatic. Some patients have a constellation of symptoms that include sudden severe aching in the chest and extremities, and vasomotor instability. When seen in a young woman, the chances are good that mitral valve prolapse will be present.[8] Coghlan studied 600 such patients and has suggested that these symptoms result from an abnormality in central (midbrain) regulation of autonomic function. Using tests that include responses to tilt-table, Valsalva maneuver, and a cold pressor test, the symptomatic patients showed a wildly oscillating heart rate, or prolonged bradycardia.[9] In other studies, higher than normal quantities of catecholamines were found in similar patients in one study,[10] but not in another.[11] Treatment with beta blockers or phenobarbital were often helpful. Some patients with mitral valve prolapse have an inherited disease of connective tissue with potential complications. Features of a high arched palate, striae, and joint laxity may suggest the Marfanoid syndrome, Ehlers-Danlos syndrome, or Marfan's syndrome and such patients may develop aortic dissection.[12]

Pleural pain is generally located on one side of the chest, is accentuated by breathing, and is generally not aggravated by movement. A common source of pain that arises from intrathoracic structures is the esophagus, particularly for that pain emanating from a hiatus hernia with reflex esophagitis. Such pain generally radiates to the anterior chest wall, may be accompanied by tenderness of the musculature of the chest wall, and is often exacerbated by recumbency. If the examiner exerts gentle pressure to the epigastrium, this maneuver frequently reproduces pain of esophageal origin.

Chest Pain Arising from Structures Inferior to the Chest. Chest pain may result from gas entrapment syndromes, biliary tract disease, peptic or gastric ulcer, pancreatitis, and subphrenic abscess.[3] A history of bowel dysfunction, weight loss, stool changes, or dietary indiscretion should provide clues to these conditions. Gastric ulcers may be present, with marked variability in history, severity, and chronicity. We have found radiographic examination of the upper gastrointestinal tract, with careful attention for gastric ulcer, essential for diagnosis when epigastric tenderness is observed, or when patients have intractable chest wall pain. Anterolateral or posterior chest pain may result from myofascial tender points in the rectus abdominis, serratus posterior inferior, iliocostalis, and other torso muscles.[14]

Chest Pain Arising from Disorders Posterior to the Chest. Chest pain may arise from herpes zoster and lesions of the dorsal spine, such as osteoporosis, tumor, Scheuermann's disease, and rarely, thoracic disc disease.[2]

Chest Pain Arising from the Chest Wall Structures. Rib trauma or fracture, metastatic tumors, and other lesions evident on radiographic examination may cause pain and local tenderness. Costochondritis is rarely a pathologic finding. However, scintigraphy has helped to identify an important group of patients. Whenever *bilateral* anterior chest wall pain and tenderness is noted in a patient under age 40, consider ankylosing spondylitis. Several such patients have been seen by us, even with normal tests of inflammation, but in whom a bone scan revealed positive findings in the costochondral joints, the sternoclavicular joints, and the sacroiliac joints. Use of gallium-67 scanning in a leukemia patient with costochondral joint tenderness was helpful in detecting a benign local inflammatory process rather than more serious disease in that patient. The follow-up scan and roentgenographs failed to demonstrate abnormality.[15] This technique is not recommended for routine use in diagnosis of costochondritis. The clinician should also consider diseases of the breasts and the regional lymph nodes. However, the vast majority of patients have benign myofascial chest wall pain syndromes.[1]

MYOFASCIAL CHEST WALL SYNDROMES

Included here are subacute and chronic painful conditions of the anterior chest wall associated with tenderness of the chest wall structures (Fig. 7–1 and Plate XIV). Swelling does not occur.

The commonly described myofascial chest wall syndromes include the costosternal syndrome, the sternalis syndrome, xiphoidalgia, and the rib-tip syndrome. Each of these descriptive syndromes is characterized by local

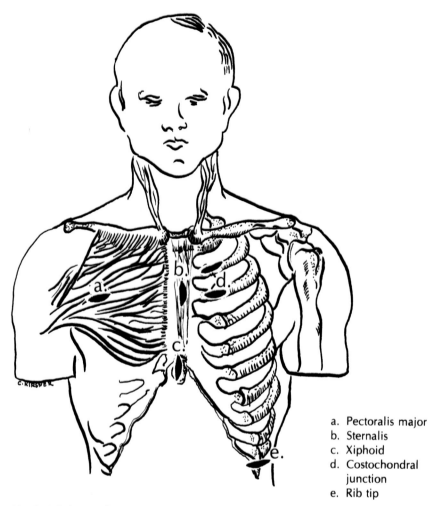

a. Pectoralis major
b. Sternalis
c. Xiphoid
d. Costochondral
   junction
e. Rib tip

Fig. 7–1. Myofascial chest wall pain: Myofascial trigger points may be found at the second or third left costo-chondral junction in the upper outer chest quadrant within the pectoralis major muscle, at the manubriosternal junction, at the tip of the xiphoid process, at the center of the sternum in the sternalis muscle, or on a lower rib tip.

chest wall tenderness with accompanying pain, of severity ranging from a dull ache to a throbbing intense discomfort. In these myofascial chest wall syndromes, pain is present at rest and during chest movement, lasts up to several hours or days, and may be related to breathing. Anxiety and hyperventilation are common accompaniments.[16] The episodes are often brief and self-limited, but occasionally myofascial chest wall pain syndrome is superimposed upon true angina and causes severe disability.[17] On occasion, nitroglycerin has relieved myofascial chest wall pain un-related to angina.[18] Although occasionally considered as one entity, *chest wall pain syndrome*,[17] most physicians prefer individual terminology, depending on points of maximum tenderness in the chest wall.[19] These syndromes require consideration for multifactorial diagnosis and treatment. These considerations will follow brief descriptions of the syndromes.

Costosternal Syndromes. This term applies to conditions involving and limited to pain in the anterior part of the chest wall. The pain sometimes radiates to the whole chest and is accentuated by deep inspiration.[20] The pains are usually intermittent, last a few days, and occur intermittently for months or years. The specific feature of costosternal syndrome is the presence of tenderness and pain reproduction during palpation at one or more costosternal junctions. Tenderness may also be noted along the nearby intercostal muscles. Relief from pain by anesthetic-corticosteroid injection of the involved costochondral joint is an additional feature of the syndrome.[20] The term "costochondritis" should be reserved for bilateral costosternal involvement by spondyloarthritis and other inflammatory rheumatic diseases.

The Sternalis Syndrome. The sternalis syndrome is the only myofascial disorder in which a trigger point gives rise to bilateral pain.[21] The trigger point is in the sternal synchondrosis, or in the sternalis muscle overlying the body of the sternum (Fig. 7–1). Pain is noted in the center of the chest wall, and usually the patient recognizes that the origin of the pain is in the chest wall region, rather than within the thorax. The symptoms tend to be less intermittent and the severity less frightening than those associated with the costosternal syndrome.

Xiphoidalgia. This syndrome is characterized by spontaneous pain in the anterior chest associated with distinct discomfort and tenderness of the xiphoid process of the sternum.[1] Pressure over the xiphoid reproduces the pain, which is intermittent, and often aggravated by eating a heavy meal, lifting, stooping, bending, or twisting. Intralesional injection with a local anesthetic can provide prompt temporary or permanent relief, and will aid in diagnosis.[22]

Rib-Tip Syndrome. This syndrome differs in that the patient presents with severe lancinating pain associated with hypermobility of the anterior end of a costal cartilage, most often the tenth rib, but occasionally involving the eighth or ninth rib.[23] The syndrome, variously called slipping rib, slipping rib cartilage syndrome, or clicking rib refers to hypermobility of a rib-tip. Digital pressure over

the involved rib may reproduce a painful clicking. The slipping rib syndrome results from recurrent subluxation of a costal cartilage, and is associated with a stabbing or lancinating pain.[24] The pain is easily confused with abdominal visceral disease.[25] Injury or indirect trauma due to lifting or twisting is often the cause.[26,27] Other features of the syndrome include pain aggravated by arm abduction, audible clicking sensation in the chest wall, and relief of pain by lying down.[27]

Physical examination includes the "hooking maneuver"—the examiner's curved fingers are hooked under the ribs at the costal margin and the examiner gently pulls the rib cage anteriorly[25] (Fig. 7–2); this reproduces the snap and pain. Excision of the involved rib has been recommended, but a steroid-local anesthetic injection into the intercostal muscles adjacent to a slipping rib may be of value. In other cases, only the rib-tip of the lower ribs is tender, and the pain is self-limited. Physical examination for myofascial chest pain should include a measurement of chest expansion. Inflammatory rheumatic disease of the chest wall (e.g., ankylosing spondylitis)

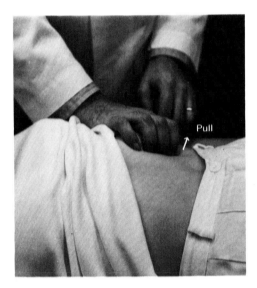

Fig. 7–2. The hooking maneuver: The examiner's curved fingers are hooked under the lower ribs, then the rib cage is gently pulled anteriorly. This reproduces a snapping sensation and pain.

restricts chest expansion to 1½ inches (3 cm) or less, and may inflame the sternocostal joints.[9]

Tests and Maneuvers for Myofascial Chest Wall Pain Syndromes. Thoracic spine motion, spinal curves, and symmetry of the chest wall and the breasts should be evaluated. Careful palpation of the supraclavicular fossae and axillae for lymphadenopathy should be performed. Palpation is best performed beginning with the acromioclavicular joints, continuing to the sternoclavicular joints, and then down each of the costosternal joints. The sternal synchondrosis, the overlying sternalis muscle, and the xiphoid process should be palpated. Xiphoidalgia must be distinguished from the deeper epigastric tenderness of gastrointestinal disease. A helpful way to distinguish these is to compare the tenderness to palpation in the epigastrium while the patient performs a partial sit-up, with the severity of discomfort during palpation while the patient is relaxed and recumbent. Xiphoidalgia and superficial lower chest wall pain are worse during the partial sit-up. Conversely, true intra-abdominal lesion tenderness is diminished during contraction of the superficial abdominal muscles, and worsens when the abdominal muscles are relaxed.

The distinguishing characteristic of myofascial chest pain is the ability to reproduce the pain state by local pressure.[17] Associated trigger points may also be found over the pectoralis muscles, the lower sternocleidomastoid area,[1] the tip of the lower costal cartilages,[23] and most commonly, the third left costochondral joint.[28] Bilateral chest wall pain may result from a trigger point in the sternalis muscle.[21] "If local pressure applied to the anterior part of the chest wall becomes a routine procedure in the physical examination of all patients with precordial pain, a surprisingly large number of cases of costosternal syndromes will be discovered."[20]

Etiology. Inflammatory rheumatic disease can cause myofascial symptoms and must be excluded. Anxiety is common in patients with chest wall pain syndrome. However, psychologic investigations suggest that pure psychogenic chest pain is uncommon.[29] Myofascial chest wall pain syndrome usually results from "misuse" activity, similar to that which causes myofascial pain in other body regions. An attack of chest wall pain may follow prolonged sitting in a slouched position or after assuming a bent-over position.[30] The pectoral muscles may be overworked in activities that require repeated adduction of the arm across the chest (e.g., stacking logs, polishing a car). A pain-spasm-pain cycle may ensue, which is aggravated by anxiety.[31] The clinician must consider household chores, job, and hobbies as possible aggravating factors. Smokers who cough are not only at risk for developing these syndromes, but often their response to treatment is less satisfactory unless smoking is curtailed (see Table 7–4).

Laboratory and Radiographic Examination. Myofascial chest wall pain has no specific laboratory abnormalities. An erythrocyte sedimentation rate is useful to exclude tumors or other inflammatory processes. A roentgenogram of the chest and an electrocardiogram are required for most patients. Calcification of costal cartilages is commonly present, and any association to the pain is speculative.[32] Scintigraphy may be considered for patients with bilateral tender costochondral joints. When costochondritis is due to a spondyloarthropathy, the scan may demonstrate involvement of symmetric costochondral joints. An upper gastrointestinal radiographic examination is often helpful. Electrodiagnostic testing of the upper extremities, on occasion, helps delineate chest wall pain that results from cervical nerve root impingement.

Differential Diagnosis. In most cases, chest wall pain syndromes can be differentiated from other more serious disorders that were discussed earlier in this chapter.[33] In one community hospital emergency room, only 7 of 50 consecutive patients seen for chest pain had coronary artery disease.[34] Myofascial chest wall pain was the cause for chest pain in the majority of the remaining patients, and in another study was responsible for approximately 2% of all office visits.[28] The patient with *psychogenic chest wall pain* presents with atypical chest pain that bears no relation to activity, time of day, or thoracic structures. The pain is usually centered over the cardiac apex. There are no discrete trigger points that reproduce the pain. Such pain frequently accompanies anxiety and depression, has an emotional precipitant, and generally does not awaken the patient.[29] A chest wall pain syndrome may be the presenting feature of the fibrositis syndrome. Such patients will demonstrate tender points in other typical locations, and have morning fatigue and aching (Chapt. 13).

Management. Most attacks of myofascial chest wall pain are self-limited, and the patient may require only reassurance.[1] For patients with subacute and chronic recurring myofascial chest wall pain, these six steps for management should be followed:

1. Exclude other organic disease.
2. Provide an explanation for the patient. The presence of a myofascial trigger point goes far to demonstrate to the patient that the pain does originate outside his head or heart. The physician should briefly describe the pain-spasm-pain cycle and its aggravation by fatigue or emotion.
3. Recognize and eliminate aggravating factors (Table 7–4). These include improper posture while sitting or working, misuse of pectoralis major muscles, and prolonged sedentary activities, such as typing. Smokers should be encouraged to quit. Often group therapy is available for this purpose.
4. Provide self-help exercises. The most helpful stretching exercise for the chest wall is the cornering exercise, or the standing push-up in a corner[35] (Table 7–5, Exercise 1). Posture correction exercises may also be necessary (Exercise 2, Table 7–5).
5. Provide for relief from pain. Pain of myofascial chest wall trigger points may be relieved either by applying a vapocoolant spray,[1,31] or by local injection with a steroid-local anesthetic mixture (Fig. 7–4). At least two thirds of

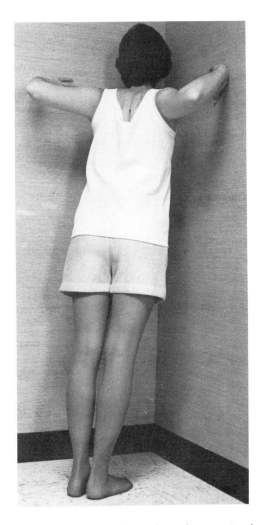

Fig. 7–3. Pectoral muscle stretching: The corner "push up" is performed with the patient standing approximately 2 feet out from the corner and both arms raised to shoulder height, hands placed on each wall, fingers pointing in toward the corner. Hands are 18 to 30 inches out from the corner to each side. The patient gently and progressively pushes into the corner until a pulling sensation is felt in the pectoral region.

the patients obtain good results with these methods.[20] Intralesional injection is best carried out with a one inch #23 needle, 1 or 2 ml of 1% local anesthetic mixed with 1 ml methylprednisolone. After careful skin preparation, the needle is used as a guide to locate the point of maximum tenderness. When multiple lesions are present, the total

Table 7–4.   Joint Protection Guide for the Chest (From Sheon RP #89)

Harmful	Helpful
■ Carrying heavy objects (e.g., logs, grocery bags) across the chest can strain muscles in the chest wall and cause sudden, severe chest pain.	■ Turn and face the object, then lift it, and use the body, not just the arms, to carry it.
■ Smoking-induced coughing aggravates chest wall pain.	■ Stop smoking!
■ Sleeping with the arms overhead can pinch nerves, which in turn can cause chest wall muscles to tighten up.	■ Sleep with the arms below the level of the chest.
■ Arching the spine backward during exercise or while working with the arms overhead (e.g., painting a ceiling) can lead to bursitis of the spine.	■ Cautiously try extension exercises; discontinue if painful. Do not arch backward while working with the arms overhead.

Table 7–5.   Exercises for Thoracic Cage Region

1. Stretching the chest: A corner pushup is performed by standing 2 feet from the corner of a room, place each hand at shoulder height, and 2 feet from the corner. Then press chest into corner until the chest muscles and ribs are stretched. Keep chin neutral like a soldier. The stretch is maintained for 20 seconds and repeated 3 times for 1 minute, and performed at least twice daily (Fig. 7–3).
2. Upper back straightening: Lean across a kitchen table or counter with abdomen, chest, and nose against surface. Place hands behind on buttock. Keep chin neutral. Draw shoulders backward. Raise the head and chest together as a block, up about 2 to 4 inches while keeping abdomen against table. Hold 10 to 20 seconds; repeat 3 to 5 times twice daily (Fig. 7–10).

dose of the 2 to 3 ml mixture can be used divided among the lesions (Table 15–4, page 298). The vapocoolant spray, Fluori-methane, may be applied as a fine thin spray at a 30 degree angle to the skin, moving in one direction only, from the tender point toward the pain zone, about 4 inches per second and for 2 to 3 sweeps per treatment.[36]

6. Project an expected outcome. Most patients with myofascial chest wall pain

who follow these management principles obtain good relief in 3 to 6 weeks. The exercises should be kept up for at least 3 weeks following relief. The patient must conscientiously avoid improper posture or repeated misuse of chest wall muscles.

When the chest wall pain syndrome and underlying arteriosclerotic heart disease coexist, careful attention to treatment of both disorders is essential. Smoking should be discontinued, since a chronic cough may cause chest wall muscle fatigue and subsequent spasm. Similarly, patients with chest wall pain superimposed upon chronic bronchitis and emphysema should stop smoking. Relaxation techniques and biofeedback training along with physical therapy are helpful. Patients with no other underlying cause for continued distress should be closely reevaluated for other causes. A trial of antidepressant medication may be rewarding. Although muscle relaxants have not proved helpful, drugs to control anxiety may be useful in an overly anxious patient. Amitriptyline and other tricyclics may be beneficial for sleep disturbances or nocturnal panic that sometimes occur in these patients. The value of analgesic compounds is limited, but prescribing the nonsteroidal anti-inflammatory agents may be worthwhile, especially if tests of inflammation suggest the possibility of a spon-

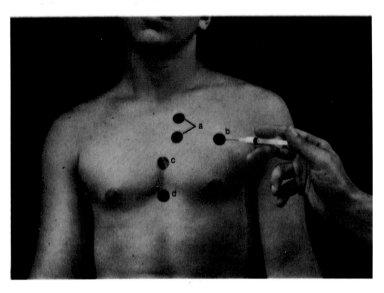

Fig. 7–4. Sites for injection: (a) second and third costochondral junctions, (b) pectoralis major muscle, (c) sternalis muscle, and (d) xiphoid process.

dyloarthritis underlying the chest pain syndrome. In some patients a therapeutic trial using a nitroglycerine compound may be rewarding. When relief does occur, it is not necessarily proof of the presence of arteriosclerotic heart disease.[17]

TIETZE'S SYNDROME[16a]

Costochondral region pain associated with *enlargement* of an upper costochondral cartilage characterizes this syndrome[16] (Fig. 7–5). Tietze's syndrome may be acute, intermittent, or chronic. The swelling is firm to bony hard, slightly elongated, or less often, round. This feature of swelling, not seen in other myofascial chest wall pain syndromes, needs emphasis. It is for this reason that Tietze's syndrome is considered separate from other chest wall pain syndromes. In approximately 80% of cases the lesion is single. Most often it occurs in the second costochondral junction, and less often in the third costochondral junction on either side.[37] The swelling is nonsuppurative, tender, and histologically reveals increased vascularity with proliferation of columns of cartilage. Cleft formation with mucoid debris is seen.[38] The

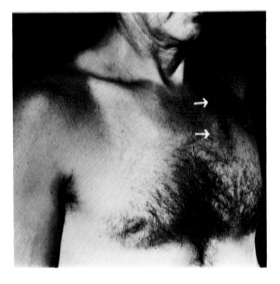

Fig. 7–5. The Tietze's syndrome lesion. Costochondral swelling is observed. (Photograph courtesy Dr. John Calabro, Worcester, Mass.)

etiology is unknown. Radiographic examination is usually not helpful, and tests for inflammation are generally normal. Differential diagnoses include mainly sepsis or tumors of the underlying rib, or pain from intrathoracic structures. Radiographic examination may be required periodically to exclude other diseases. Although spontaneous remission generally occurs, months or years may elapse before improvement is noted. Biopsy of the rib may be required for reassurance. We have found local injections with a corticosteroid-anesthetic mixture effective. Patients with persistent symptoms may be helped by local physical therapy, including hot or cold applications, and nonsteroidal anti-inflammatory drugs.

JUVENILE KYPHOSIS (SCHEUERMANN'S DISEASE)

During puberty a child may be noted to have a slouched appearance, and may be

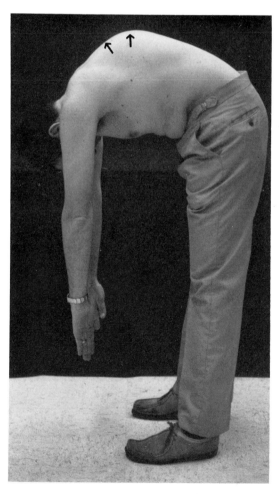

Fig. 7–6. Dorsal kyphosis may be a result of Scheuermann's disease or may be simply a postural deformity, the adult round back.

brought to the physician for "poor posture." The child may or may not complain of discomfort. One cause of the kyphosis of adolescence is an epiphysitis of the dorsal vertebrae, accompanied clinically by forward-sloping shoulders, and a round back (Fig. 7–6). Most commonly, the disease appears in the early years of the second decade of life, but may first be detected in adulthood.

The kyphosis of Scheuermann's disease is accompanied by vertebral abnormalities that can be seen on roentgenographs as vertebral end-plate irregularities, and wedging of the vertebral body.[39-43] In one study of 500 children, aged 17 and 18, 56% of males and 30% of females had roentgenographic evidence of previous Scheuermann's disease.[44] This high incidence requires further substantiation. Tight hamstrings was significantly related to the disorder in males. Nonspecific kyphosis, such as adult round back, which is a postural deformity, occurs commonly in young persons, but vertebral abnormalities are not seen.[40] Juvenile kyphosis with epiphysitis (Scheuermann's disease) is accompanied by pain in up to 60% of patients, and scoliosis in 30 to 40% of patients.[40] The pain is often worse with rest and after prolonged activity, and is characterized by a dull ache in the mid-dorsal spine region between the scapulae, or diffusely in the mid-back region. This pain usually does not awaken the patient. There are no associated neurologic signs or symptoms.

Avascular necrosis of the vertebral end plate, herniation of intervertebral disc material, metabolic, endocrine, and vitamin deficiency factors have all been implicated in causation of this entity.[39] The central artery to the vertebral end plate, which usually is obliterated by the age of six, has been noted to persist in patients until age 13 in Scheuermann's disease. The persistence of this vessel beyond the normal time span is thought to lead to irregularity of the vertebral end plate.[43] In a recent investigation of the pathology of two patients with Scheuermann's disease, Bradford noted bone, cartilage and disc to be normal on histologic and electron microscopic study.[41] There was no definite evidence of avascular necrosis. However, gross examination revealed wedging and collapsing of the vertebral body with a normal disc width. Breaks in the vertebral end plate were found with protrusion of disc material into the bony spongiosum.[45] Bradford speculates that perhaps osteoporosis plays a role, although the etiology still remains unknown.[41]

No abnormalities have been noted in calcium or phosphorus values, or in tests for inflammatory processes. As noted, character-

istic radiographic features include vertebral end-plate irregularity, Schmorl's nodes, and anterior wedging of the involved vertebrae[39,40] (Fig. 7–7).

Juvenile ankylosing spondylitis must be considered in the differential diagnosis of Scheuermann's disease. A history of iritis, heel pain, or synovitis of lower extremity joints in a male suggests HLA-B27 associated spondyloarthropathies. Leukemia, hemangioma of the vertebra, juvenile osteoporosis, and osteomalacia must be considered. These disorders which may have spinal involve-

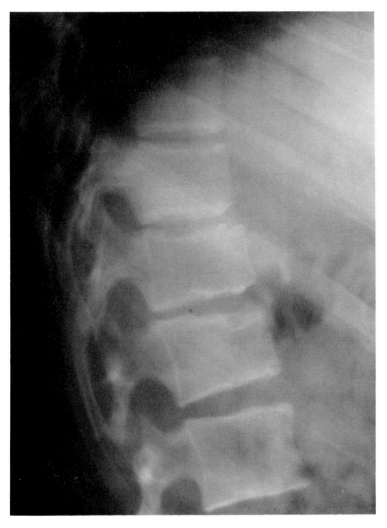

Fig. 7–7. Radiographic features of Scheuermann's epiphysitis include vertebral end-plate irregularity, herniation into the vertebral body, and anterior vertebral wedging. (Courtesy of Toledo Hospital.)

ment, are usually readily identified by characteristic radiographic features.[42]

Management. Management includes advising parents to stop nagging the child just to "straighten up."[42] All patients should be taught an exercise program to strengthen the extensor muscles of the dorsal spine. Hyperextension exercises should be performed at the same time as pelvic tilting. This is best performed by having the patient bend over a table or ironing board flexing the hips, with the chest and abdomen in contact with the tabletop. While in this position, the patient raises the head and shoulders thus hyperextending the dorsal spine. This position is held for 10 to 30 seconds and performed for 6 to 10 repetitions twice daily. Shoulder shrugging and scapular abduction exercises may help reverse the forward inclination of the shoulders (see Table 4–5). If the kyphosis is greater than 40 degrees, a cosmetically significant deformity is noted. It is wise to refer the patient to an orthopedist who may prescribe a Milwaukee brace to improve the kyphosis and prevent the need for surgery.[39,42,46] Improvement in the kyphotic deformity is likely if treatment is begun early in the course of the disease.

OSTEOPOROSIS AND OSTEOMALACIA (OSTEOPENIA)

Osteoporosis commonly presents as back pain with segmental radiation in the distribution of the contiguous nerve roots. Sitting often aggravates the pain. The patient may be disturbed by muscle spasm during the night. Dorsal kyphosis, "dowager hump," and loss of height may be noted; T-12 and L-1 are the most common vertebrae involved.[40] Occasionally, radiographic evidence of osteoporosis and vertebral compression fracture may be observed in asymptomatic individuals.[40] Limb fracture or periodontal disease often precede the spinal complaints.[47–51] In postmenopausal osteoporosis trabecular bone loss occurs during the first 10 years after menopause; whereas cortical bone loss continues linearly and indefinitely by endosteal absorp-

tion. The rapid trabecular bone loss may lead to fractures before the age of 65, whereas the insidious cortical loss leads to femoral neck fractures after age 65.[52]

Etiology. The etiology of osteoporosis is uncertain and complex. Many patients have a combination of both osteoporosis and osteomalacia.[42] Accordingly, the term osteopenia of bone may be preferred. Osteoporosis, characterized by loss of osteoid and mineral, is contrasted to osteomalacia, in which the primary defect is related to mineral loss alone. Factors strongly considered causative in the etiology of osteoporosis include estrogen deficiency, age, genetic factors, physical disuse, and steroid therapy.[53–58]

Riggs and Melton[52] suggest two distinct syndromes of osteoporosis: Type I osteoporosis consists of a small subset of postmenopausal women under age 65 and some men. Type II osteoporosis occurs in a large proportion of women or men older than 75 years of age. The distal limb and vertebral fractures is typical of the Type I osteoporosis and is due to loss of trabecular bone. Fractures of the hip, proximal humerus, femur, pelvis, and proximal tibia are typical of Type II osteoporosis with loss of cortical bone. Decreased parathyroid hormone and decreased estrogen may occur in Type I, and increased parathyroid hormone may occur in Type II osteoporosis. Increased parathyroid hormone may be in response to decreased calcium absorption caused by impaired metabolism of 25-hydroxyvitamin D to 1,25-dihydroxyvitamin D.[50,52,59–61] Postmenopausal osteoporotic women were noted to have lower total body calcium levels, had undergone earlier menopause, smoked more cigarettes, had lower levels of estrone, estradiol, testosterone, 25-hydroxyvitamin D, 24,25-dihydroxyvitamin D, and 1,25-dihydroxyvitamin D than did age-matched control women.[62] Younger women who had oophorectomy during young adulthood had findings of bone loss nearly as great as that seen in older postmenopausal women.[63] These findings support the contributions of estrogen deficiency in some patients who develop osteoporosis.

Additional considerations in men included a relationship of osteoporosis to smoking and drinking, whereas obesity was protective.[64] The involved women tend to be northern European, short, and have thin skin and a higher rate of dental loss. The possibility that a subset of women might have osteogenesis imperfecta was raised.[65]

Laboratory and Radiographic Examination. Wedging, collapse, codfish deformity, Schmorl's nodes, vertebral end-plate irreg-

ularity and general demineralization are noted on radiographs to some degree in all patients with osteoporosis[48] (Fig. 7–8). Pseudofractures (Looser zones or Milkman's lines) (Fig. 7–9), although pathognomonic for osteomalacia, occur in less than 10% of such patients; bone biopsy is the only definite way to diagnose senescent osteomalacia.[54] Bone scans,[53] determination of serum calcium, phosphorus, alkaline phosphatase, and vitamin D levels (if available), and measures of

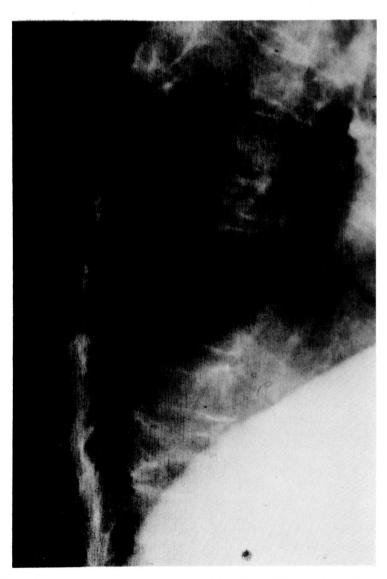

Fig. 7–8. Radiographic features of osteoporosis include wedging of the vertebra anteriorly with vertebral collapse, vertebral end-plate irregularity, and general demineralization. (Courtesy of Toledo Hospital.)

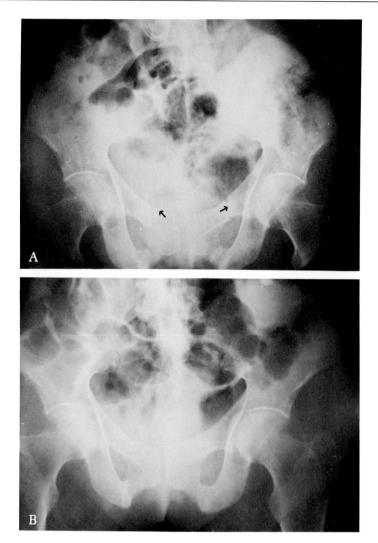

Fig. 7–9. *A,* Pseudofractures (Looser zones or Milkman's lines) are evident on the pubic rami, and, *B,* they readily disappear following treatment as seen in the follow-up roentgenograph.

thyroid function are useful in excluding some of the many causes of osteopenia.[54]

Primary osteoporosis must be a diagnosis of exclusion. The clinician must consider all disorders that can cause secondary osteopenia. Among the important entities to be excluded are primary or metastatic malignant disease, multiple myeloma, and causes of osteomalacia, such as malabsorption syndrome and drug-induced disease as seen in patients on long-term phenytoin (Dilantin) therapy.[40,48,54,57,66] Furosemide, used widely for treatment of hypertension and edema is cal-

ciuric, whereas the thiazides tend to conserve calcium.[67]

Bone biopsy, dual-photon absorptiometry, computed tomography[68–70] and radiographic photodensitomitry are techniques that may provide further information useful for epidemiology, etiology, and for individualized treatment.

Management. The goals of management of osteopenia are to alleviate symptoms and arrest disease progression.[48] Although there is only limited evidence that any presently available treatment can restore bone toward normal, dietary and physical methods of treatment may be useful. Additional therapy is aimed at preventing further loss of calcification and stimulating bone formation rather than simply symptomatic care.[48] Exercise, especially daily walks, is a recommended means of retarding progression of osteoporosis.[56,71] Severe pain from fractures may require bracing to allow ambulation. Prolonged bracing immobilizes the spine and can accentuate the osteoporotic process. Accordingly, bracing for pain relief should be discontinued when symptoms permit. Patients should avoid carbonated beverages at mealtime, since these retard calcium absorption. Other dietary recommendations include maintaining ideal weight and eating foods high in calcium, such as dairy products. Postmenopausal women and persons with lactase deficiency should have elemental calcium intake of 1000 to 1500 mg/day.[72] An extension exercise program can be helpful to alleviate back pain[73] (see Exercise #2 Table 7–5 and Figure 7–10).

Other current recommendations for treatment of various forms of osteoporosis include estrogen, calcium, vitamin D; and fluoride only in cases of recurrent fractures.[51,54,58,72,74] Calcitonin has also been shown to increase total body calcium and may be of benefit in patients with osteoporosis. Vertebral compression fractures were not prevented from occurring or progressing in one controlled study.[75] Calcitonin requires daily parenteral administration and may be accompanied by local irritation.[75] Patients with mixed osteoporosis and osteomalacia, and patients who have steroid induced osteoporosis may benefit from the addition of vitamin D in doses of 50,000 units 1 to 3 times per week.[48,54,76,77] Patients on long-term corticosteroid treatment may be given this treatment regimen for the prevention of bone loss secondary to the chronic steroid use.[77,78] 1,25-dihydroxyvitamin D may result in *worsening* of osteoporosis since this vitamin can result in stimulation of bone *resorption*.[51]

The use of estrogen is suggested in the first 2 years of menopause. Dosage is important. Ethinyl estradiol in doses below 15 μg per day were associated with a net loss of bone (measured by sequential change in cortical diameters of metacarpals), whereas doses of 25 μ or more per day were associated with a net gain in cortical bone.[79] Weiss et al. noted a 50 to 60% lower risk of fracture in women who had used estrogens for 6 years or longer than women who did not use estrogen.[80] The value of these agents versus these agents alone and fluoride were the subject of a controlled study. The use of calcium alone or with vitamin D or estrogen; these agents plus fluoride; and a no treatment group were compared. New fractures (rate per thousand person years) were: 834 in untreated patients; 419 in those given calcium with or without vitamin D; 304 in those given fluoride with calcium with or without vitamin D; 181 in those given estrogen and calcium with or without vitamin D; and 53 in those given fluoride, estrogen, and calcium with or without vitamin D.[81]

The use of fluoride has been associated with bone pain in the lower limbs. These patients were studied prospectively by O'Duffy et al. who found that symptoms began about 3 months after starting fluoride therapy. Swollen ankles were noted in 4/5 patients. Scintigraphy revealed abnormal uptake in tarsal bones, tibias, and femurs. These findings suggest intense bone remodeling and was improved only when fluoride treatment was discontinued.[82] Increased microfractures of bone has also been a concern of fluoride treatment.[74] In a previous report of 36 patients studied prospectively, 15 had major adverse reactions using sodium fluoride in doses of 40 to 60 mg daily.[83] Fluoride use should be limited to 6 months of therapy.

A costoiliac impingement syndrome may develop following multiple vertebral fractures. In such patients who have significant loss of height of the trunk, the lowest rib may become impinged against the iliac crest. This results in pain in the region of the twelfth thoracic vertebra and radiates to the posterolateral trunk. In 6 patients, surgical resection of the rib provided pain relief. No further impingement occurred in follow-up of 5 to 34 months.[84]

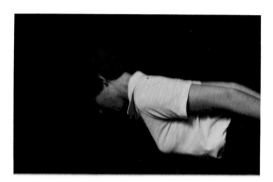

Fig. 7–10. Extension exercise for the upper back.

HERNIATED DORSAL INTERVERTEBRAL DISC

Although this disorder represents less than 1% of all patients undergoing operation for spinal disc disease,[55,56] a herniated dorsal intervertebral disc must be considered in the differential diagnosis of thoracic back pain. Patients with thoracic disc protrusion rarely have night pain, and there usually is no paraspinal muscle spasm. The patients do have radicular pain and sensory findings that can be intermittent or constant. Pain complaints include a dull diffuse backache. Of these patients, 50% have weakness or spasticity of the lower extremities.

Love and Schorn reviewed their experience with 61 patients in whom surgery verified thoracic disc protrusion.[55] Duration of symptoms before surgery was 1 to 2 years; gradual worsening of symptoms including pain, numbness, weakness of the lower extremities, and rarely, urinary retention or spinal shock occurred; 50% had features of bilateral spastic paralysis. Slight atrophy of the small muscles of the hand (T-1 protruded disc), or atrophy of lower extremity muscles were only seen occasionally; reflexes at the knee and ankle were often hyperactive. Positive Babinski reflexes occurred in half of the patients. Spinal fluid findings were often normal, and cerebrospinal fluid protein was elevated above 50 mg/100 ml in less than half of the patients.

Roentgenograms of the spinal column occasionally revealed calcification of the tho-racic intervertebral disc, which proved to be the offending disc in every instance. Only one myelogram was normal among those studied. Computed tomography and electrodiagnostic studies were not available. Lesions found at surgery included seven instances in which the disc eroded through the anterior dura; in one case a spicule of disc material actually penetrated the spinal cord. Two cases of hematomyelia of the cord and two cases of posterior infarction of the cord at the level of the protruded disc were encountered.[85] Unfortunately, patients with a severe neurologic deficit were not improved by surgical intervention. A wide complete laminectomy of two or more vertebrae was the procedure of choice recommended by Love and Schorn.[85] Ransohoff[87] and others[88] have shown that the surgical failures resulted because of the posterior surgical approach. They recommend the anterior or anterolateral approach, which has significantly improved the outcome.

REFERENCES

1. Wehrmacher W: The painful anterior chest wall syndromes. Med Clin N Am 42:111–118, 1958.
2. Edmeads J: Pain arising from thoracic nerves, nerve roots and spinal cord. *In* Chest Pain: An integrated diagnostic approach. Edited by DL Levene. Philadelphia, Lea & Febiger, 1977.
3. Saibil FG, Edmeads J: Pain arising from extrathoracic structures. *In* Chest Pain: An integrated diagnostic approach. Edited by DL Levene. Philadelphia, Lea & Febiger, 1977.
4. Myers G, Freeman R, Scharf D, et al: Cervicoprecordial angina: Diagnosis and management. Am J Cardiol 39:287, 1977 (Abstract).
5. Nachlas W: Pseudo-angina pectoris originating in the cervical spine. JAMA 103:323–325, 1934.
6. Levene DL, Davies GM, Saibil FG: Chest pain arising from intrathoracic structures. *In* Chest Pain: An integrated diagnostic approach. Edited by DL Levene. Philadelphia, Lea & Febiger, 1977.
7. Wooley CF: Where are the diseases of yesteryear? Circulation 53:749–751, 1976.
8. Spiera H, Swerdlow F, Meller J: A musculoskeletal syndrome associated with mitral valve prolapse. (Abstract E55) Arth Rheum 28(4) [Supp], 1985.
9. Coghlan HC, Phares P, Cowley M, et al: Dysautonomia in mitral valve prolapse. Am J Med 67:236–244, 1979.
10. Gonzalez ER: The 'nonneurotic' approach to mitral valve prolapse. JAMA 246:2113–2120, 1981.
11. Chesler E, Weir EK, Braatz GA, Francis GS: Nor-

mal catecholamine and hemodynamic response to orthostatic tilt in subjects with mitral valve prolapse. Am J Med 78:754–760, 1985.

12. Perloff JK: Evolving concepts of mitral-valve prolapse. N Engl J Med 307:369–370, 1982.

13. Gelfand ML, Kronzon I, Decarolis P, Winer HE: Mitral valve systolic click syndrome. Am Fam Phys 21:135–141, 1980.

14. Simons DG, Travell JG: Myofascial origins of low back pain—1. Principles of diagnosis and treatment. Postgrad Med 73:66–108, 1983.

15. Miller JH: Accumulation of Gallium-67 in costochondritis. Clin Nucl Med 5:362–363, 1980.

16. Pinals RS: Traumatic arthritis and allied conditions. In Arthritis and Allied Conditions. 10th Ed. Edited by DJ McCarty. Philadelphia, Lea & Febiger, 1985.

16a.Tietze A: Uebver eine eigenartige Haufung von Fallen mit Dystrophie der Rippenlenorpel. Klin Wehnschr 58:829–831, 1921.

17. Epstein, SE, Gerber LH, Borer JS: Chest wall syndrome: A common cause of unexplained cardiac pain. JAMA 241:2793–2797, 1979.

18. Master AM: The spectrum of anginal and noncardiac chest pain. JAMA 187:894–899, 1964.

19. Hench PK: Nonarticular rheumatism. In Rheumatic Diseases: Diagnosis and Management. Edited by WA Katz. Philadelphia, JB Lippincott, 1977.

20. Wolf E, Stern S: Costosternal syndrome. Arch Intern Med 136:189–191, 1976.

21. Pace JB: Commonly overlooked pain syndromes responsive to simple therapy. Postgrad Med 58:107–113, 1975.

22. Sklaroff HJ: Xiphodynia—another cause of atypical chest pain: six case reports. Mt Sinai J Med 46:546–548, 1979.

23. McBeath AA, Keene JS: The rib-tip syndrome. J Bone Joint Surg 57-A:795–797, 1975.

24. Davies-Colley R: Slipping rib. Br Med J 1:432, 1922.

25. Heinz GJ, Zavala DC: Slipping rib syndrome: Diagnosis using the "hooking maneuver." JAMA 237:794–795, 1977.

26. Holmes JF: A study of the slipping rib cartilage syndrome. N Engl J Med 224:928–932, 1941.

27. Ballon HC, Spector L: Slipping rib. Can Med Assoc J 39:355–358, 1938.

28. Benson EH, Zavala DC: Importance of the costochondral syndrome in evaluation of chest pain. JAMA 156:1244–1246, 1954.

29. Billings RF: Chest pain related to emotional disorders. In Chest Pain: An integrated diagnostic approach. Edited by DL Levene. Philadelphia, Lea & Febiger, 1977.

30. Miller AJ, Texidor, TA: "Precordial catch," a neglected syndrome of precordial pain. JAMA 159:1364–1365, 1955.

31. Travell J, Rinzler SH: Pain syndromes of the chest muscles: Resemblance to effort angina and myocardial infarction. and relief by local block. Can Med Assoc J 59:333–338, 1948.

32. Lovshin L: Personal communication.

33. Greenfield, S, Nadler MA, Morgan MT, Shine KI: The clinical investigation and management of chest pain in an emergency department: Quality assessment by criteria mapping. Med Care 15:898–905, 1977.

34. Mohan LA: Personal communication.

35. Swezey RL: Arthritis: Rational Therapy and Rehabilitation. Philadelphia, WB Saunders, 1978.

36. Travell JG, Simons DG: Myofascial Pain and Dysfunction. The Trigger Point Manual, Baltimore, Williams & Wilkins, 1983.

37. Levey GS, Calabro JJ: Tietze's syndrome: Report of two cases and review of the literature. Arth Rheum 5:261–269, 1962.

38. Cameron HU, Fornasier VL: Tietze's disease. J Clin Pathol 27:960–962, 1974.

39. Bradford DS, Moe JH, Winter RB: Kyphosis and postural roundback deformity in children and adolescents. Minn Med 56:114–120, 1973.

40. Benson DR: The back: Thoracic and lumbar spine. In Musculoskeletal Disorders. Edited by RD D'Ambrosia. Philadelphia, JB Lippincott, 1977.

41. Bradford DS, Moe JH: Scheuermann's juvenile kyphosis. Clin Orthop 110:45–53, 1975.

42. Winter RB, Hall JE: Kyphosis in childhood and adolescence. Spine 3:285–308, 1978.

43. Turek SL: Orthopaedics: Principles and Their Applications. 4th Ed. Philadelphia, JB Lippincott, 1984.

44. Fisk JW, Baigent ML, Hill PD: Scheuermann's disease: clinical and radiological survey of 17 and 18 year olds. Am J Phys Med 63:18–30, 1984.

45. Hilton RC, Ball J, Benn RT: Vertebral end-plate lesions (Schmorl's nodes) in the dorsolumbar spine. Ann Rheum Dis 35:127–132, 1976.

46. Levine DB: The painful low back. In Arthritis and Allied Conditions. 10th Ed. Edited by DJ McCarty, Philadelphia, Lea & Febiger, 1985.

47. Krook, L, Whalen JP, Lesser GV, Berens DL: Experimental studies on osteoporosis. Methods Achiev Exp Pathol 7:72–108, 1975.

48. Hahn BH: Osteopenic bone disease. In Arthritis and Allied Conditions. 10th Ed. Edited by DJ McCarty. Philadelphia, Lea & Febiger, 1985.

49. Khairi MR, Johnston CC: What we know—and don't know—about bone loss in the elderly. Geriatrics 33:67–76, 1978.

50. Aaron JE, Gallagher JC, Anderson J, et al: Frequency of osteomalacia and osteoporosis in fractures in the proximal femur. Lancet 1:229–233, 1974.

51. Raisz LG: Clinical strategy in osteopenia. Hosp Pract 13:11–12, 1978.

52. Riggs BL, Melton LJ: Evidence for two distinct syndromes of involutional osteoporosis. Am J Med 75:899–901, 1983.

53. Mundy GR: Differential diagnosis of osteopenia. Hosp Pract 13:65–72, 1978.

54. Avioli LV: What to do with "post-menopausal osteoporosis"? Am J Med 65:881–883, 1978.

55. Avioli LV: Management of osteomalacia. Hosp Pract 14:109–114, 1979.

56. Aloia JF, Cohn SH, Ostuni JA, et al: Prevention of involutional bone loss by exercise. Ann Intern Med 89:356–358, 1978.

57. Finneson BE: Low Back Pain. 2nd Ed. Philadelphia, JB Lippincott, 1981.

58. Jowsey J, Riggs BL, Kelly PJ, Hoffman DL: Effect of combined therapy with sodium fluoride, vitamin D and calcium in osteoporosis. Am J Med 53:43–49, 1972.

59. Raisz LG, Kream BE: Medical Progress: regulation of bone formation. N Engl J Med 309:29–89, 1983.
60. Slovik DM, Adams JS, Neer RM, et al: Deficient production of 1,25 dihydroxyvitamin D in elderly osteoporotic patients. N Engl J Med 305:372–374, 1981.
61. Kumar R, Riggs BL: Vitamin D in the therapy of disorders of calcium and phosphorus metabolism. Mayo Clin Proc 56:327–333, 1981.
62. Aloia JF, Cohn SH, Vaswani A, Yeh JK, Yuen K, Ellis K: Risk factors for postmenopausal osteoporsis. Am J Med 78:95–100, 1985.
63. Richelson LS, Wahner HW, Melton LJ, Riggs BL: Relative contributions of aging and estrogen deficiency to postmenopausal bone loss. N Engl J Med 311:1273–1275, 1984.
64. Seeman E, Melton LJ, O'Fallon WM, Riggs BL: Risk factors for spinal osteoporosis in men. Am J Med 75:977–983, 1983.
65. Shapiro JR: Imperfect osteogenesis and osteoporosis. N Engl J Med 310:1738–1740, 1984.
66. Newcomer AD, Hodgson SF, McGill DB, et al: Lactase deficiency: Prevalence of osteoporosis. Ann Intern Med 89:218–220, 1978.
67. Norenberg DD: Furosemide, hypertension, and osteoporosis. JAMA 241:237–238, 1979.
68. Lane JM, Vigorita VJ: Current Concepts Review—Osteoporosis. J Bone Joint Surg 65:274–278, 1983.
69. Heath H III: Progress Against Osteoporosis. Ann Intern Med 98:1011–1013, 1982.
70. Whyte MP, Bergfeld MA, et al: Postmenopausal osteoporosis. Am J Med 72:193–201, 1982.
71. Krolner B, Toft B, Nielsen SP, Tondevold E: Physical exercise as prophylaxis against involutional vertebral bone loss: a controlled trial. Clin Sci 64:541–546, 1983.
72. Consensus Conference: Osteoporosis. JAMA 252:799–802, 1984.
73. Sinaki M, Mikkelsen BA: Postmenopausal spinal osteoporosis: flexion versus extension exercises. Arch Phys Med Rehabil 65:593–596, 1984.
74. Marx SJ: Restraint in use of high-dose fluorides to treat skeletal disorders. JAMA 240:1630–1631, 1978.
75. Gruber HE, Ivey JL, Baylink DJ, Matthews M, et al: Long-term calcitonin therapy in postmenopausal osteoporosis. Metabolism 33:295–303, 1984.
76. Wallach S: Management of Osteoporosis. Hosp Pract 13:91–98, 1978.
77. Hahn BH, Hahn TT: Reduction of steroid osteopenia by treatment with 25 OH vitamin D and calcium. Abstract presented to Fortieth Annual Meeting Am Rheum Assoc, Chicago, 1976.
78. Sherk HH, Bellin H: Combined anticonvulsant osteomalacia and Paget's disease: a case report. Orthopedics 3:987–989, 1980.
79. Horsman A, Jones M, Francis R, Nordin C: The effect of estrogen dose on postmenopausal bone loss. N Engl J Med 309:1405–1407, 1983.
80. Weiss NS, Ure CL, et al: Decreased risk of fractures of the hip and lower forearm with postmenopausal use of estrogen. N Engl J Med 303:1195–1202, 1980.
81. Riggs BL, Seeman E, Hodgson SF, et al: Effect of the fluoride/calcium regimen on vertebral fracture occurrence in postmenopausal osteoporosis: comparison with conventional therapy. N Engl J Med 306:446–450, 1982.
82. O'Duffy JD, Wahner HW, Johnson KA, Muhs J, Riggs BL: Sodium fluoride (NaF) bone lesions in postmenopausal osteoporosis (PMO). (Abstract #9) Arth Rheum 27: (No. 4) [Supp], 1984.
83. Riggs BL, Hodgson SF, Hoffman DL, et al: Treatment of primary osteoporosis with fluoride and calcium: Clinical tolerance and fracture occurrence. JAMA 243:446–449, 1980.
84. Wynne AT, Nelson MA, Nordin BEC: Costo-iliac impingement syndrome. J Bone Joint Surg 67B:124–125, 1985.
85. Love JG, Schorn VG: Thoracic-disk protrusions. JAMA 191:627–631, 1965.
86. Fidler MW, Goedhart ZD: Excision of prolapse of thoracic intervertebral disc. J Bone Joint Surg 66B:518–522, 1984.
87. Ransohoff J, Spencer F, Siew F, et al: Transthoracic disc protrusions causing spinal cord compression. Neurosurg 31:459–461, 1969.
88. Perot P, Munro DD: Transthoracic removal of midline thoracic disc protrusions causing spinal cord compression. Neurosurg 31:452–458, 1969.
89. Sheon RP: A joint protection guide for nonarticular rheumatic disorders. Postgrad Med 77(5):329–338, 1985.

8

The Low Back

Ever since man assumed upright posture, back pain has been an accompaniment of life. Low back pain is the most perplexing and most frequent orthopedic problem of man,[1] and is the most poorly understood. Fahrni goes so far as to suggest that "good posture" is a major cause of disc disease.[2] He prefers the Oriental stooping position and he is supported by the fact that degenerative disc disease is seen in a smaller percentage of Oriental skeletons compared to Northern European skeletons. Although degenerative joint disease may be detected within the articulations of the low back, fibrofatty nodules may be palpated in the presacral soft tissues, or a "classic sciatica" history may be obtained, no assumption can be made between these features and the cause of pain in a particular patient.[3] Sciatica is a symptom and not a disease.[1] It may result from herniation of the nucleus pulposus (ruptured disc), from extrinsic problems in the pelvis or thigh such as an entrapment neuropathy, or from a myofascial pain syndrome.[4,5] Often multiple etiologic factors are operating in an individual patient. Secondary gain, misuse injury at work or at home, or psychologic factors may predispose toward chronicity. Three times as many workdays are lost due to back pain than the number of workdays lost due to strikes![6]

Until recently, any consideration for back pain has centered around a structural concept such as discogenic pain, degenerative disease of the spine, facet joint disturbance, nerve entrapment and spinal stenosis, or vertebral bony disorders. As the sciences of epidemiology, ergonomics, industrial psychology, rheumatology, neurosurgery, and orthopedics investigate and interreact, we learn that previous held concepts and classification methods failed to address the majority of patients with back pain.[7,8] This subject will be presented as viewed from the perspectives of these disciplines. This chapter begins with the symptom complex (descriptive) syndromes, and the investigations that attempt to identify a basis for causation.

Occurrence of Back Pain. As mentioned, back pain is important to industry as a leading cause for time away from work. In 1982, 580,000 workers were treated in emergency rooms for industrial injuries; low back pain was the largest subset. In 1980, one fifth of all workplace injuries and illnesses resulted from back disorders.[9] In England, back pain was second only to bronchitis in causing time lost from work.[10] In Sweden, 1% of all workdays are lost on account of back pain each year.[11] Overall, 80% of adults in Western countries will eventually suffer from back pain.[12,13] In the office experience of one American family practitioner, 11% of men and 9.5% of women reported low back pain in a 3-year period.[14] In another study, among those with back pain, 80% suffered longer than 2 weeks, and most had a family member who had suffered persistent pain.[15] Attempts to gather data have many biases. For example, the definition of backache can influence data.[16] Women seek medical attention for backache more often than men, but may tolerate the pain better, so that surgical procedures are less often performed in them.[17] The severity of back symptoms leads to a disproportionate use of medical care, unrelated to the severity of the medical condition.[18]

Contributing Social and Environmental Factors. Ergonomics, also called human engineering, is the study of the complex relationships between people and their occupational, domestic, and leisure activities.[19] Review of such studies reveals a significant correlation of low back pain to persons between age 35 and 55, and duration of pain to increasing age. Back pain is more likely to be seen in relation to lower social class, drug and alcohol abuse, divorce, family problems, and lower education.[17] Prolapsed lumbar intervertebral discs may be more common before age 40. They are more frequently seen in relation to driving motor vehicles whether for work or pleasure, due to lack of support in the vehicle seats, mechanical factors associated with accelerating or decelerating the vehicle, and extension of the driver's leg in the direction of the floor pedals rather than flat on the floor.[13] Use of cruise control may be beneficial! Other risk factors outside the workplace include chronic cough and bronchitis, insufficient physical exercise, sport activities of baseball, golf, bowling; and spring and fall seasons.[13]

Psychological Factors. In our society, until recently, prolonged illness was devoid of any significant social pressure.[20] Presently, anyone with persistent pain is suspected of harboring either malingering or psychosocial factors. Yet, malingering is rarely found to be causally related. More often, neurotic depression, disturbed affect, and hypochondriasis are detected in these patients. Patients whose psychologic profile determination revealed hypochondriasis were more likely to have brief pain relief from manipulation therapy compared to others.[21] Service industries employ more highly motivated individuals than manufacturing and may result in more stress related illnesses among which back pain is a consideration. Although patients with low back pain comprise 17% of all disabled persons, only 1.6% of them request handicapped services, 48% take no medications at all, only 20% see a specialist, 20% consult osteopaths, and 6% seek assistance of faith healers.[22] Thus these patients do not overuse the health care system. Controlled studies suggest that a poorer intellectual capacity, less ability to establish emotional contacts, and an aloof attitude were more frequent in back pain patients.[17] Using a Sickness Impact Profile, Deyo and Diehl re-

cently reported findings in 80 back pain patients during their first walk-in clinic visit and then after 3 weeks. The findings correlated with anxiety and psychiatric problems, which improved as the patient improved.[23] Perhaps the person is psychologically impaired by the disease, and the patient then seeks medical care. Tonelli et al. in a prospective study to assess neurotic traits among 19 patients with herniated disc disease of longer than 6 months noted no effect of neuroticism on surgical outcome; nor were those patients with emotional distress or depression more complaining of their pain than others.[24] A controlled study of women with backache attending a family practice clinic revealed no greater anxiety or depression symptoms or other psychologic problems when compared with other patients.[25] In another study comparing back pain patients with those having facial pain, no difference was noted in pain estimate, level of depression, or the ability to experience physical pleasure (anhedonia).[26] In a study of biofeedback for the control of muscle tension, manic, depressive, and agitated patients could achieve better relaxation with this technique than could the control group.[27]

Occupational Factors. Nearly 2% of the nation's workforce suffer a compensable back injury each year, with significant cost to the nation's economy.[28] Workplace injuries are often not the primary pathogenetic factor in low back pain, only the setting in which underlying disease becomes manifest.[16] The relation of back pain to driving has been mentioned. In addition, back pain may occur in the workplace in relation to slipping accidents,[29] manual handling and lifting tasks,[16,19] improper seated work postures,[19,30] "heavy" dynamic work loads such as lifting, pulling, pushing, carrying, prolonged sitting, bent-over posture, excessive bending or twisting, and frequent lifting. Exposure to vibrations as when riding a train, bus, or subway vehicle is associated with back pain.[13,17] The importance of job satisfaction and stress were found equally important to the occurrence of a back injury as lifting or handling loads.[31,32]

Buckle[33] reported that in a group of workers

who attributed back pain to a particular activity at work, there was no significant relation between the accident record and the onset of pain. Rather, a direct correlation of back pain to the distance driven per year by these workers was noted when compared to their coworkers who were without back pain.[33] In a Swedish study, covariance analysis of 10 variables among workers with back pain revealed only 3 with a direct association to back pain. These were overtime work, monotonous work, and a high degree of lifting.[11] Magora[34] found the earliest age of onset of low back pain occurred among bank clerks, heavy industry workers, farmers, and nurses. Also, a high incidence of low back pain correlated with prolonged sitting, or being unable to sit at all during the work day. Repeated brief sitting was associated with the least incidence of low back pain.[35] When workers returned to work, future disability was studied and found to correlate with persistent pain in the leg, duration of original disability longer than 5 weeks, more than two previous symptom attacks, an injury caused by a fall; additional correlates included physical signs of more than 15 degrees restriction in straight leg raising (SLR), pain on SLR, weakness of trunk flexors, pain or weakness in hip flexors, and back pain induced by passive knee flexion with the patient prone.[36]

Pre-employment Status. Industrial physicians recognize that pre-employment radiographic examination and history are not reliable predictors of work capability. Snook et al.[37,38] developed a psychophysical method for determining ideal weights and workloads for men and women. They established a workload acceptable to the worker, based on strength and psyche. Chaffin et al.[39,40] used a rating scale for each job by measuring the workload, the distance lifted from the floor, and the distance forward from the front ankle. They also used an isometric lifting test. By rating the jobs to the strength of the individual workers, a determination was made about whether the person and the job were matched. These investigators found that 3 times more back injury occurred when the strength of the individual did not match the job performance, or if the individual had far more capability than the job required. Back pain occurred in laborers as well as in sedentary workers.

Anthropomorphic Factors. Studies relating backache with obesity, height, weight, body build, muscularity, and leg or spine structure have produced conflicting data. Most studies, on the other hand, agree that tallness, large frame, poor posture, and decreased abdominal and trunk strength contribute to the back pain.[13,17,41,42] Degrees of back muscle strength is felt not to correlate with future back pain.[43]

Back pain is most often the result of a regional disease of the low back,[44] but may occur as part of a systemic disease. Consider systemic disease if the patient is in an older age group, has worse symptoms while lying down, has fever or other systemic complaints, or has pain localized to a point more lateral than the usual location of the myofascial trigger points.[44] A history of early morning back stiffness of gradual onset and physical findings of limitation of spinal movement in a young man would suggest inflammatory spinal disorders.[45]

Is the complaint of back pain a surgical emergency? Findings that signify danger are listed in Table 8–1.

These signals should alert the clinician to consider urgent surgical consultation for such emergencies as intraspinal bleeding, infection, tumor, or massive disc herniation.[44]

Table 8–1. Danger Signals in Back Pain

Bladder or bowel dysfunction or impotence
Weakness of ankle dorsiflexion
Ankle clonus
Color change in the extremity
Considerable night pain
Constant and progressive symptomatology
Fever and chills
Weight loss
Lymphadenopathy
Distended abdominal veins
Buttock claudication

PATHOPHYSIOLOGY OF LOW BACK PAIN

Since 1934, when Mixter and Barr described the ruptured disc as a cause for sciatica[46] most etiologic considerations for back pain have focused on anatomic findings or radiographic abnormality. Today we believe that many cases of back pain have little direct correlation to any structural abnormality evident on roentgenographs. Nevertheless, it is important to consider the known and demonstrable abnormalities that can give rise to back pain.

The spinal unit consists of a three-joint complex comprised of two posterior apophyseal joint articulations and the vertebral body with interposed disc.[47,48] (See Anatomic Plates III, IX, and XV.) Pathologic changes may be due to apophyseal joint synovitis or degeneration, injury or degenerative changes within the articular disc, apophyseal joint laxity, or traumatic subluxation. The result is entrapment of the nerve root as it exits through this complex. Also, stenosis of the spinal canal or additional new instability of articulating units above or below the level of involvement are also causative. Chronic low back pain resulting from these structural changes include mechanical low back pain or the posterior joint syndrome (the facet syndrome), the classic herniated nucleus pulposus (ruptured disc) syndrome, and spinal stenosis.[3,47,48] "Lumbosacral strain" in many instances is misused as a wastebasket term.[3]

In 1933 Ghormley emphasized the importance of abnormalities of the posterior facet joint (zygapophyseal joint) as a cause for back pain.[48] The posterior facet joints are innervated by the posterior rami of two spinal nerve levels. Proof that these joints were capable of causing symptoms resulted from studies in which instillation of hypertonic saline into a facet joint produced low back pain, pain radiating into the trochanteric area, and pain radiating down the posterolateral thigh. Furthermore, a local anesthetic injection of the facet joint restored normality.[48]

The introduction of pressure transducers into the nucleus pulposus of humans while assuming various positions and tasks revealed complex forces occurring in the human spine.[49] Pressure in the third lumbar disc was investigated in these experiments. Measurements while the person was standing were used as a standard and the intradiscal load in other body positions was compared. Sitting increased the load by 30%, walking by 15%, coughing by 50%, jumping by 50%, bending 20 degrees forward by 85%, lifting a 20-kg weight with the knees bent by 300%, and lifting a 20-kg load with the knees straight by 500%.[50] Sitting with a backrest inclined greater than 90 degrees reduced the load on the lumbar L-3 disc by 10 to 20%.[51] Lumbar disc pressure also correlated positively to body weight.[49]

The role of abdominal and chest musculature in back support was investigated using an inflatable corset and a measuring balloon placed within the stomach. This demonstrated that 30 to 50% of lumbar disc and thoracic disc pressures could be reduced by tightening abdominal and chest muscles while performing various activities and assuming different positions.[52–54] The abdominal muscles minimize torquing and bending, and shearing stresses in the lumbar spine, thus protecting the lumbar spine.[53] Improper lifting (back bent—legs straight) can result in generating 1000 to 2000 lbs/in.[2] of intradisc pressure. If the annulus of the lumbar disc has been previously injured the disc can rupture at 700 lbs/in.[2,54] The thoracolumbar trunk may be considered a hollow chamber. If the pressure of this chamber is increased by compression of abdominal musculature, the cylinder can withstand greater stress.

Trunk muscle strength and fatigue have been the subject of more recent studies which affirm the importance of good muscle tone.[42,55] Using an encapsulated transmitter (a radio pill) and with electromyographic data, measurement of trunk stress and intradiscal pressures during the performance of several occupational tasks were performed by healthy student volunteers during activities that required spinal movement and trunk stress.

Lumbar disc pressure and myoelectric back muscle activity during effort correlated best with symptoms.[17,41,56] These studies support the concept of the trunk as a cylinder, and the role of trunk muscles during spinal stress and work. Gracovetsky et al. used an optimized model of the lumbar spine based on data from a weight lifter performing a "dead-lift" exercise. The study results suggested that in handling heavy loads the stress at each intervertebral joint is identical, and with maximal voluntary effort the weight lifter does not exceed 67% of the ultimate strength of his tissues.[57]

Howes and Isdale examined 102 patients with backache for hypermobility.[58] Measurement included determination of spinal rotation, flexion and extension utilizing the length of the spine during these various maneuvers. In the study, 19 patients, all females, were found to be hypermobile, and only 2 of these 19 had another cause for back pain. Hypermobility as a cause of limb pain has been discussed elsewhere in this book. Whether hypermobility is a significant cause for backache requires further study.

Low back pain may bear a relationship to the lumbosacral lordotic angle (normal = 120 degrees).[1] Because a mobile spine is adjoined to the fixed sacrum, lumbosacral region strain may occur following sudden body movements. This strain occurs commonly in the female with increased lumbar lordosis, in whom L-5–S-1 disc-space narrowing is often seen. However, in other reports, pelvic lateral tilt, scoliosis, kyphosis, and lumbar lordosis did not correlate with the presence of back pain.[44] Disc degeneration, as evidenced by discography, also correlated poorly with low back pain. Rather, pain probably results only if the vertebral end plate is also fractured.[59] Fissures and tears of lumbar discs is common with advancing age.[60] The occurrence of multiple fissures led Jayson to speculate that a systemic disease process might be operative in cases of degenerative disc disease.[61] Pressure studies suggested that only discs that are already fissured will undergo rupture from external trauma. Based on these findings it was postulated that a disc that prolapses after some heavy work would have likely prolapsed anyway. The particular incident only precipitated its onset early.[61] Although the pain appears to originate in the spinal musculature, more likely the pain is referred from ligaments or articular structures.[6] The posterior thoracolumbar fascia covers the posterior aspects of the back muscles; the fascia provides a series of accessory posterior ligaments that anchor the L2 to L5 spinous processes to the ilium and resist lumbar flexion. The posterior fascia attaches to the posterior-superior iliac spine and posterior segment of the iliac crest.[62] Presumably, the injury of the fascia can become a source for a myofascial trigger point.

"Soft tissue incompetence" is a category that Mooney[7] uses to describe that large group of patients to whom this chapter is dedicated. These patients have what we call "myofascial back pain" and they lack neurologic, orthopedic, roentgenographic, and thermographic abnormality. But they have intermittent loss of lumbar motion, palpable spasm, and typical trigger or tender points.

Spinal mobility includes ventroflexion, extension, lateral flexion, and rotation. Movement is restricted by various ligaments, and other skeletal structures. The "stiffness" of aging is often the result of degenerative expansion of the apophyseal joints and spur formation, disc degeneration, and ligamentous changes. Yet the very old who are without osteoporosis tolerate inactivity or sitting much better than those in midlife. We infer from this that much of midlife back pain results from muscle and fascial structures.

Reactive muscle spasm occurs in stages. Spasm is no more common than strain or fatigue but is more persistent with average duration lasting 3 weeks; it is involuntary. The muscle cannot be passively stretched. This stage may proceed into *hypertonia*. Muscles in hypertonia come under voluntary control but increased tone may persist for years if the provocative source is not removed. The final stage may be *physiologic adaptation* after prolonged disuse. Elastic muscle fibers are thought to be replaced by inelastic fibrous strands. In addition, the skin, subcutaneous tissue, fascia, and muscle sheaths also deteriorate.[63] Although a plausible concept, no histologic features that support this hypothesis have been presented.

THE PAIN SYNDROMES

Clinical Presentation. Today, pain of myofascial origin is considered a leading cause for back pain. The syndromes described in this chapter are presented as if they occur individually. More often, they are superimposed on other back disorders. At onset of back pain, the features may first appear to represent mechanical low back pain; later, sciatica may become evident; and finally a chronic pain state with a remarkable limitation of spinal motion may result. Thus the syndrome presentation may change with time. However, most patients with back pain have self-limited problems that the clinician can readily assist. Aggravating factors are well recognized and can be changed. Thus, the physician has an obligation not only to relieve pain, but also to prevent recurrences by providing education in back care.

Whether chronic persistent pain progresses from an acute back disorder, and whether or not precipitating injurious events play a role in the progression to chronicity is not known.[22] As mentioned, roentgenographic abnormalities of the low back do not always correlate with future back pain or disability. Thus the presence of low back pain and a structural abnormality may have no relation one to the other. For the present time, a simple diagnosis of "myofascial low back pain" can be provided for patients with a dominant muscular component in the absence of some discernible cause. The terms "lumbar insufficiency" and "lumbago" have been applied similarly, but are less attractive nomenclature.

Patients with low back pain, can be categorized by mode of clinical presentation into (1) those with intermittent acute low back pain that seems to be of structural origin (me-chanical low back pain); (2) those with sciatica (pain that radiates from the back to a leg, usually from the buttock to below the knee on the posterior or posterolateral aspect); (3) those with myofascial back pain—a persistent distressing backache worse after rest; and (4) those with psychogenic back pain that fluctuates with internal psychic stress and is out of proportion to physical features. A brief description of the syndromes is presented, followed by a general discussion of the back examination, differential diagnosis, and treatment.

Mechanical Low Back Pain

Back pain resulting from a mechanical cause should be suspected when pain is related to posture, minor trauma, or excessive use.[6] Mechanical low back pain is episodic or intermittent and is aggravated by those actions that demand more from the supporting back structures; this pain is relieved by rest and recumbency. Most patients with this type of back pain are involved in handling and lifting tasks.[16] Often, patients with mechanical backache will describe previous "catches"— attacks that immobilize the patient in a slightly bent forward position. Such attacks are generally self-limited, last for about 4 days, and are thought to arise in the posterior articulations. Signs accompanying the pain include unilateral muscle spasm and a spinal "list" in which the patient is pulled slightly to one side. However, a list also suggests herniation of a nucleus pulposus. Flattening of the lumbar spine is similar to that seen in ankylosing spondylitis. Limb strength and reflexes remain normal.[6]

Other patients present with extremely variable symptoms, best described as a dull ache in the low back, aggravated by activity and improved with rest.[65] These patients suffer subacute episodes of worsening with radiation to one or both thighs. "Lumbosacral strain,"[1,3] "the posterior joint syndrome," or "the facet syndrome"[48] have no distinguishing features that differ from the symptoms and signs already mentioned. However, these terms do serve to point out the importance of the posterior joints, the lumbosacral ligaments, and other deep structures in the development of low back pain and spasm. The facet syndrome with compression of nerve roots in association with osteoarthritis of the posterior spinal articulations has the added feature of nerve root compression.[48]

Physical examination reveals variable degrees of tenderness of the low back musculature and tightness of the hamstrings and sacrospinalis muscles (observed during straight leg raising and forward bending maneuvers). Neurologic examination is normal.

Mechanical low back pain may occur in middle age as an acute self-limited process with frequent recurrences, only to disappear in late age, or it may progress to the totally invalid "low back loser."[66] Acute low back pain accounts for approximately 2% of all office visits to physicians, with the sexes equally involved.[67] The acute painful self-limited low back attack must not be dismissed with only symptomatic care. Such attacks may be considered as "mechanical backache" when a posture or related strain is thought to be the cause.[6] The physician is then obligated to consider the patient's work position and tasks that can cause recurrences. Table 8–2 provides a list of both helpful and harmful ways the back is used. Other conditions that may predispose to recurrent mechanical low back strain include faulty posture, structural disturbances such as spondylolisthesis and disc degeneration, all of which can be helped.[65] Spinal curvature, scoliosis, does not seem to predispose to acute low back pain.[68] Specific strains or injuries are documented in only 20% of low back pain patients, and in 80%, no evident cause is elicited on careful history.[67] Of ambulatory care for acute low back pain, 90% is satisfactory for pain relief, yet almost half the patients have recurrences within 4 years. No significant differences in outcome were noted in relation to sex or age.[67]

In summary, mechanical low back pain often results from a breakdown in the supporting soft tissue structures, abnormalities of the posterior apophyseal joints, or injury to spinal ligaments that assist in the maintenance of the upright spinal position. This may result from postural deficits, improper work habits, or a job or task inappropriate to the muscular control of the individual.[40] The clinical features include intermittent, subacute, or acute episodes of pain with limitation of spinal motion, sometimes related to a recent specific injurious task; physical signs include limitation of spinal motion, or listing and tightness of the hamstring and sacrospinal muscles. (Management is discussed later in this chapter.)

Sciatica and Other Nerve Entrapment Syndromes

Sciatica, as previously mentioned, is a symptom complex that occurs as a result of many entities afflicting the low back.[4] The symptoms include pain and neuritic features such as numbness, tingling, and burning. The neuritic manifestations often occur at a location distant from the area of pain. Any activity that increases intra-abdominal or intrathoracic pressure, such as lifting, pushing, bending forward, coughing, sneezing, or the act of defecating may aggravate sciatica. This history should alert the clinician to consider an intraspinal cause. Sciatica is also aggravated during motion that hyperextends the spine. Symptoms of sciatica that occur spontaneously during sleep strongly suggest an intraspinal pathology, such as tumor or infection. In most cases, the symptom of sciatica is an intermittent aggravation and often is layered upon chronic persistent back pain. When the sciatica symptom complex is not aggravated by coughing, sneezing, or defecating, and the examination reveals normal neurologic findings with no limb weakness, the term "pseudosciatica" is appropriate. It suggests that the cause lies outside the spinal canal, often the result of bursitis or myofascial pain.

Mooney and Robertson[48] demonstrated the posterior apophyseal (facet) joints as a source of sciatic pain radiation. In 15 patients with chronic back pain and sciatica, and in 5 control patients, they performed arthrography using fluoroscopic localization of the facet

Table 8–2. Aggravating Factors for the Low Back[233]

Harmful	Helpful
■ Having weak abdominal muscles puts a strain on the low back.	■ If possible, perform exercises that strengthen the abdominal muscles and then *use* these muscles. Always keep them contracted.
■ Shoveling snow, weeding the garden, or lifting heavy objects can cause an acute attack of back pain, often referred to as "a catch in the back."	■ Lie on the back and elevate the legs with a sofa cushion placed under the ankles, not the knees; place moist heat packs under the back, then do numerous knee-to-chest lifts.
■ Bending over with the knees locked can injure the back.	■ Always bend at the knees, not at the waist.
■ Twisting at the waist while holding large or heavy objects can cause back strain, as can constantly carrying an object, such as a young child, to one side of the body.	■ Turn or rotate the entire body by moving the feet. Draw the object to the chest, lift it with the arms held stiff, and use the thigh muscles for strength. Hold the object centered in front of you.
■ Standing for prolonged periods, especially on a concrete surface, rapidly tires the back muscles.	■ Place one foot atop a 2 × 4 × 8-in. (about 5 × 10 × 20-cm) wood block for a while and then alternate, thus transferring body weight from one foot to the other. Wear cushion-soled shoes when working or walking on concrete.
■ Having one leg that is more than 0.5 in. (1.3 cm) shorter than the other should not be overlooked as a cause of back pain.	■ Have shoes for the foot of the shorter leg built up.
■ Sitting for too long can strain the back.	■ Sit on a bar stool; doing so is uncomfortable and promotes frequent changes of position. Break up desk work and card games by standing up and moving around every 30 minutes. Use cruise control, if available, when driving long distances.
■ Doing strenuous physical work or engaging in a sports activity on an occasional or weekend basis can lead to back pain.	■ Do trunk-stretching warm-up exercises before engaging in any strenuous activity.

Table 8–2. *Continued*

Harmful	Helpful
■ Sleeping on the stomach or flat on the back can cause backache.	■ Sleep on one side or on the back with the knees and feet elevated with a cushion or pillow.
■ Sitting or falling hard often results in pressure injury to the coccyx, or tailbone.	■ Protect the point of tenderness at the tip of the coccyx by using a foam-rubber or sponge-like cushion that is at least 3 in. (about 8 cm) thick and the size of a seat cushion. Cut a 3-in. circle out of the center of the cushion with a bread knife. For at least a month following injury, place the cushion under the tailbone whenever seated or doing exercises on the floor.
■ Bending over with the knees locked is a very common cause of pain in the buttock region. Persons who can touch the floor with their palms are likely to bend improperly.	■ Always bend at the knees, not at the waist.
■ Applying pressure to the sciatic nerve, such as occurs with a ruptured disk, direct injury, constriction of the spinal canal (spinal stenosis), or muscle spasm adjacent to the nerve, can result in sciatica. Sciatica is a symptom complex of pain, numbness, and tingling radiating from a buttock to below the knee. Another cause of sciatica is bursitis at the side of the hip. Here again, bending over with the knees locked is a common causative factor.	■ Take proper care of the back by strengthening and using the abdominal muscles to support the back, attaining and maintaining ideal weight, avoiding prolonged periods of sitting or standing, wearing cushion-soled shoes when working or walking on concrete, assuming proper rest and sleep positions, and performing trunk-stretching exercises before engaging in strenuous activities.
■ Carrying a large wallet in a back pocket can cause sciatica. Similarly, wearing a tight belt, leaning over a drafting table, or improperly positioning a seat belt can put pressure on a nerve, causing numbness, tingling, and a burning sensation in the lateral hip and thigh region.	■ Check for pressure placed on the pelvic bones by a wallet, belt, or workbench and, if present, remedy the situation. Learn to wear seat belts correctly.

joints at L3–4, L4–5, and L5–S1. In each of the patients, the instillation of dye resulted in deep localized backache followed by pain radiation into the posterolateral leg. Injection at L3–4 tended to be associated with a more lateral pain zone. Increased myoelectric activity in the hamstring muscles was detected. Pain occurred in the control patients as well, but tended to go only to the knee area in contrast to the patients, in whom pain referral was more distal in location.

Herniation of the nucleus pulposus (ruptured disc) may result in pain in either the back or leg alone, or in both the back and leg, whereas sciatica that results from entrapment neuropathy often spares the back. Sciatica accompanied by pain in the anterior groin and hip suggests herniation of an L-4–5 nucleus pulposus. Patients with proven nucleus pulposus herniation usually have had episodic back pain preceding rupture. The back pain may improve when sciatica develops.[3] The intermittency of symptoms contrasts with the more chronic pain experienced by patients with intraspinal tumors. Non-disc causes of sciatica (see Table 8–3) should be

Table 8–3. Non-Disc Causes of Sciatica[3]

A. Entrapment Neuritis
  1. Obturator neuritis
    a. obturator hernia
    b. osteitis pubis
  2. Meralgia paresthetica
    a. arthritis
    b. psoas abscess
    c. traction injury
    d. obesity
    e. external pressure
  3. Lumbar spinal stenosis
  4. Spinal degenerative joint disease
    a. Apophyseal joint spur formation
    b. Facet syndrome
    c. Root sleeve fibrosis
  5. Ankylosing spondylitis
  6. Sacral cysts and tumors
B. Trauma
  1. Iatrogenic injections
  2. Contusion
C. Sciatic Neuritis (rare)

suspected when physical examination has failed to demonstrate positive signs of spinal disease (reflex change, motor weakness) or if the sciatica is unrelated to activities that increase intra-abdominal or intrathoracic pressure (lifting, pushing, bending), or movements that hyperextend the spine. Not all herniated lumbar discs result in pain. Of 108 cases of disc disease in which the patients suffered no pain, but presented with only abnormal neurologic findings and weakness, pain subsequently occurred in only 36% of these "silent disc disease" patients who were observed for an average of 5 years before surgical intervention occurred. These patients did not have as good a surgical result because, when pain was absent, delay in diagnosis resulted in more advanced neurologic damage.[69]

Entrapment neuropathy of the sciatic nerve may occur from direct injury when sitting on a hard surface or horseback riding, with pressure occurring just below the gluteal border where the sciatic nerve lies superficially.[70] Bilateral sciatic nerve symptoms following prolonged unicycling has been reported.[71] Pseudosciatica can be due to trochanteric bursitis and other myofascial pain disorders of the pelvis. Relief may follow injection of the involved soft tissue lesion with an anesthetic-corticosteroid combination.[5,72]

A not uncommon cause of sciatica is spasm of the piriformis muscle, an external rotator of the thigh. The piriformis muscle fills the greater sciatic foramen.[73] Pain in the buttock and point tenderness in the sciatic notch, as well as during rectal examination, strongly suggest a piriformis myofascial trigger point with secondary sciatica.[74,75] Spinal stenosis can cause piriformis spasm. When associated with spinal stenosis, symptoms are bilateral, whereas in the piriformis syndrome alone, the symptoms are unilateral. Most patients report buttock pain rather than back pain, pain worse after sitting and at night, and improvement with walking. Neurologic examination is normal.[76] The Trendelenberg test for diagnosis of this condition was modified by Hallin as follows: The patient stands with the back to the examiner who is seated. The examiner's hands are placed on the patient's iliac crests, and thumbs on the posterior iliac spines. The patient is asked to walk in place. If there is weakness of hip abduction, the pelvis drops to the opposite side and the upper trunk may shift to the same side. The pelvic tilt then is easily observed. Palpation reveals tender induration of the piriformis deep in the buttock between the proximal end of the greater trochanter and the sacrum.[76,77] Rectal palpation may disclose exquisite tenderness within the piriformis muscle in the lateral rectal wall. A local anesthetic-corticosteroid injection, carried out through the buttock over the sciatic notch, may provide relief.[74] The piriformis syndrome is also a common presentation in loose jointed individuals who can easily bend over and lay their palms to the floor with legs straight. Perhaps they strain the muscle by performing tasks with their back bent and knees straight and with excessive spinal rotation. Then upon returning to the upright position, the piriformis and gluteal muscles are strained.

The sciatic nerve may rarely become trapped in the posterior thigh region with symptoms of numbness in the posterior leg, calf, and lateral foot. Pain may be noted in the posterior thigh. Entrapment is due to nerve constriction by a myofascial band running across the posterior aspect of the nerve. Electrodiagnostic testing usually establishes the zone of constriction.[78] Surgery to release the constriction is required for relief.

Another form of neurovascular entrapment is related to spinal stenosis. Stenosis may result from degenerative changes of the spine or from any cause that narrows the spinal canal (e.g., developmental and dysplastic disorders, spondylolisthesis, Paget's disease, fluorosis, and postoperative bone hypertrophy).[65,78–83] Characteristic symptoms include nerve root irritation and vascular embarrassment.[83a] Walking results in buttock pain or ache, paresthesia and loss of coordination of the lower limbs. Relief occurs after sitting, but is often followed by numbness and tin-

gling in both lower extremities. Symptomatology may range from intermittent claudication to symptoms that mimic a herniated nucleus pulposus. Night pain occurs in the upper thigh regions. Symptoms are intermittent at first, but frequently become progressive until the patient is required to become sedentary. The patient sometimes discovers relief by bending forward, such as by leaning across a table. Physical examination reveals flattening of the lumbar curve; however, tests for nerve root irritation (straight leg raising, examination for reflexes, and determination of sensation) are often normal.[84] The back is often flexed during walking. Hyperextension of the spine during physical examination aggravates the pain and may suggest the disorder.

Myelography and computed tomography are utilized in diagnosis.[83a] The risks of surgical intervention and subsequent long-term complications demand careful consideration and exclusion of all other treatable disorders before labeling a patient with the diagnosis of spinal stenosis.[47,82,85,86]

Myofascial back pain (see below) is a common cause of pseudosciatica. A spinal percussion test, performed in the midline above the level of suspected disc herniation, is usually positive when lumbar disc disease is present. In contrast, a diagnosis of myofascial pain is suggested if the sciatic radiation is reproduced when the percussion is over the erector muscle to the side of the spine. A therapeutic intralesional injection, as described below, can often assist in diagnosis.

Myofascial Back Pain

Variously called fibrositis of the low back, tension myositis, or the "low back syndrome," this condition may occur as the sole cause of a painful low back or may be layered upon other disease of the low back. Myofascial back pain may involve the gluteal fascia, the iliocostalis, sacrospinalis, and other muscles, or an interspinous bursa[87] (Fig. 8–1). Pain is a constant dull aching that waxes and wanes; it is worse when at work, when cold, or while sitting; yet is improved with heat, walking,

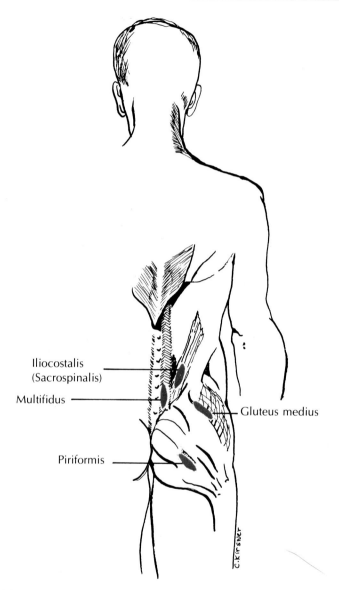

Iliocostalis
(Sacrospinalis)

Multifidus

Gluteus medius

Piriformis

Fig. 8–1. Myofascial trigger points of the low back region: Trigger points arising in the erector muscles, the gluteal fascia and the presacral fascia are common in patients with low back pain.

and bedrest. The condition may be acute or chronic, and may not have physical characteristics of spasm, listing, or limping.[1] Nevertheless, this disorder affects up to 80% of patients who come to the general practitioner with acute low back pain and in whom no other cause is evident.[67,88]

Myofascial back pain occurs in the third to fifth decade of life and is rarely preceded by a single definitive injury. Repeated minor trauma of sedentary living, misuse strain,[89] or a chronic pain-spasm-pain cycle[64] are probably operational. Myofascial back pain[89] certainly may be layered upon degenerative disc disease or apophyseal joint disease and may be synonymous with the "facet syndrome." By definition, this regional low back pain syndrome has a myofascial trigger point, which when palpated reproduces or accentuates the patient's pain. Episacroiliac fibrofatty nodules (lipomas) may co-exist. True sciatica is rare; if the pain has radiated to a leg, palpation of the myofascial trigger point reproduces the pain radiation. The most common sites of involvement are the origin of the sacrospinalis overlying the sacrum (multifidus triangle), the origin of the gluteus maximus adjacent to the posterior superior iliac spine, over the sacroiliac joints particularly beneath an epi-sacroiliac nodule, or bilaterally at the origin of the gluteal fascia.[1] The patient may adopt a protective attitude of flexion during the 3 or 4 days of increased pain and spasm.[65]

Simons and Travell[77] reviewed the various muscle trigger points and their zones of pain referral. The thoracolumbar erector group, the iliocostalis, longissimus thoracic, semispinalis, and the multifidus tend to refer pain downward toward and into the buttock; the iliocostalis thoracis may also refer pain into the lower anterior chest and abdomen, and into the scapular region. The deeper muscles refer pain toward the midline. In the experience of Simons and Travell, the quadratus lumborum is the most overlooked source of myofascial low back pain. The muscle lies deep but is palpable by examining the patient as follows: the patient lies on his uninvolved side, reaching high overhead with the uppermost arm to grasp the table edge, and dropping the uppermost thigh and knee backward on the table. The muscle is then taut, nearer the surface and can be palpated from the 12th rib to the iliac crest near to the midline. Press inward toward the lumbar transverse processes. Pain is referred into the buttock and lateral thigh regions. Aggravating factors include a short leg, standing on an uneven surface, or sitting unevenly as a result of pelvic asymmetry (small hemipelvis). The iliopsoas muscle may be the source of pain distributed along the lumbar spine close to the midline and into the anterior thigh. The taut muscle is discovered when performing the Ober test (see page 208).

Gluteal trigger points are common and often cause pseudosciatica. They may result from bending with straight knees and then using the back as a lever to straighten back up. Often the patient has joint laxity. Some have called it the "iliac crest syndrome" when the posterior superior iliac crest is the point of maximum tenderness; local infiltration with an anesthetic provides relief.[90] The gluteus minimus may refer pain into the lateral hip and down the side of the leg.

In children with spastic contracture of the hamstrings, a backward tilt of the pelvis occurs, resulting in limited anterior flexion of the spine. Pain in the low back and sciatica are common complaints. The Schober test (see below) and the finger-to-floor test are very restricted, as is straight leg raising. Although the syndrome can result from a herniated disc, most cases are of unknown cause and should be treated conservatively.[91]

The episacroiliac lipomas, as described by Ries,[92] are common soft fleshy nodules occurring over the sacroiliac joints at the insertion of the erector spinal muscles[43] (Fig. 8–2). In one study, these lipomas were found in 16% of a "normal" population (1000 persons), and of these, only 10% had back pain.[92] Their relation to pain is uncertain, although they are found in the vicinity of local pain and tenderness.[86,93] Injecting the tender lipomas and adjacent tissues with procaine and corticosteroid often provides prompt pain relief.

Psychogenic Back Pain

Psychogenic back pain and true malingering are rare, occurring in less than 2% of patients presenting with low back pain.[44] In these instances the patient's history is vague, and the patient often places emphasis on blaming others for her plight.[1] The term "compensation neurosis" is a rather ambiguous term, yet these patients often continue disabled after their claims for financial gain are settled.[1] The real question is how much are the symptoms related to anatomic disease and how much is psychologic. In such circumstances the physician must rule out organic diseases as quickly as possible, set goals for the patient, and obtain the help of a psychologist. Blumer states "To define chronic pain in the absence of a somatic lesion as 'psychogenic pain disorder' (American Diag-

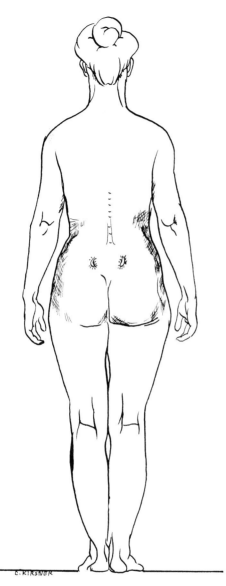

Fig. 8–2. Episacroiliac lipomas: These fleshy fibrofatty nodules commonly occur over the sacroiliac joints at the insertion of the erector muscles.

nostic and Statistical Manual—DSMIII), or as 'psychalgia' (International Classification) represents a negative and unsatisfactory approach." He described the "pain-prone disorder", which occurs mostly in women of all socioeconomic classes and ages. The features include:

—Somatic complaints: continuous pain of obscure origin, hypochondriasis and preoccupation, desire for surgery.

—"Solid citizen": denies conflicts, idealization of self and family, compulsive work or relentless activity.

—Depression: (after pain) fatigue, lack of initiative, inability to enjoy social life, leisure, or sex. Insomnia, depressed mood, despair.

—History: family history of alcoholism and depression, past abuse by spouse, crippled relative, relative with chronic pain.

These patients may present with perplexing backache.[94] Chronic persistent pain is discussed more fully in Chapter 14.

The patient called a "low back loser" by Sternbach[66] has the following characteristics: a history of previous physical labor and poor education; false denial of depression with a history of loss of appetite, decreased libido, poor sleep patterns, and test results two or more standard deviations above the normal mean on depression scales of the MMPI (Minnesota Multiphasic Psychologic Inventory Assessment); and a life style of invalidism. The patient perceives herself more ill than rheumatoid arthritis patients on the Cornell Medical Index scale. These patients are homebound and their illness perception is as hard to break as chronic alcoholism. During history taking, these patients are likely to "play games" with the clinician and frustrate the diagnostic evaluation. Psychologic assessment of patients begins with the first physician encounter, which should include the patient's social, occupational, and marital history. A Back Pain Classification Scale is reported of value in identifying patients with significant psychologic disturbance. Thirteen pain terms are utilized.[95] Other psychologic scales are under study.[96]

The psychodynamics of chronic back pain have received considerable investigation. Prospective studies have revealed no relation between a psychologic profile and future outcome or disability.[97] Positive answers to two questions at the outset of a treatment program are good predictors of a bad outcome: (1) "Has your appetite decreased recently?" or (2)

"Has your sexual interest diminished?"[98] Although the MMPI has not been a reliable predictor of the results of surgery, the MMPI may be a useful warning device in undertaking treatment of patients with chronic back pain.[98,99]

MacNab described the "racehorse syndrome," which applied to tense, hard-working, hyper-reactive persons who tend to hyperextend their spines, and the "razor's edge syndrome," which signified persons on the razor's edge of emotional stability who present outlandish appearances and complaints.[100] Persons suffering from anxiety may confuse "hurting" with "harming."[100] Careful examination, followed by reassurance, is necessary for care.

History and Physical Examination

In taking a history of a patient with low back pain the clinician must consider the age of the patient, history of previous back pain, aggravating factors in home or job performance, the presence of litigation or other secondary gain factors, and the general demeanor of the patient.[99] Pain localization is important, as is the distance and direction of the pain radiation. The pain history is often better evidence for localization than is sensory nerve testing.[99] The clinician should elicit which activities reproduce the pain, which aggravate the pain, and which alleviate the pain. Has there been a decrease in the level of work activity to a more sedentary life, with resultant loss of muscle tone?

The clinician must ask five basic questions of the patient with low back pain in order to "suffer vicariously" as the patient suffers and thus entertain the various modalities of diagnosis and treatment.[101–103]

Where is the pain? Many clinicians recommend the use of a pain drawing (Fig. 8–3). Is the pain perceived as deep, or superficial?

When does it hurt: continuously or intermittently, unchangingly or does it wax and wane? At night, does it awaken the patient from sleep? Is it worse upon arising? when walking, bending, reaching overhead, or sitting? Has it happened in the past? When was the first episode? How long has this episode been present?

How and *Why*: is it aggravated or started? Definite injury history? After certain movements or after coughing, sneezing, defecating? After driving a certain distance? After a particular sport activity?

What gives relief? How long does it take before the pain settles down? What is the disability on the job, hobby, housekeeping chore?

The pain drawing provides a permanent record of the location, quality, type, depth and intensity of pain.[103] This can assist in decision making (Table 8–4). It can also suggest psychological disturbance.[105]

The symptom of stiffness should be considered separately from pain. Stiffness that begins insidiously and occurs during the night or early morning hours may suggest inflammatory diseases of the spine (e.g., ankylosing spondylitis).[45] In addition to stiffness, characteristic clinical findings suggestive of ankylosing spondylitis include: Insidious onset, symptoms more than 3 months' duration, age less than 40 years, and pain improvement with motion.

A history of aching, numbness, and tingling radiating posteriorly or posterolaterally into the lower extremity below the knee (sciatica), or pain and burning that radiate anteriorly into the groin or anterior hip region, is often present in herniated disc disease. Aggravation by coughing, sneezing, or straining at defecation also suggests intraspinal disease. Certain symptoms may suggest a diagnosis or location of disease origin: night pain is often a result of intraspinal tumors or disease within abdominal or retroperitoneal structures; chills or fever suggest septic causes of back pain; changes in bowel and sexual function or urination suggest lesions of the cauda equina; and claudication followed by numbness and tingling suggests spinal stenosis. Spinal stenosis often causes the patient to stop walking because of aching in the buttock and calf regions; numbness and tingling may occur in one or both lower extremities. Relief in these

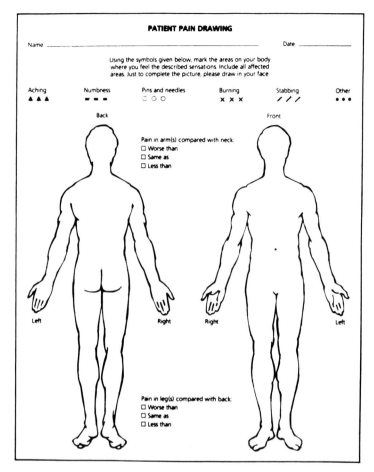

PATIENT PAIN DRAWING

Name _____   Date _____

Using the symbols given below, mark the areas on your body
where you feel the described sensations. Include all affected
areas. Just to complete the picture, please draw in your face.

Aching	Numbness	Pins and needles	Burning	Stabbing	Other
▲ ▲ ▲	▬ ▬ ▬	○ ○ ○	× × ×	╱ ╱ ╱	● ● ●

Back   Front

Pain in arm(s) compared with neck:
☐ Worse than
☐ Same as
☐ Less than

Left   Right   Right   Left

Pain in leg(s) compared with back:
☐ Worse than
☐ Same as
☐ Less than

Fig. 8–3.   Pain drawing for documenting back pain history[104] (with permission).

patients may occur with bending forward, such as leaning over a table.[107]

Hadler points out that before our first worker's compensation laws were passed, all backache was ascribed to soft tissue injury. Since then, despite 50 years of debate, only rarely can we ascribe a given backache to a particular disease of the back.[108] But we must decide whether the pain is arising in the back or referred from elsewhere, whether we must have radiologic studies, whether we can embark upon a conservative plan of treatment, or if urgent surgical consultation is needed. The physical features must be carefully determined, and objective findings of spasm, deformity, weakness, or neurologic deficit must be delineated.

Physical examination begins with obser-vation of the appearance of the patient while sitting, rising, standing, walking, and bending. Observing the patient undressing can be helpful. Structural abnormalities can only be demonstrated with the patient completely disrobed. The examiner proceeds to search for such objective findings as back or pelvic asymmetry, unequal leg length, spasm, scoliosis, loss of range of motion, loss of muscle mass, weakness, or abnormal reflexes. The value of the back examination lies in its use as a screening method for disease identification, not severity or prognosis.[109,110] In fact the reliability of the examination is directly related to keeping it simple and basic.[110,111] Interobserver error has demonstrated little value to the sensory nerve examination when compared to pain drawings; the sensory ex-

Table 8–4. Decision Chart: The Low Back

Problem	Action	Further Action
1. Acute recurrent No neurologic loss Spinal motion restricted No major trauma	CONSERVATIVE CARE Correct aggravating factors Provide pain relief Trigger point injection Vapocoolant spray Prescribe exercises, rest Traction/supports/relaxants	
2. Acute onset with sciatica with weakness Reflexes normal	Electrodiagnostic study if >6 weeks Roentgenographs if age >50 years Antidepressants if indicated	Rheumatology/Physiatry Consultation Bone Scan CT Scan Electrodiagnostic study
3. Chronic Backache Myofascial trigger points present Rest aggravates, movement helps	Add Manipulation Rule out Fibrositis syndrome Bone scan if persistent	
4. Chronic Backache with Stiffness Morning Stiffness Onset under age 40 3 months duration Limited lumbar motion/chest expanse	Rule out spondyloarthropathy	
5. Acute or subacute with weakness with reflex loss Positive Spinal Punch or root signs	Urgent consultation with surgeon	Neurosurgical or Orthopedic consultation Vascular study
6. Danger Signs present Night pain, paralysis Fever, weight loss Bladder/bowel dysfunction Color change in limb Constant and progressive symptomatology	Immediate action or consultation	

amination findings correlated poorly to final diagnosis;[110] neurologic deficits had little relation to outcome.[109] Pes planus should be noted. Mobility can be observed as the patient bends over. Can the patient touch the palms to the floor with legs straight? This is an important clue to hypermobility. Scoliosis, when evident, should be described as occurring to the right or left, depending on the convexity direction of the curve.[65] Using a tape measure the examiner measures the chest circumference at the breast line, after expiration and again after inspiration. A difference of two or more inches is normal.[112] Restriction of chest expanse may suggest ankylosing spondylitis or other inflammatory disease of the spine or rib cage. The spinal curvatures are examined with forward flexion, extension, and lateral flexion (Fig. 8–4). The examiner notes rigidity, spasm, pain, or listing of the body to one side. Symmetric loss of spinal motion may occur in degenerative disease of the posterior joints and ankylosing spondylitis, whereas asymmetric loss of movement suggests disc disease; this is not a hard-and-fast rule.[6,65] One objective way to measure mobility of the lumbar spine is the modified Schober test: With the patient standing erect, mark the skin in the midline at the level of the lumbosacral junction in line with the "dimples of Venus" (at the level of the posterior superior iliac spines); place another mark 10 cm above the first; and a third mark 5 cm below the first mark. Ask the patient to bend forward as if to touch his toes. Then measure the distance between the upper and lower marks. Normal is greater than 5 cm after subtracting 15 cm.[113,114,114a] In addition to ankylosing spondylitis, less common disorders associated with loss of motion include diffuse idiopathic skeletal hyperostosis (DISH), the rigid spine syndrome,[115] and severe myofascial pain disorders. With the patient bent over a table, myofascial trigger points are palpated, and pain reproduction is sought[63] (Fig. 8–5).

While the patient is bent over the examining table with knees flexed, firm percussion in the center and to each side of the lumbar vertebrae may reproduce sciatica[65] (Fig. 8–6). In our experience, a positive percussion test is as good an indicator of lumbar disc disease as a positive supine straight-leg-raising maneuver (Fig. 8–7) or a reflex change. Tenderness in the sciatic notch in patients with sciatica is often due to herniated nucleus pulposus (ruptured disc), but may also occur in the piriformis or other myofascial syndromes.

While the patient is supine on the examining table (lying on his back), the examination continues with careful palpation of the abdomen. Auscultation for bruits over the abdominal, iliac, and femoral vessels is performed. Examination of range of hip movement, and straight-leg-raising (Lasègue's sign), with comparison of the opposite side, is carried out (Fig. 8–7). Most commonly, straight-leg-raising is limited by tightness of the hamstring muscles rather than by sciatic nerve irritation, and is poorly correlated with the presence or absence of herniated disc disease. Shortening of the hamstring muscle itself is a frequent cause of low back pain.[1]

The classic features of herniated nucleus pulposus with sciatica are pain in the buttock, characterized by aching, and nonburning pain radiating into the posterior thigh and calf, or into the posterolateral thigh and lateral foreleg. Paresthesia may be noted all the way to the heel, or within a zone of the lateral foreleg. The pain distribution rarely extends down the entire nerve trunk, but when the S-1 nerve root is compressed, the pain often radiates into the posterior gluteal fold and down the posterior thigh into the calf and heel. Maneuvers that stretch the nerve trunk include straight-leg-raising (Lasègue's sign), and the reversed straight-leg-raising test.[6] The straight-leg-raising test is usually performed with the patient lying flat on his back with the uninvolved knee bent 45 degrees, and that foot resting on the table. The involved leg is raised straight up, while the ankle is kept at 90 degrees of flexion (Fig. 8–7). Generally, if hamstrings are not tight, straight-leg-raising can reach 90 degrees of upright vertical position.[107] When this test is positive, pain and tingling are reproduced;

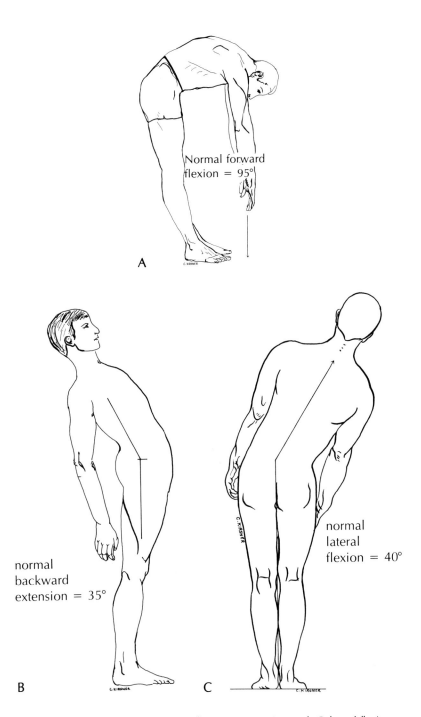

Normal forward
flexion = 95°

A

normal
backward
extension = 35°

B

normal
lateral
flexion = 40°

C

Fig. 8–4. Normal ranges of spinal movement in, *A*, flexion, *B*, extension, and, *C*, lateral flexion.

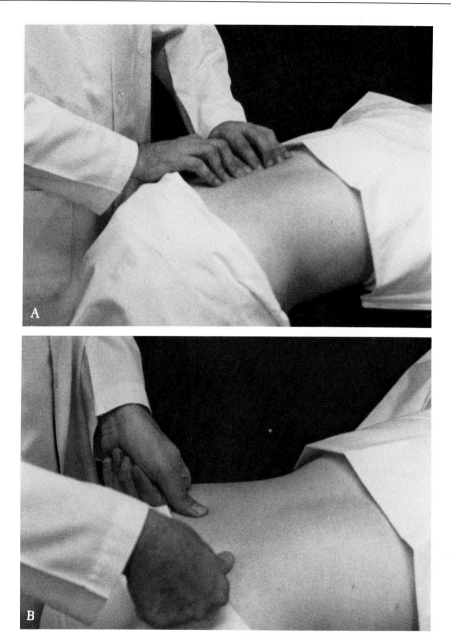

Fig. 8–5. Physical examination for myofascial trigger points is best performed with the patient lying across an examining table with knees bent. This relaxes the hamstrings and allows careful palpation for the trigger points that reproduce the pain: *A,* erector muscles, and, *B,* presacral fascia, gluteal fascia, and episacroiliac nodules.

this test is nonspecific, and any type of irritation of the sciatic nerve may cause a positive result. Dorsiflexion of the foot increases the pain during the straight-leg-raising maneuver. If medial hip rotation is added during straight leg raising the reliability is also improved.[36] Perhaps more reliable is the straight leg raising test performed while the patient is seated: the leg is passively raised as the patient bends forward while seated on a firm chair. Reversed straight-leg-raising is performed while the patient is lying on his

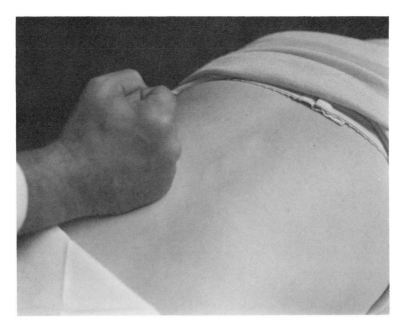

Fig. 8–6. Firm spinal percussion should be performed over each vertebra in the midline and to the symptomatic side as well as the side opposite. A positive test occurs with pain reproduction in the symptomatic hip or limb. A positive test is highly suggestive of herniated nucleus pulposus (ruptured disc).

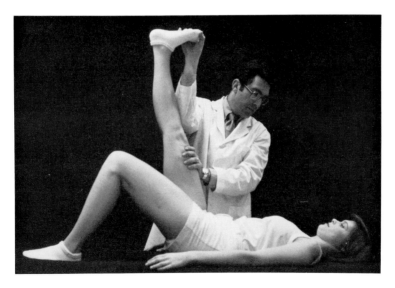

Fig. 8–7. The straight-leg-raising maneuver (Lasègue's sign): After gradually raising the straight leg to the maximum tolerated position, the foot is then drawn to a 90 degree angle. Paresthesias are accentuated if the sciatic nerve has been irritated. Tightness of the hamstrings may result in a false position straight-leg-raising maneuver.

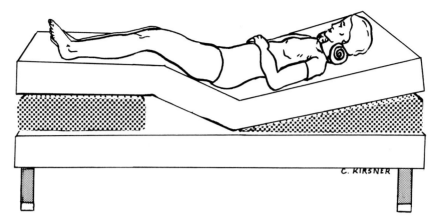

Fig. 8–8. The semi-Fowler bed position: A helpful resting position for patients with back pain.

stomach with his legs raised backwards, one at a time. Pain over the involved nerve root may be reproduced regardless of which leg is posteriorly raised.[107]

Range of hip movement should always be performed to exclude muscle spasm referred from intrinsic hip disease (Fig. 9–1). Special maneuvers to increase intraspinal pressure, using jugular compression (Naffziger's test), may prove useful in some patients. Sensory deficits to pinprick testing may not be as valuable as the patient's description of pain pattern and radiation. When the L-5 nerve root is compressed, pain radiates into the posterolateral hip, and numbness and tingling may be noted in a lateral zone of the foreleg.[99] Impingement of the L-3–4 nerve roots is associated with depression of the knee jerk; impingement of the first sacral nerve root is associated with depression of the ankle jerk, and impingement of the L-5 nerve root may be associated with depression of the posterior tibial tendon reflex.[65] Asymmetric hamstring reflex (for L-5 nerve root) may be determined with the patient prone. The examiner percusses the conjoint tendon of the semitendinosus and biceps femoris muscles at the ischial tuberosity and notes muscle contraction at the popliteal region.[116] The pain is often complicated by reflex spasm, which results in pain during rest and flattening of the lumbar spine. Trigger points may be present, and atrophy is usually not evident. Limb

strength and circumference above and below knee should be determined and compared. The dominant side is usually 1 to 2 cm larger than the other. Peripheral pulses are palpated. The physical examination is not complete until strength has been determined in the lower extremities. Gait abnormalities should be noted. Inability of the patient to walk on her toes or heels provides evidence of weakness in the gastrocnemius or tibialis anterior muscle groups, respectively. Foot and toe dorsiflexion testing against the examiner's resistance picks up more subtle weakness of involved muscle groups. Limb length measurement should be performed. Rectal and pelvic examinations are carried out to complete the examination. Table 8–5 provides a review of examination techniques in the various body positions. Table 8–6 reviews the usual findings of various nerve root disturbances.

If malingering is suspected, two tests may be helpful. When the patient has weakness of a limb, have the patient lie on his back, the examiner standing at the foot of the examination table. Grasp both of the patient's legs and hold the legs up from the table about 6 inches with the patient's heels supported on your palms. Now ask the patient to lift the uninvolved leg. When this is attempted, the opposite leg should depress the examiner's hand. Now reverse the procedure and ask the patient to lift the involved limb. If the patient

Table 8–5. Back Examination[102,117]

Position	Test	Impairment
Standing	Alignment	Scoliosis; pelvic asymmetry
Standing	Trendelenberg	Hip muscle weakness
Bending	Schober test	Spasm, arthritis, DISH, disc degeneration
Extension	Pain aggravation	Facet joint disease
Twisting actively	Range of motion	Discogenic pain, muscle spasm
Twisting passively	Psychogenic response	Should be pain free
Stand up on toes ten times	Plantar flexion	S1
Walking	Gait	Weakness, cerebellar dysfunction, pes planus
Kneeling	Ankle reflex*	S1
Sitting with feet on floor	Toe/ankle dorsiflexion	L5
Sitting with feet on floor	Toe/ankle dorsiflexion	Malingering if cogwheel action is noted
Sitting with feet on floor	Abduct hip with resistance	Piriformis muscle irritation
Sitting with legs hanging free	Knee reflex*	L4
Arising from chair	Quads, hip extensors	Muscle weakness
Bending forward over table	Palpation	Spasm, episacroiliac nodules, trigger points, piriformis syndrome
Bending forward over table	Percussion	Intraspinal impingment (disc or tumor)
Lying supine	Hip, abdominal exam	Referred pain disorder
Lying supine	Straight leg raising	Sciatic nerve root irritation; tight hamstrings
Lying supine	Leg length	Structural disorder
Lying on side, hip extended and knee flexed	Ober test	Hip flexor contracture, psoas muscle, fascia lata contracture
Lying on side upper leg extended	Hip abduction	L5
Lying on side upper leg flexed	Trochanteric bursitis	Pseudosciatica
Lying prone (on abdomen)	Hip extension	L2, 3, 4 (Pain); S1 (Weakness)
Lying prone (on abdomen)	Hamstring reflex	L5
Lying prone (on abdomen)	Reversed SLR	L4, 5, S1

*Hyperreflexia: Test for Babinski, other signs of segmental cord compression above lesion.

Table 8–6. Neurologic Table for Low Back Disorders[117]

Nerve Root	Sensory Loss	Motor Weakness	Reflex Change
L2	Proximal lateral thigh	Iliopsoas	Normal
L3	Distal anteromedial thigh	Hip adduction	Normal
L4	Medial calf	Foot dorsiflexion, quadriceps	Normal Knee jerk
L5	Lateral calf, first toe web	Toe extension	Hamstring
S1	Lateral dorsal and plantar foot	Foot eversion, stand on toes	Ankle jerk

is not making a true effort, the opposite limb will not reflexly try to depress that palm. Another technique, described as the Burns test[117] is done by asking the patient to kneel on a chair and bring his buttocks as close to his heels as he can. This, of course, relaxes the sciatic nerve. The patient is then told to hold onto the chair with his left hand and reach to the floor with his right hand. Because the sciatic nerve is relaxed, and the patient's back is supported, no pain should result and the patient should be able to reach within 5 cm of the floor, even when sciatic nerve impingement is present. In malingering patients, however, pain will be described, and motion limited.

In an effort to determine the predictive value of various physical findings, Biering-Sorensen examined 920 patients and followed them prospectively for 12 months. The examination included abdominal and trunk strengths and tests of endurance. Of those with a past history of back pain, the findings that were predictors of future back pain were tightness in the hamstrings, and lack of endurance of back muscle strength. First occurrence of back pain correlated with spinal laxity, lack of trunk muscle strength, and lack of trunk muscle endurance. Patients who had a past history of back pain but without occurrence in the study period were noted to have leg length inequality, obesity, and tallness.[118]

A careful history and physical examination may suggest more than one condition causing low back pain; however, in most cases only one condition predominates. Often myofascial trigger points with accompanying muscle spasm are aggravating degenerative disease of apophyseal joints or other structural disorders.

Examinations for purposes of disability determination do not have to be difficult if the examination includes appropriate consideration for objective information. The Code of Federal Regulations defines *disability* as the inability to engage in any substantial gainful activity by reason of any medically determinable physical or mental impairment or im-

pairments which can be expected to result in death or which have lasted, or can be expected to last, for a continuous period of not less than 12 months. *Impairment* is defined as an impairment that results from anatomic, physiologic, or psychologic abnormalities which are demonstrable by medically acceptable clinical and laboratory diagnostic techniques. Statements of the applicant, including his own description of his impairment (symptoms) are, alone, insufficient to establish the presence of a physical or mental impairment. *Disability determination:* primary consideration is given to the severity of the individual's impairment, age, education and work experience. Medical considerations alone (including the physiologic and psychologic manifestations of aging) can justify a finding that the individual is under a disability where his impairment is one that meets the duration requirement and is listed.[108] Payment is made for the amount of "disease" whereas illness may be independent, according to Hadler. He accepts low back pain as a disease, but the *illness impact* on behavior may result from such other factors as life style, quest for medical attention, and other attributes.[108] Illness is how we perceive our disease. According to Hadler, the physician should not have a role in judging whether a particular injury arose out of or during work; neither can we determine causality with any degree of precision.[119] Unfortunately, the physician is given the task of stating causality in industrial cases. As has been pointed out, more than an injury is often involved when disability occurs. Impairment can be considered as an anatomic or functional loss, and disability as the loss of capacity to work in gainful employment. The physician has to assist in:

1. the determination of compensability, a subjective assessment;
2. determining the termination of the healing period (when no further medical recovery is feasible), also subjective;
3. and the degree of permanent impairment.[120] The AMA guidelines for rating disability (permanent impairment) use

only objective determinants. Most orthopedists use this guide but also add other attributes that are subjective.[120] Problems lie in the fact that injury may result from "normal" work in which the repetitive task or activity results in rapid degeneration of tissue, or when a structural disorder is additive to job stress, or when injury is not really definable and separate from other underlying or predisposing causes.[119]

In a study of 160 patients with low back disorders, a simple yes/no questionnaire of nine activities was used to provide an index of loss of function. In addition, the pain pattern, Schober test, straight leg raising test, signs of nerve root compression, previous back surgery, duration of attack, and evidence for fracture provided a physical impairment score. From these data, the predictive value of the results were tested in 30 patients following an acute attack of back pain or sciatica. This technique, presently under investigation, may provide a better guide to severity of back pain and sciatica.[121] In another study patients with pain intolerance, with inability to cope with pain, and who have psychological symptoms, had reduced spinal mobility and restricted straight leg raising compared to other back pain patients.[122] Thus, pain intolerance may lead to increased muscle spasm and loss of spinal movement.

Laboratory and Roentgenographic Examination

Tests of inflammation, particularly erythrocyte sedimentation rate, should be utilized to aid in excluding underlying tumor or inflammation, such as ankylosing spondylitis or diverticulitis. Urinalysis, blood counts, serum acid and alkaline phosphatase, serum protein electrophoresis, HLA B27 determination, and other tests should be performed as appropriate.

Exclusion of tumor, sepsis, effects of trauma, or congenital abnormalities are some reasons for performing radiographic examination of the spine. Routine roentgeno-graphic back examination should be reserved for persons with a history of major trauma; those with physical examination abnormality, older age, or those whose medication or treatment could result in skeletal disorders (e.g., steroids).[123,124] Only 16% of radiographic studies contribute to diagnosis in patients with backache.[109,123] In one study, findings of joint space narrowing, sclerosis and spur formation bore no relation to type of work, absence from work, sex, race, or sport activity. The findings correlated only with age.[125] In another study of 292 men, with back pain graded as none, mild, or severe, the finding of transitional vertebrae, Schmorl's nodes, disc sign, disc space narrowing at L3–4, and L5–S1, and spurs was similar in all three symptom groups. Traction spurs are those in which the spur points directly anterior or away from the disc space and is separated from the adjacent osseous end plate by 3 to 5 mm. When a traction spur was noted to be present and when disc space narrowing was limited to L4–5 interspace, then these findings were significant in relation to symptoms of severe low back pain.[126] When indicated, roentgenographic examination of the lumbar spine for basic assessment should include anteroposterior (AP) and lateral views of the lumbosacral spine, and a true AP view of the pelvis. Additional views that may be helpful in certain circumstances include sacroiliac joint films, and left and right oblique views of the spine. Attempts to prove spinal instability with flexion-extension roentgenographs have not been reliable.[127] The addition of side-bending views may improve reliability but further study is needed.[128] Spurs and other evidence of degenerative changes of the articular structures are so prevalent[129,130] that the clinician should interpret the relationship of radiologic findings to symptoms with caution.[44]

Osteoarthritis with marginal vertebral and apophyseal joint spurs is likely to be significant if the neuroforamina are encroached upon. Osteoarthritis, if severe, does result in limitation of spinal motion.[1] Most patients with proved herniation of the nucleus pulposus have normal roentgenograms.[1] Congenital deformities of the low lumbar and lumbosacral spinal areas are seen in up to 30% of radiographic surveys.[1] Changes in the neural arch, abnormality of the transverse process of the fifth lumbar vertebra, with or without sacralization, or a spina bifida occulta often are unrelated to symptoms.[51] Rarely, after trauma, symptoms may occur in relation to such structural changes in younger individuals. Roentgenographic examination may also reveal squaring of the vertebral bodies, erosion, sclerosis characteristic of ankylosing spondylitis, and other spondyloarthritides.[6] Spinal roentgenographic examination reveals the occasional abscess, with soft tissue swelling adjacent to an involved disc and its adjacent vertebra. Specialized radiographic techniques include tomograms and computed tomography for determining the size of the spinal canal and for identifying tumors.[131] Scintigraphy is of value in diagnosis of adolescent sport injuries to the pars interarticularis in which a stress fracture might have occurred;[132] or if inflammatory arthritis of the spine, osteoporosis with fracture, osteomalacia, osteomyelitis, disc space infections, tumor, or Paget's disease are suspected.[133] Computed tomography has been helpful in diagnosing many diseases of the spine including herniated disc, facet degeneration, and spinal stenosis.[134] When compared to myelography in cases of herniated disc, both may be necessary. Myelography was accurate in 83% and computed tomography in 72% of 122 patients who had surgically confirmed disorder.[135] Magnetic resonance imaging can be particularly helpful in the diagnosis of disc degeneration, disc space infection, and soft tissue lesions.[136] Arthrography of facet joints with instillation of steroids and local anesthetic agents using fluoroscopic control has been advocated for diagnostic study.[136a] Dory[137] notes that the articular capsule nearly always bursts following the procedure! Others state that arthrography findings do not differentiate a pain producing joint from a normal one; the subjective response to an anesthetic facet joint injection must serve as the

diagnostic end point.[138] Less expensive techniques include routine and pulsed-echo ultrasound, if available.[139]

An exciting new factor in consideration of back disability is the determination of HLA B27. This test should be considered for patients under age 40 with spinal distress that has an insidious onset, a duration greater than three months, is accompanied by morning stiffness, and is improved with exercise.[45] In such individuals, particularly in the absence of radiographic abnormalities, a B27 determination may support a working diagnosis of spondyloarthritis.[44] A chemical battery of tests should be obtained in patients with persistent back pain and disability. Cushing's syndrome, Paget's disease, tumor, hematologic disorders with marrow encroachment, and osteomalacia are some of the systemic disorders that chemical and blood count determinations might reveal. A urinalysis should be part of the back examination. A Westergren sedimentation rate is an inexpensive and excellent screening test for the presence of tumors, infection, and inflammatory diseases of the spine. For older patients, in whom the sedimentation rate elevation may be nonspecific, the C reactive protein test may be more helpful.

An EMG may be falsely normal if performed too early after onset of symptoms. This test cannot detect nerve compression until demyelination has occurred. Later it may help confirm nerve root compression. Electromyography and nerve conduction studies may be helpful in patients with atypical sciatica, nerve root entrapment syndromes, peripheral neuropathy, and herniated nucleus pulposus. Motor nerve conduction velocities, H reflexes and F responses occur depending upon levels of electrical stimulation. Motor unit activity is zero electrically at rest; with contraction, electrical activity is seen. Fasciculations represent discharges of the entire motor units, fibrillations and positive sharp waves may signify denervation. The reliability of electrodiagnostic testing is correlated with the clinical expertise of the electromyographer.[104] If danger signals for spinal cord compression are present, do not wait for an electrodiagnostic determination; get surgical consultation promptly. Elective contrast myelography is reserved for patients with atypical pain, or for localization of the site of pathology, preceding operative intervention. Discography is still a controversial diagnostic procedure.[3] Thermography has had great technical enhancement in recent years but remains a tool of uncertain value. Certainly it does not stand alone in the diagnosis of back pain etiology.[140]

Most patients have acute or subacute soft tissue injury as the predominant etiology of their back pain. The *best test* may be injecting a myofascial trigger point with a local anesthetic-corticosteroid, in association with a back exercise program, as a test as well as a treatment. Rapid relief of pain by this method may be more revealing than a roentgenogram of the back.

Differential Diagnosis

In addition to what we have discussed, the following points are stressed again. Systemic infections cause few local findings on back examination, and local tenderness is rarely significant. Weight loss, fever, and elevation of the erythrocyte sedimentation rate should raise suspicion for an infectious origin of low back pain. Fractures, congenital spinal deformities, spondylolysis, spondylolisthesis, the spondylarthritides, Paget's disease, osteitis condensans ilii, osteoporosis, osteomalacia, tumors, and infections are disorders that are suggested by clinical and radiographic examination. Intraspinal neoplasms, including ependymoma, neurofibroma, or metastatic tumors, usually cause constant pain without relief when the patient is recumbent. See Table 8–1, Danger Signs for the Low Back, and Table 8–4, the Decision Chart. Rare causes for stiffness of the spine include alkaptonuria, interspinous bursitis (Brastrup's syndrome), and Forestier's disease.[141] Benign bone tumors, such as giant cell tumors, hemangioma, and osteoma, are rare. Don't forget herpes zoster as a cause for unilateral back pain. Back pain may be re-

ferred from the hip, and physical examination should detect the limitation of hip motion. Hip pain often limits the patient's ability to cross the leg while putting on a stocking.[65,142]

Many disorders can cause *referred pain* in the back. Peptic ulcer disease produces pain localized near the midline of the lower thoracic region, kidney disease causes flank pain with radiation into the groin, and neurofibromatosis (with café-au-lait spots) may cause sciatica-like pain that radiates into the legs.[107] Pelvic disease and aortic aneurysms may first cause low back pain. Renal colic (stone) often refers pain into the testicle, in addition to producing back distress. Retroperitoneal fibrosis may raise the erythrocyte sedimentation rate, and prostatitis or pyelonephritis may cause a dull persistent ill-defined back pain.

Management

Treatment for back pain varies with acuteness, mode of onset, duration, and etiology. The earlier a comprehensive evaluation and treatment are introduced, the greater the likelihood that the individual can return to an improved state of function, regardless of the site or severity of injury.[143] Spontaneous improvement occurs in many back disorders. Conversely, psychogenic and compensation factors are known to prolong disability. Psychopathology may be more complex in the back-injured individual than in the extremity-injured individual, yet even in these persons, the outcome tends not to be influenced by the psychopathology.

Aggravating factors that may cause recurrences should be sought (see Table 8–2). No significant relation of back pain to jogging is noted. Runners do demonstrate increased mineral content of bone, somewhat more spur formation, and more apparent sclerosis of the spine than others.[144] Beals suggests that we inquire whether the patient has a fear of returning to a former job, or has vocational dissatisfaction for any reason.[143] Other recognizable aggravating factors to be determined include lifting, stooping, bending, prolonged sitting, stair climbing, use of high-heeled shoes, and strains resulting from occupational sources or new hobbies.[3] Nachemson has stressed consideration for the strain involved in lifting with the knees straight instead of flexed, and the back flexed instead of straight.[51] (In nearly all cases of gluteal fasciitis a history of lifting with straight knees can be obtained.)

Proper sitting and sleeping positions should be provided. Keegan has performed a roentgenographic study for the determination of proper posture and sitting.[145] No sitting position was found to achieve vertebral alignment comparable to erect standing. However, the best results that could be obtained occurred when the trunk-thigh angle was 105 degrees or greater. Thus, the upright portion of the chair should be tilted slightly backward from the vertical position, the seat should be convex, and support for the lumbar region should be present across the back of the chair. Sitting forward or backward from this position increases lumbar flexion and thereby increases lumbar disc compression. The height of the chair should allow frequent changes in position, the distance of eye level to a work surface should be approximately 16 inches (eye glasses are set for this distance). There should be an open space beneath the seat of the chair to allow knee flexion beyond 90 degrees.[145] The patient's feet should be able to touch the floor or footrest. The end of the seat should be approximately 5 inches from the posterior aspect of the knee. The seat fabric should be porous. The height of the table or work surface may have to be adjustable also, allowing the arms to be comfortable as the patient sits back. Patients who work on concrete floors or walk with a heavy heel-strike may benefit from use of viscoelastic shoe inserts.[146]

Back schools have become popular recently. These programs teach groups of patients symptomatic management as well as prevention. Ergonomic analysis of job tasks can be provided. Patients have a fair degree of satisfaction with this approach,[147,148] but they must be able to comprehend the information.[149,150] In one study, employment status doubled after back school education.[149] However, patients with acute back pain do not benefit.[19] Back schools should provide followup reinforcement of the behavior modification. The physician should also perform this task for patients who have attended a back school.

Proper resting position for patients with back pain should reduce lumbar lordosis. Such a position is provided by the semi-Fowler position (Fig. 8–8). This position is achieved by having the patient lie on her back with a thin pillow under her head, with the thighs and legs elevated on cushions, pillows, or blankets.[1,51,151] Use of a bed pan actually *increases* lumbar lordosis and disc pressure, and is more aggravating than allowing the patient to use a bedside commode.[3,6] Proper bed rest as the *only treatment* of low back pain resulted in good pain relief in patients so treated and followed for 8 years. In this group, only 9% subsequently came to surgery, and only 44% required any other medical treatment.[152] However, elderly persons can be harmed by bedrest. Osteoporosis with compression fractures, thrombophlebitis, and disuse quadriceps atrophy may follow such treatment.

Use of pelvic traction is often subjectively beneficial. Because enormous forces are necessary to distract the lumbar spine, the traction serves the purpose of providing rest.[153] It may have a placebo effect. We place the patient in a semi-Fowler position (head of mattress elevated 45 degrees, foot of mattress elevated 15 to 25 degrees). This places the low back into a more convex position; 15 to 30 pounds of traction are applied as much of the time as is tolerated. If the treatment program provides relief, the duration in traction during daytime is progressively shortened. Traction, however, should never be the only treatment of back pain.[154,155] In our experience, if bed traction aggravates sciatica, a ruptured disc of significant size will often be present on myelogram.

The use of corsets is controversial. The corset may be utilized for the patient who is unwilling to remain in bed; however, there are no controlled data on their use.[44] If a corset is used, it should provide abdominal compression and be utilized only briefly. The patient should learn to depend on stronger abdominal muscle tone for back support.[1,3,63,65,99] In general, fewer than 5% of patients with back disease follow through on wearing the corset after purchase.[156] A back brace differs from a corset in having horizontal rigid elements, producing more restriction of spinal motion. A brace is utilized predominantly for patients with osteoporosis and vertebral compression fractures, or for post-traumatic vertebral fractures.[3] The lumbosacral corset with a heat-moldable plastic insert has been in wide use recently. In one 8-week study the corset relieved symptoms to a greater degree when the insert was included than when the binder alone was provided.[157] We use the support in older patients with osteoporosis, those with lumbosacral junction anomalies, or in young patients with joint laxity until they develop good abdominal tone with exercise. Patients with chronic or repeated pain occurrences should be referred for a back protection program provided by a physical or occupational therapist.

Therapeutic exercise is the cornerstone of management of the painful low back (see Table 8–7 Exercises for the low back). Although their value in controlled studies is unproved, exercises nevertheless remain an extremely important and useful part of management in the experience of most physicians.[7] Exercises that specifically strengthen the abdominal muscles are of reasonably established value.[158] Also, good quadriceps power allows the legs to assist in lifting. Inversion exercise in which the patient is suspended upside down using a commercial frame, has proved dangerous because inversion doubles intraocular pressure.[159] Headache may be a troublesome complication. The most sensible exercises are those that provide some back protection. These include exercises that develop abdominal strength (Fig. 8–9), provide posture correction (Figs. 2–7 and 8–9) and pelvic tilting[44,99,160,161] (Fig. 8–10) (see Exercises 1 to 8, Table 8–7). The

addition of lateral rotation of the trunk to the curl up gave a high activation of the oblique muscles when tested electrically and is helpful[162] (see Exercise 2, Table 8–7). Ten second holds and ten repetitions performed twice daily are recommended. The Williams flexion exercises have proved useful in over 30 years of experience, yet theoretically these exercises increase disc pressure.[44] The knee-chest exercises are helpful, whether performed while lying on the back or sitting (Figs. 8–11, 8–12).[163] Tight hamstring muscles and Achilles tendons can accentuate lumbar lordosis and should be stretched[3] (Fig. 8–13). General torso-stretching is an excellent warm-up maneuver (Fig. 8–14). As the patient achieves increased abdominal strength, she should reinforce conscientious continued voluntary contraction of the abdominal muscles throughout daily activities.[158,161] A "trapeze" exercise that is helpful for some patients is performed by gripping a chinning bar overhead. Knees are drawn up from below, and the weight of the pelvis stretches the low spine region; a chinning bar is available at athletic supply stores (Fig. 8–15).[153]

Extension exercises have been advocated for patients with limited lumbar movement associated with muscle spasm (see Exercise 11, Table 8–7). Used 5 times daily, McKenzie reported that 80% of patients could abort an attack and felt generally improved.[164] Another technique we use is described in Exercise 12, Table 8–7. This is particularly useful in patients with an adult round back or thoracic kyphosis.

Group exercise has been developed for the YMCA by Kraus et al. who reported results in 12,000 enrollees who completed a 6-week program. Pain and trunk strength improved in 80% of patients irrespective of whether surgical procedure had been performed in the past. Success was directly proportional to maintenance of strength.[165] In another program, a group exercise included flexion exercises, pool therapy, and back school education for patients receiving compensation, half of whom had previous back surgical pro-

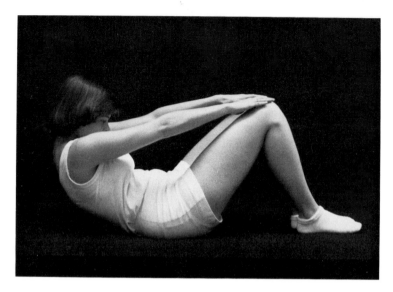

Fig. 8–9. Abdominal strengthening exercise is properly performed when the knees are kept bent and the patient does not sit up fully. Rather, the patient raises the trunk approximately 6 inches from the table. This contracts the superficial abdominal muscles without bringing the psoas muscle into play.

cedure; this resulted in 72% becoming employed 6 months later. Half the patients had symptoms longer than 3 months before entry.[166] A small study compared flexion versus extension exercise in young persons with backache, and the results favored extension exercises.[167]

A study comparing results in back management offered by physicians or physical therapists was reported. When physical therapists were given primary care management for low back pain, their results were as good as that of physician management in a prospective study. Whereas the physician prescribed more analgesics, relaxants, bed rest and less physical therapy, the opposite was true of the physical therapists. Both groups showed similar results in the number of new symptoms, days of symptoms, and disability. Patients with greater psychologic disturbance did better with the physical therapist![168] On the other hand, a prospective trial comparing treatment with corsets, traction, manipulation, and exercise added sequentially at 1-month intervals revealed no benefit at 4 or 16 months.[169]

Which exercise for which patient? A patient in severe pain must have relief before active exercises can be attempted. The therapist may begin with gentle stretching exer-

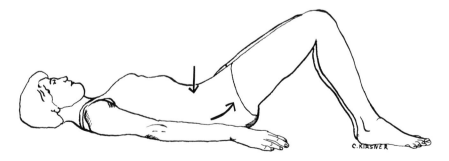

Fig. 8–10. Pelvic tilt exercise: To correct the lumbar lordosis, the abdominal muscles and gluteal muscles are contracted, and the lumbar spine is flattened.

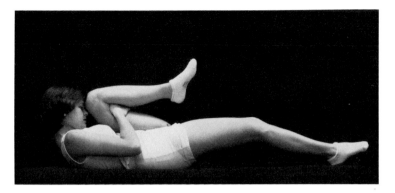

Fig. 8–11. The knee-chest exercise: Stretching of the low back muscles and fascia is obtained through these mobilizing exercises. One and then both knees are drawn toward the chest, the sacrum is lifted up, and the patient should perceive a pulling sensation in the low back tissues.

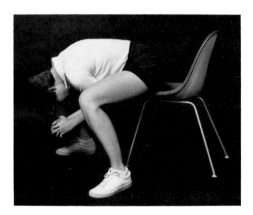

Fig. 8–12. Knee-chest exercise performed while seated on a chair: If standard knee-chest exercise (Fig. 8–11) does not provide a pulling sensation in the low back (perhaps due to hypermobility of the hip), the exercise should be attempted while the patient is seated as shown above.

cises and relaxation techniques.[170] Once pain is controlled, the exercise can begin. In our experience there are no predictors. Each patient has to be individualized and, with trial and error, most patients find that they do better with a particular set of exercises. We begin with posture correction, including neck erector and shoulder elevator strengthening when needed (see Figs. 2–6 and 2–7). All patients are instructed in the abdominal curl-up, pelvic tilt, and trunk stretch (except for those with joint laxity). Patients with restricted back motion on examination are also instructed in the trapeze hanging stretch (see Exercise 10, Table 8–7). Those who have limited lumbar motion due to spasm are shown extension exercises as well. The physical therapist should be permitted to individualize the home exercise program. Many patients are also started in water aerobic classes, group exercise, and a back school or individual back protection instruction.

Satisfactory results may also require proper resting position with the knees flexed, while lying on the back, with the thighs elevated with pillows; exercises to correct posture and strengthen the abdomen; recognition and correction of improper habits of sitting, lying, lifting; and, when necessary, use of vocational rehabilitation measures (see Table 8–2, Joint Protection).

Pain relief begins with reassuring the patient that you have found no structural damage that would cause lifelong pain. Conversely, the examination should convey to the patient the fact that they can improve. Changes in daily living habits, posture improvement, weight control and other physical improvements will be helpful. Pain relief is only an adjunct to the exercise and behavioral changes that must occur. For acute attacks of pain, particularly in patients with discogenic or facet joint (mechanical) associated backache, teach the patient to lie down on the floor and elevate legs up on a chair whenever an attack comes on. Then begin abdominal curlup, knee chest, and extension exercises.

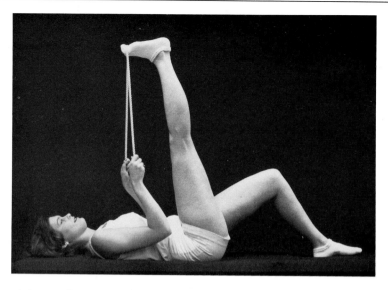

Fig. 8–13. Straight leg stretching: Tightness in the hamstring muscles, gastrocnemius, soleus, and Achilles tendon may be stretched progressively using a 4-ft length of rope looped across the ball of the foot. The extremity is pulled gradually toward the maximum tolerated upright position and held for 1 min during which further stretching may be accomplished.

Ice massage to trigger points can be beneficial but requires the assistance of another person. Similarly, vapocoolant spray can be used. Fluorimethane sprayed in a slow sweep from the trigger point to the pain zone, and not more than twice, while the patient performs a muscle stretching exercise, may break the pain-spasm-pain cycle.[77] Manipulation can provide striking pain relief but again requires a hands-on other person. Manipulation has received increasing attention and will be discussed later (p. 195).

Oral medication has a limited role in the treatment of back pain,[156] yet the use of muscle relaxants at night has had some advocates.[172] Cyclobenzaprine, a tetracyclic with more rapid action, is of value when muscle spasm is present. Gradual buildup of dosage from 10 mg bid to qid or 10 mg in AM and 20 to 30 mg in the evening can be helpful. There

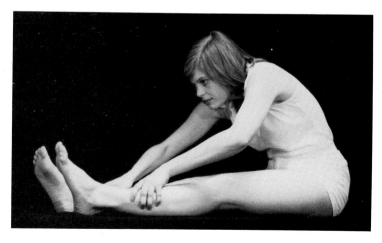

Fig. 8–14. Trunk stretching exercise: An excellent warm-up exercise to stretch posterior trunk and leg muscles before performing sport activities or more selective exercises.

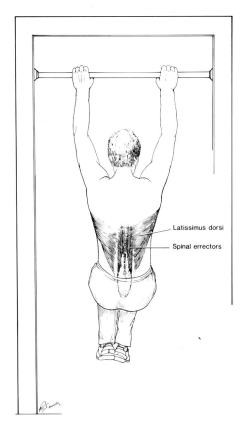

Latissimus dorsi

Spinal errectors

Fig. 8–15. The trapeze exercise: Using a chinning bar placed in a doorway, the patient grasps the bar overhead and draws the knees up. The weight of the lower body stretches the musculature and soft tissues about the lumbar spine region. The patient should spend a minute or two repetitively holding this position as long as grasping permits.

is a growing recognition of the value of mood altering drugs, such as amitriptyline, in providing improvement.[99,156,172,173] Use of tricyclic antidepressants for nocturnal sedation as well as depression has been helpful for most patients with *chronic* back pain. These agents should be started slowly, and may be given every 2 hours for 2 or 3 doses each evening (e.g., 8 PM, 10 PM, midnight). This regimen decreases the side effects, including morning hangover and daytime dry mouth. A prospective study of chronic backache in which amitriptyline was tested against atropine used as a placebo was reported by Pheasant et al. The patients had pain duration of at least 1 year, and had failed even after ex-

ercise and back school education. No injections were permitted during the study. MMPI scales normalized, and the analgesic use dropped by 50% in the treatment group.[174] Nonsteroidal anti-inflammatory agents may be helpful in some patients with chronic myofascial back pain, especially those with associated degenerative arthritis of the posterior apophyseal joints. Benefit is related to analgesic or anti-inflammatory effects. Naproxen, diflunisal and placebo were compared in 37 patients with backache of at least 3 months' duration. Appropriate dosages of the two test medications were provided and physical therapy was permitted. Visual analog scales and descriptive scales for pain assessment were used. Naproxen, but not diflunisal, relieved pain on movement, and both relieved night pain when compared with the placebo.[175] Diflunisal, 250 mg qid seems well tolerated and helpful in the elderly patient, in our experience. *There is no place for long-term oral corticosteroids in any myofascial disease of the low back.*

Myofascial trigger point injection has also proved itself over the course of time. Steindler,[176] in 1938, advocated the use of local anesthetic injections of trigger points within the soft tissue of the low back, and claimed lasting relief in the vast majority of patients with low back pain. He emphasized the importance of using the needle as a probe; contact of the needle with the trigger point must reproduce the patient's pain before injection. We have found local corticosteroid-anesthetic injections helpful in providing lasting benefit (Fig. 8–17). The corticosteroid-anesthetic should be a long-acting preparation. Injection into a painful trigger point is no different than injection for bursitis or tendinitis.[156] The trigger point injection provides pain relief, which allows the patient to pursue corrective exercises and to return to normal function quickly.[3,48,63,72,99,156,176,177]

The efficacy of local intralesional injections of an anesthetic or corticosteroid has received increased study. Bourne reported ten year results of injections of triamcinolone acetonide 10 mg and 1 ml 1% lidocaine into the

Table 8–7. Exercises for the Low Back

A. Flexion exercises:
   1. Abdominal strengthening: Lie on floor with knees bent; place arms across chest. Exhale, roll the upper trunk up about 3 to 6 inches but keep chin and neck straight. If hiatus hernia is present, start with pillows under head and chest. Hold for 30 seconds and begin breathing while holding the position, repeat 3 to 10 times (Fig. 8–9).
   2. Rotator stretch: Lie on floor, knees bent, hands behind head. Curl upward to situp and at same time twist right elbow to left knee and return to floor: repeat with left elbow to right knee.
   3. Pelvic tilt: Stand against a wall with back to wall, or lie on the floor with knees bent. Place hand behind back at waistline. Squeeze abdomen as if to have a bowel movement and at the same time tighten buttocks to rock pelvis forward (sort of like a belly dancer doing a pelvic grind); you should feel the low back flatten backward against your hands. Hold position for 5 to 20 seconds, repeat for 1 to 2 minutes twice daily (Fig. 8–10).
   4. Hip and low back flex: Lie on back, both knees bent. Hook elbow under one leg and draw knee to chest, hold ten seconds; then repeat with other side, and then both knees to chest at the same time. Repeat exercise twice daily (Fig. 8–11).
   5. Knee chest flexion exercise: Lie on back on a firm surface (floor or board on top of a bed), draw both knees slowly toward chest, curl head and shoulder up toward knees. Do not bring head forward first, bring head and shoulders up together, otherwise, the front neck muscles will feel a strain. Now rock buttock upward. Hold ten seconds, repeat 10 times. Repeat exercise twice daily (Fig. 8–11).
   6. Knee to chest exercise can also be performed while seated on a chair, with knees spread apart, feet on the floor. The arms are extended forward and down through the knees toward the floor, with the shoulders and chest approaching the knees until a pull is felt in the buttocks or low back muscles. This position is held while breathing for 10 to 20 seconds and repeated 6 times. Repeat exercise twice daily (Fig. 8–12).

B. Hamstring and Pelvis Exercises:
   7. Hamstring stretch: Lie on back with legs bent at knee, feet to floor. Raise one leg straight up, place a 4-foot length of rope looped under toes and pull leg straight up. Slowly increase the pull and direct leg higher or toward head. Hold 1 minute with increased forward pull each 10 seconds. Then repeat with other leg. Repeat exercise twice daily (Fig. 8–13).
   8. Trunk flexion/stretch: Sit on floor, legs straight. Keep knees straight, exhale and reach forward, grasp forelegs, breathe and pull trunk forward while bending elbows outward. Hold for 30 seconds, repeat 3–6 times. Repeat exercise twice daily (Fig. 8–14).
   9. Pretend you are holding a pencil between the cheeks of the buttocks. Squeeze buttocks hard, hold 10 seconds. Repeat often throughout the day.
   10. Trapeze (chinning bar) stretch: Obtain a chinning bar and fit it into a doorway. Grasp and hang by hands, draw knees up toward chest. Hold as many seconds as possible; let go and then repeat for 1 to 2 minutes, two or more times a day (Fig 8–15).

C. Extension exercises:
   11. Back extension: Lie on stomach, press the top half of body up with arms as extended as possible, with legs and pelvis kept against floor. Do 10 repetitions, 4 or 5 times per day (Fig. 8–16).
   12. Upper back straightening: Lean across a kitchen table or counter with abdomen, chest, and nose against surface. Place hands behind on buttock. Keep chin neutral. Raise the head and chest together as a block, up about 2 to 4 inches while keeping abdomen against table. Hold 10 to 20 seconds; repeat 3 to 5 times twice daily (Fig. 7–10).

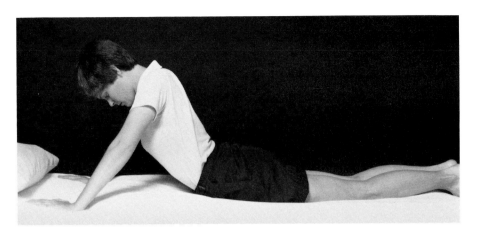

Fig. 8–16. Technique for passive extension exercise.

point of maximum tenderness in 22 patients with myofascial back pain of 10 years' duration. Pain relief for a minimum of 5 weeks per injection was the minimum requisite for "success". Over the 10-year period the average patient received a total of 44 mg of triamcinolone. Results of injection for myofascial pain of nonspecific origin in the sacroiliac region was 51% good, 28% fair, and 21% failure. For myofascial pain in other areas of the back, the results were 52%, 24%, 24% respectively. In patients with myofascial pain associated with degenerative disc disease, the results were 41%, 18%, and 41% respectively. Overall, these 22 patients had a total of 115 trigger points injected with a 77% good or fair result.[178] A controlled study compared the effects of long-acting local anesthetics versus saline solution; patients were assessed by a subjective pain scale, effect of pain on physical activity, limitation of movement, and effect of pain on mood and sleep

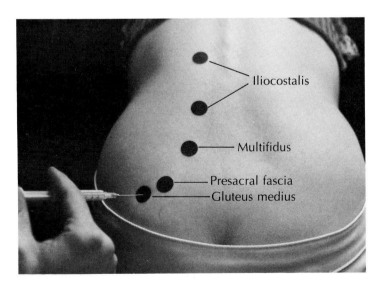

Fig. 8–17. Myofascial trigger point injection: Using the needle as a probe, the points of tenderness are located. Following skin penetration, aliquots of a corticosteroid-local anesthetic mixture are injected. Needle length varies with the size of the patient and ranges from a 1½-in. No. 22 needle to a 4-in. No. 20 spinal needle. Often both sides require injection at the same time, but we seldom exceed a volume of 5 ml.

at the following intervals: before, 15 minutes after, 24 hours after, and 7 days after injections. Benefit was noted in both groups only at 15 minutes; but the treatment group had significant pain relief and global improvement at each assessment. Bupivacaine, 0.5% and up to 36 ml per patient visit, was used;[179] no adverse reactions were reported. However, cardiac sensitivity and other reactions to bupivacaine are being reported with increasing frequency. In a random controlled study of 30 patients, Sonne et al.[179a] reported good to excellent results in 9 out of 14 patients injected with methylprednisolone in 1% lignocaine; only 3 out of 15 patients injected with saline showed good to excellent results. One to three injections of the iliolumbar ligament were performed; results were assessed at two weeks.

No prospective controlled data comparing intralesional corticosteroid treatment alone or mixed with a local anesthetic, with a local anesthetic alone have been reported. Oral steroids are not effective. In our experience, patients with pain of 3 months' duration or longer will often have relief of symptoms for 3 weeks or more when a maximum of 20 mg methylprednisolone or triamcinolone mixed with a local anesthetic is injected per lesion. Do not exceed a total of 60 mg of steroid at one sitting. We do not inject more than 6 times per year. Most patients will require 1 to 3 injections per lifetime (20 years of followup thus far!). Intrathecal or facet joint injections with corticosteroids give similar results but require fluoroscopic control[137a] and are not established as superior to simple percutaneous trigger point injections. Lynch and Taylor[137a] used arthrography following facet joint injection to determine that the joint was injected. Only the intra-articular injections were effective in providing relief of pain. The presacral fascia and sacroiliac joint areas often contain trigger points and use of a #20 3.5 inch spinal needle may be required. Piriformis syndrome may similarly benefit from such injection therapy. Steroid injection may be tried in patients with spinal stenosis. Using the needle as a probe (2 inch #20 or 3.5 inch

spinal needle), injecting beneath the transverse processes of L4 and L5 and into the sacroiliac joints on each side may provide prolonged relief. Although epidural steroids have been advocated one report failed to demonstrate efficacy.[180] Bupivacaine, 1 to 4 ml (0.5%) may also provide relief, but up to 12 injections are required.[181,182]

The patient with low back pain associated with episacroiliac lipoma may have substantial and lasting pain relief by an injection of the lipoma and adjacent tissue.[86,92]

Outcome and Additional Suggestions

Most causes for low back pain are poorly understood at this time, and exacerbation and remissions of symptoms are the rule. Return to the previous accepted level of function represents a "satisfactory outcome." This, of course, is modified by age and other health situations.[156,183] Outcome often depends on the motivation of the patient and good communication between all involved parties (employer, insurer, physician, attorney, patient, and the patient's family).[156]

The importance of a comprehensive program was reported by Reed and Harvey in 1964.[183] In this study, medical, psychologic, sociologic, and vocational evaluations were performed on 185 persons, all of whom were on welfare although previously employed. Of these, only 69 patients were felt likely to be employable full-time; 31 of these 69 welfare recipients did become fully employed; in addition, 16 became part-time employees. Interestingly, 33 other patients left the evaluation program prematurely because they had obtained full-time employment. Only 4 were felt to be malingering. In another series of 100 chronic low pain patients, 80% were reportedly improved; however, of those previously working, only 3 actually returned to work.[156] Yet in most series, less than 2% of patients with back pain are malingering. These 2 reports, a decade apart, offer conflicting return-to-work results. The later report had the poorer result. Is this a result of greater financial support of illness in the more recent decade?

In another study, ambulatory care provided relief in 90% of patients at follow-up.[67] Over the 4-year period of evaluation, surgery was unnecessary for any patient, yet 44% did have recurrences. In those patients with established disc disease, 74% had recurrences of pain, and sciatica alone was not of prognostic value.[67]

The injured worker can benefit from *work hardening*. This program is supervised by an occupational therapist. The patient is guided through highly structured simulated work tasks. Work hardening may help the patient achieve a level of productivity that is acceptable in the competitive labor market.[184] The program requires a therapist trained in this program, which was developed at Rancho Los Amigos Hospital, Downy, California.

Runners occasionally develop herniated lumbar disc disease. Guten followed 10 such patients and reported that the runner who developed the back problem tended to be between 30 and 50 years old, had changed his running style, and in 3 of 10 there was a previous history of disc disease. Only 2 required laminectomy; 8 returned to active running, 1 became a marathon bicyclist and only 1 was unable to return to active sport activities.[185]

Subacute and chronic back pain often respond to a comprehensive treatment program, and the methods outlined are available to any practitioner. Additional new measures receiving attention include transcutaneous nerve stimulation, implantable stimulators, acupuncture, spinal manipulation, biofeedback training, and special inpatient "pain center" therapy. Transcutaneous nerve stimulation, TENS, was of short term benefit in patients with postsurgical back pain, benefit did not last beyond 2 months.[186] Acupuncture (recommended by Osler 50 years ago!)[44] has come and gone in the treatment of low back pain in this country. When the acupuncture therapist provided *no suggestion* of benefit to the patient, only 4% of the patients had lasting relief.[187] This failure of acupuncture was confirmed by others.[188] The use of TENS and other forms of physical therapy will be discussed in Chapters 14 and 16.

Manipulation of the spine has been utilized for nearly a century, and a major segment of the patient population with chronic back pain utilizes this treatment. Finneson details seven types of manipulation that include thrusting, hyperextension, rotation, torsion, and pelvic rock;[3] in general, rotational and mobilizing types are also used.[189–191] Increasing interest in the various "hands on" forms of therapy has led to numerous books and articles describing the techniques. Swezey recently provided a comprehensive review of this subject including massage, traction, mobilization, and manipulation.[153] Current orthopedic literature is accepting manipulation as a valid treatment.[1,3,156,192] Doran and Newell reported the results of osteopathic manipulation versus standard medical care in 456 patients with painful limitation of spinal movement, unassociated with overt disc herniation or vertebral lesions.[191] After 3 months, nearly all patients in both therapeutic groups improved, so that no conclusions could be drawn. Analgesics were of little help. Almost all of the patients were back to work, but 44% still had pain interfering with their work regardless of the treatment modality. Similarly, studies comparing outcome from manipulation versus routine medical care gave results that were comparable.[190,193,194] Jayson et al. noted improved results of mobilization and manipulation compared to placebo physiotherapy in a randomized study of 188 patients. However, the benefit noted at 2 months had disappeared at 3 months, and at 1 year the results were no different. It did not matter whether the patient was referred from a family doctor or from an orthopedist.[195] Similar findings were reported in another study of hospitalized patients.[196] In another study manipulation fared slightly better than sham treatment.[197] When manipulation was compared with massage, immediate benefit with manipulation occurred; but no difference was noted later, at discharge.[198]

The Chiropractic Low Back Pain Study, Inc. reported results of a prospective series of 576 patients treated by 23 chiropracters. Sciatica was present in 78 patients. Manipulation had been used previously in 167 patients. The type of manipulation was not specified. Diagnoses ranged from minor structural change to spinal stenosis. Good to excellent symptomatic response was achieved in 75% of patients; they had an average of 19 visits and required an average of 43 days until maximum benefit.[199] Most reports suggest that the effectiveness of manipulation treatment for low back pain is best for patients with acute pain with no leg pain or neurologic deficits. Improvement in spinal motion and straight leg raising also are noted.[200] Spondylolisthesis was associated with more prolonged treatment.[199]

Indications for surgical intervention for low back pain have altered considerably in the last decade. Selection for surgery and a successful outcome are based upon a definite diagnosis that can be helped by a specific surgical therapy (e.g., laminectomy, fusion, abscess drainage). Probably fewer than 5% of patients with herniated nucleus pulposus require surgical intervention. Surgical results parallel the size of defect seen on myelograms (i.e., the larger the defect, the greater the chance for a good outcome). The severity of a patient's pain is a poor indicator for surgical outcome. Surprisingly, surgical outcome has not correlated well with psychopathology as evidenced by personality inventory determination.[201] Resumption of normal activity postoperatively was 16 days when no secondary gain was present, compared to 36 days if secondary gain was evident. Also, surgical failures were twice as common in those having secondary gain.[202]

Caudal blocks, epidural blocks, epidural steroids, radiofrequency denervation, and posterior rhizotomy have been advocated but are investigational in the opinion of many authors and clinicians.[82,180,203,204,205] Complications following epidural steroid therapy include bacterial meningitis, anesthetic toxicity, steroid toxicity, and improper needle placement.[206]

Chemonucleolysis with chymopapain has been approved for selected patients with established herniated nucleus pulposus. Criteria for diagnosis includes at least four of the following five features:

1. Leg pain greater than back pain
2. Paresthesia localized to a dermatome
3. Straight leg raising reduced 50% or more or positive tibial nerve sign
4. Two or more neurologic findings: atrophy, motor weakness, reflex loss, diminished sensory appreciation
5. Radiographic evidence of abnormality

Chymopapain has adverse reactions, including anaphylaxis. Only experienced surgeons who carefully screen patients for the procedure should be given referrals. In their hands beneficial results up to 80% have been reported.[207] Chymopapain was compared with placebo in a double-blinded randomized study.[208] Thirty-one of 53 placebo treated patients failed to benefit, whereas 40 of 53 treated patients were improved. Of the placebo failures, all were then given chymopapain and 91% improved.[208] In another randomized prospective study without selection, less success with chymopapain was reported; those treated with chymopapain had a 52% failure rate, whereas those operated upon had an 11% failure rate.[209]

Chronic back pain is seldom due to a single structural disorder. More often social and psychologic factors equally contribute to "injury." We discussed Sternbach's description of the "low back loser" (p. 172). Treatment requires that the patient must want to recover. The patient must have goals that she wishes to achieve.[66]

Pain centers are utilizing multiple treatment modalities in an inpatient setting. The eight points of treatment listed by Gottlieb are:[210] biofeedback relaxation, self-control techniques to handle stress and anxiety, patient-regulated medication, case conferences, physical therapy education, vocational rehabilitation, patient education, and a therapeutic milieu. Some critics of pain clinics view them as a graduate school for professional pain patients![211]

A comprehensive back therapy program requires active patient participation. Structural causes for pain, if present, are treated with anesthetic blocks or corticosteroid-anesthetic blocks and injections. In one such program,[212] patients participate in daily activities under the direction of a psychologist, a physical therapist, an occupational therapist, a recreational therapist, and a physician. The patient has an appointment list and must keep the appointments or does not obtain a weekend pass. Should the patient fail on the initial program, she then enters "operant conditioning" in an inpatient facility for 4 to 6 weeks of therapy. This "operant unit" has a "performance and reward" concept. Each bed is connected to a monitor that records the duration of time the patient is up and about. Activity quotas are provided each patient. A psychologist is in charge of such a unit. The patient does obtain positive reinforcement support for demonstrating improvement. Such improvement includes decreased dependency on drugs other than psychotropic agents. Discharge goals are set by the patient in group therapy sessions. Patients, also in group therapy, learn to recognize manipulative factors of chronic pain complaints and their effect on interpersonal relationships. A ten-month follow-up revealed that 70% of the patients had increased their activity or were working. In an 80-month followup of 36 patients in a similar pain clinic program, despite verbal reports of continued pain, most patients reported they were coping much better with back pain, and displayed a marked reduction in their utilization of medical resources.[213] However, most of these patients still regard themselves as failures, and require rewards for the smallest improvements.[212] It should be obvious to the physician that a pain center must provide a multi-faceted program. "Center" programs that provide only one or two modalities, such as biofeedback training or acupuncture, do not suffice and can only delay comprehensive care.

Most patients with low back pain require supportive and preventive therapy. They usually do not have a complex esoteric disease. A treatment regimen, readily provided in an outpatient setting, includes (1) recognition and modification of aggravating factors sometimes through the use of vocational guidance personnel or an occupational therapist, (2) physical therapy and exercise to restore proper soft tissue support for the spine, (3) relief from pain with mild analgesics, nonsteroidal anti-inflammatory drugs, ice massage, vapocoolant spray and stretch, or with local soft tissue injections using an anesthetic-corticosteroid mixture, (4) proper instructions in rest, with or without a corset or traction, and (5) possible use of mood altering drugs for nocturnal sedation and for altering pain perception. Even the patient with chronic, longstanding back pain can be helped in most instances by the personal physician (see Chapter 14). Most patients with "chronic benign pain" have back pain. If pain persists longer than 6 months, then the measures described in Chapter 14 deserve consideration.

PAIN SYNDROMES OF THE PELVIS

Osteitis Condensans Ilii

For a long time this entity has been erroneously considered a radiographic curiosity detected in asymptomatic persons. Sclerosing densities occur on the iliac side of the pelvis. This is usually readily distinguishable from radiographic features of ankylosing spondylitis in which the lesion involves both the sacrum and ilium. Blaschke, however, reviewed 109 patients with the finding of osteitis condensans ilii and discovered that a third suffered from sciatica, two thirds of them had a diffuse fibrositis syndrome, and nearly half the patients had elevation of the erythrocyte sedimentation rate.[214] The symptoms often are self-limited and may respond to nonsteroidal anti-inflammatory agents. HLA B27 typing is reported positive in 25% of these patients.[215] Findings of osteitis condensans ilii may be seen in patients with familial chondrocalcinosis and calcium apatite deposition disease. Two involved families, reported by Arturi et al.,[216] with a total of 9 affected persons demonstrated osteitis condensans ilii (3/

9), costal cartilage calcification (7/9), intervertebral disc calcification (4/9) and articular calcifications.

Osteitis Pubis

Inflammation on each side of the periosteal bone of the symphysis pubis is detectable clinically by local direct point tenderness, and radiographically by erosion, sclerosis, and widening of the symphysis pubis (Fig. 8–18). This disorder may result from regional spread of sepsis following surgery of the prostate or bladder, or herniorrhaphy. However, it often occurs insidiously without any known provoking cause. The vast majority of patients are females in the third to fourth decades of life. The presentation consists of pain in the low anterior pelvis with radiation into the adductor muscles of both thighs. The patient may assume a duck-waddling gait. Local tenderness with reproduction of accentuation of pain by pressure over the symphysis pubis is diagnostic. Tenderness may occur before radiographic changes are evident. Later, the radiographic features of bone rarefaction and erosion with separation of the symphysis pubis and subsequent new bone repair are revealed.[217]

Osteitis pubis may be secondary to ankylosing spondylitis, chondrocalcinosis,[217,218] or polymyalgia rheumatica.[220] When the condition is associated with arthritis, pain frequently has no relation to radiographic change. Subluxation and irregularity were correlated with number of children born (in the females) and not to arthritis.[218] Often the condition is self-limited, and symptomatic benefit may be obtained from use of nonsteroidal anti-inflammatory agents,[221] or local corticosteroid injections into the tender regions of the symphysis pubis (Fig. 8–19), if sepsis has been excluded. Use of a sacral belt to stabilize the pelvis has also provided symptomatic benefit. Obviously, radiographic progression suggests osteomyelitis, and surgical consultation should then be obtained.[217]

Traumatic osteitis pubis, *the gracilis syndrome*, is a fatigue fracture of the bony origin of the gracilis muscle at the pubic symphysis. Surgery, in one case, suggested the lesion resulted from an avulsion fracture.[222] Similarly, osteitis pubis may result from injuries of the adductor longus muscle origin. Pain usually radiates to the perineal region or to the adductor region of the thigh. Athletic activities associated with traumatic osteitis pubis include fencing, basketball, track, hockey, soccer, and bowling. A bony lesion on the lower margin of the pubis at the symphysis is often the only roentgenographic

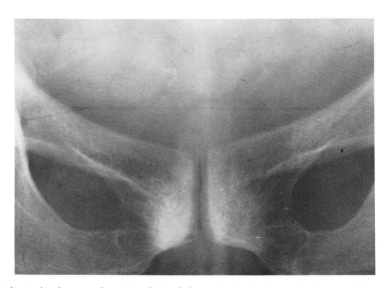

Fig. 8–18. Radiographic features of osteitis pubis include erosion, sclerosis, and widening of the symphysis pubis.

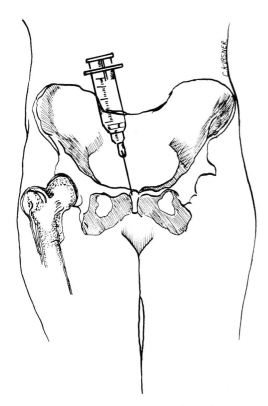

Fig. 8–19. Injection for osteitis pubis: After proper preparation a 1½-in. No. 22 or No. 23 needle is used as a probe. The corticosteroid-local anesthetic mixture is injected at the proximal symphysis pubis region along the bony surface. Strict aseptic technique is essential.

finding. Spontaneous relief has been reported; others recommend local corticosteroid injection; surgical procedure is recommended only if symptoms persist beyond 6 months and a definite lesion is evident.[222]

Coccygodynia

This disorder may occur secondary to low back disorders with referred pain to the coccyx region; from visceral, rectal, or genitourinary disturbances with regional muscle spasm; from local myofascial injury with point tenderness at the sacrococcygeal joint; or from local inflammatory or post-traumatic lesions involving the coccyx and its ligamentous attachments.[65,223,224] A lumbar disc herniation of the nucleus pulposus may result in pain in the coccyx region. Percussion over the L-4

often reproduces such pain. The most common aggravating factor is improper sitting posture.[225] Local treatment measures include injection with a local anesthetic-corticosteroid into soft tissue at the level of vertebra, if a spinal percussion test is positive. Local myofascial injury with point tenderness at the sacrococcygeal joint may be benefited by a local anesthetic-corticosteroid injection directly into the tender area. Use of a 3- or 4-inch thick, soft, foam rubber cushion with a 3-inch hole cut out of the center provides additional comfort. The cushion may prevent a pain-spasm-pain cycle. A silastic or water filled cushion has also been helpful. Surgical resection of a radiographically normal coccyx has not been necessary. Persistent pain raises suspicion for a lumbar disc herniation.

Aching discomfort in the rectum, pelvis, coccyx, or lower back with radiation to the legs and pain during defecation or during sexual intercourse may result from presumed spasm of the piriformis, levator ani, and coccygeus muscles.[224] The symptoms are often aggravated by sitting longer than 30 minutes and are relieved by lying down. Anxiety and fatigue are other aggravations. Tenderness upon rectal examination with reproduction or accentuation of pain occurs when the gloved examining finger palpates the involved muscle. Neurologic examination is normal and there are no radicular features. Rectal massage of the muscles in the lateral rectal walls surrounding the coccyx (the piriformis, the levator ani, and the coccygeus) performed 4 to 6 times over a 10-day period is recommended. The massage is carried out with a gentle stroking of the lateral and posterior rectal walls within reach of the examiner's fingers. The underlying muscles are massaged continually with gradual increased pressure. Relief occurs in approximately two thirds of patients.[223,224] Careful assessment for underlying disc disease is important in those who fail to benefit. We have tried the tricyclic anti-depressants without benefit in these patients. The *levator syndrome*, in which coccygodynia and a sensation of a high, vague pain in the rectum is associated with tenderness of the left levator muscle, may respond to high-voltage electrogalvanic stimulation. This can be administered by rectal probe that is commercially available.[226,227]

Ischial (Ischiogluteal) Bursitis

"Weaver's bottom" or "tailor's bottom" represents pain in a bursa overlying the ischial prominence, and irritation of the sciatic nerve may coexist.[228] The patient often has exquisite pain when sitting or lying. Such patients often are given floor exercises to do and find them painful. Point tenderness with pain reproduction is suggestive. Occasionally we have seen similar pain accompany silent prostatitis in males, in association with ankylosing spondylitis, or in Reiter's syndrome. Rectal examination for prostate irritation should be considered in patients with atypical symptoms. Ankylosing spondylitis or other spondyloarthritides should be excluded. Local anesthetic-corticosteroid injection and use of a 3-inch foam rubber cut-out cushion is helpful. The cushion should have two holes cut for the ischial prominences. Each hole should be about 3 inches in diameter and about 3 inches apart. This condition is intractable, and may last many months. Exercises should be done while lying on the cushion. These consist of stretching (Fig. 8–14) and knee to chest (Fig. 8–12). When injecting the bursa, warn the patient to call out if neuritic pain occurs, since the sciatic nerve is nearby and should *not* be injected.[228] A 2 inch #20 needle with 20 mg methylprednisolone and procaine is used.

ENTRAPMENT NEUROPATHIES

Abdominal Cutaneous Nerve

The patient is often a teenage girl who notes a dull burning pain with sharp exacerbations. The pain radiates transversely across the lower abdomen to the mid-line, and often the patient can localize the origin of pain with one finger.[229,230] The abdominal cutaneous nerves arise from the thoracoabdominal nerve trunks and divide into anterior, lateral, and posterior branches. The nerves pass through a tough fibrous ring in the abdominal wall. Traction of the nerve against this ring may result in a burst of pain. In some patients the nerve is overstretched and angulated as a result of spinal, rib, or other skeletal structures. Symptoms may also result from abdominal distention, but often no apparent cause is found.[229,330] The nerve is easily put under tension and angulated within the abdominal wall's fibrous ring. Most cases involve the anterior cutaneous branch at the rectus margin. Examination with careful palpation of the rectus abdominis usually localizes and reproduces the pain at the fibrous ring. Local anesthestic injection of the region is both diagnostic and therapeutic.[229]

Obturator Nerve

Often following a pelvic fracture, osteitis pubis, or development of an obturator hernia, the patient notes pain and paresthesia in the groin that travels down the inner aspect of the thigh; these symptoms are aggravated during passive or active hip motion.[231] Local nerve block is necessary to establish the diagnosis.

Ilioinguinal Pain Syndrome

Chronic pain across the low anterior pelvis, perineum, groin, thigh, or testicle may result from cicatricial adhesions which entrap the ilioinguinal nerve following herniorrhaphy, appendectomy, urologic or gynecologic surgery. Treatment with local injection, nerve block, TENS, tricyclics, or biofeedback are not often helpful. The condition can arise from faulty posture associated with hip or spine disease in which gait must rely heavily on abdominal muscle support.[232]

REFERENCES

1. Duthie, RB, Ferguson AB: Mercer's Orthopedic Surgery. 8th Ed. Baltimore, Williams & Wilkins, 1973.
2. Fahrni WH: Conservative treatment of lumbar disc degeneration: Our primary responsibility. Orthop Clin N Am 6:93–103, 1975.
3. Finneson BE: Low Back Pain. 2nd Ed. Philadelphia, JB Lippincott, 1981.

4. King JS, Lagger R: Sciatica viewed as a referred pain syndrome. Surg Neurol 5:46–50, 1976.

5. Swezey RL: Pseudo-radiculopathy in subacute trochanteric bursitis of the subgluteus maximus bursa. Arch Phys Med Rehabil 57:387–390, 1976.

6. Matthews JA: Backache. Br Med J 1:432–434, 1977.

7. Mooney V: The syndromes of low back disease. Ortho Clin N Am 14:505–515, 1983.

8. Nachemson AL, Andersson GBJ: Classification of low back pain. Scand J Work Environ Health 8:134–136, 1982.

9. Leads from the MMWR. JAMA 249:2300–2301, 1983.

10. Editorial: Back pain—what can we offer? Br Med J 1:706, 1979.

11. Svensson HO, Andersson GBJ: Low-back pain in 40- to 47-year-old men: Work history and work environment factors. Spine 8:272–276, 1983.

12. Kelsey JL, White AA III, Pastides H, Bisbee GE Jr: The impact of musculoskeletal disorders on the population of the United States. J Bone Joint Surg 61A:959–963, 1979.

13. Kelsey JL, White AA III: Epidemiology and impact of low-back pain. Spine 5:133–142, 1980.

14. Frymoyer JW, Pope MH, Constanza MC, et al: Epidemiologic studies of low back pain. Spine 5:419, 1980.

15. Crook J, Rideout E, Browne G: The prevalence of pain complaints in a general population. Pain 18:299–314, 1984.

16. Hadler NM: Industrial Rheumatology: Clinical investigations into the influence of pattern of usage on the pattern of regional musculoskeletal disease. Arth Rheum 20:1019–1025, 1977.

17. Andersson GBJ: Epidemiologic aspects on low-back pain in industry. Spine 6:53–60, 1981.

18. Yelin E, Kramer J, Epstein W: A national study of medical care use by persons with four rheumatic conditions: effect of symptoms, social and demographic factors. (Abstract #A117) Arth Rheum 25 (No. 4) [Supp], 1982.

19. Hayne CR: Ergonomics and back pain. Physiotherapy 70:9–13, 1984.

20. Gyllenhammar PG: Volvo awards speech. Spine 5:97–98, 1980.

21. Hoehler FK, Tobis JS: Psychological factors in the treatment of back pain by spinal manipulation. Br J Rheum 22:206–212, 1983.

22. Wood PHN: Back pain in the community. Clin Rheum Dis 6:3–16, 1980.

23. Deyo RA, Diehl AK: Measuring physical and psychosocial function in patients with low back pain. Spine 8:635–642, 1982.

24. Tonelli L, Falasca A, Argentieri C, Andreoli M, Merli GA: Influence of psychic distress on short-term outcome of lumbar disc surgery. J Neurosurg 27:237–240, 1983.

25. Becker LA, Karch FE: Low back pain in family practice: A case control study. J Fam Pract 9:579–582, 1979.

26. Marbach JJ, Richlin DM, Lipton JA: Illness behavior, depression and anhedonia in myofascial face and back pain patients. Psychother Psychosom 39:47–54, 1983.

27. Blue LA, Blue FR: Effects of biofeedback on muscular tension in selected personality states. J Psych 101:11–14, 1979.

28. Klein BP, Jensen RC, Sanderson LM: Assessment of workers' compensation claims for back strains/ sprains. J Occup Med 26:443–448, 1984.

29. Manning DP, Shannon HS: Slipping accidents causing low-back pain in a gearbox factory. Spine 6:70–72, 1981.

30. Grandjean E, Hunting W, Pidermann M: VDT workstation design: preferred settings and their effects. Human Factors 25:161–175, 1983.

31. Griffin AB, Troup JDG, Lloyd DCEF: Tests of lifting and handling capacity. Their repeatability and relationship to back symptoms. Ergonomics 27:305–320, 1984.

32. Seamonds BC: Extension of research into stress factors and their effect on illness absenteeism. J Occup Med 25:821–822, 1983.

33. Buckle PW, Kember PA, Wood AD, Wood, SN: Factors influencing occupational back pain in Bedfordshire. Spine 5:254–258, 1980.

34. Magora A: Investigation of the relation between low back pain and occupation. Scand J Rehab Med 6:81–88, 1974.

35. Magora A: Investigation of the relation between low back pain and occupation. Indus Med Surg 41:5–9, 1972.

36. Troup JDG, Martin JW, Lloyd DCEF: Back pain in industry: a prospective survey. Spine 6:61–69, 1981.

37. Snook SH, Irvine CH, Bass SF: Maximum weights and work loads acceptable to male industrial workers: A study of lifting, lowering, pushing, pulling, carrying, and walking tasks. Am Ind Hyg Assoc J 31:579–586, 1970.

38. Snook SH, Ciriello VM: Maximum weights and work loads acceptable to female workers. J Occup Med 16:527–534, 1974.

39. Chaffin DB, Park KS: A longitudinal study of low-back pain as associated with occupational weight lifting factors. Am Ind Hyg Assoc J 34:513–525, 1973.

40. Chaffin DB: Human strength capability and low-back pain. J Occup Med 16:248–254, 1974.

41. Davis PR: The use of intra-abdominal pressure in evaluating stresses on the lumbar spine. Spine 6:90–92, 1981.

42. Addison R, Schultz A: Trunk strengths in patients seeking hospitalization for chronic low-back disorders. Spine 5:539–544, 1980.

43. Pederson OF, Petersen R, Staffeldt ES: Back pain and isometric back muscle strength of workers in a Danish factory. Scand J Rehabil Med 7:125–128, 1975.

44. Quinet RJ, Hadler NM: Diagnosis and treatment of backache. Sem Arth Rheum 8:261–287, 1979.

45. Calin A: Back pain: Mechanical or inflammatory? Am Fam Phys 20:97–100, 1979.

46. Mixter JW, Barr JS: Rupture of the intervertebral disc with involvement of the spinal canal. N Engl J Med 211:210–215, 1934.

47. Kirkaldy-Willis WH: Five common back disorders: How to diagnose and treat them. Geriatrics 33:32–41, 1978.

48. Mooney V, Robertson J: The facet syndrome. Clin Orthop 115:149–156, 1976.

49. Nachemson A, Morris JM: Lumbar discometry: Lumbar intradiscal pressure measurements in vivo. Lancet 1:1140–1142, 1963.

50. Nachemson A, Morris JM: In vivo measurements of intradiscal pressure: Discometry, a method for the determination of pressure in the lower lumbar discs. J Bone Joint Surg 46A:1077–1092, 1964.

51. Nachemson A: Towards a better understanding of low-back pain: A review of the mechanics of the lumbar disc. Rheumatol Rehabil 14:129–143, 1975.

52. Morris JM, Lucas DB, Bressler B: Role of the trunk in stability of the spine. J Bone Joint Surg 43A:327–351, 1961.

53. Farfan HF: Muscular mechanism of the lumbar spine and the position of power and efficiency. Orthop Clin N Am 6:135–144, 1975.

54. Bartelink DL: The role of abdominal pressure in relieving the pressure on the lumbar intervertebral disc. J Bone Joint Surg 39B:718–725, 1967.

55. Suzuki N, Endo S: A quantitative study of trunk muscle strength and fatigability in the low-back-pain syndrome. Spine 8:69–74, 1983.

56. Ortengren R, Andersson GBJ, Nachemson AL: Studies of relationships between lumbar disc pressure, myoelectric back muscle activity, and intraabdominal (intergastric) pressure. Spine 6:98–103, 1981.

57. Gracovetsky S, Farfan HF, Lamy C: The mechanism of the lumbar spine. Spine 6:249–262, 1981.

58. Howes RG, Isdale IC: The loose back: An unrecognized syndrome. Rheum Phys Med 11:72–77, 1971.

59. Hirsch C: The mechanical response in normal and degenerated lumbar discs. J Bone Joint Surg 38A:242–243, 1956.

60. Hilton RC, Ball J, Benn RT: Annular tears in the dorsolumbar spine. Ann Rheum Dis 39:533–538, 1980.

61. Jayson MIV: Back pain: Some new approaches. Med J Aust 1:513–516, 1979.

62. Bogduk N, Macintosh JE: The applied anatomy of the thoracolumbar fascia. Spine 9:165–170, 1984.

63. Russek AS: Biomechanical and physiological basis for ambulatory treatment of low back pain. Orthop Rev 5:21–31, 1976.

64. Bonica JJ: Management of myofascial pain syndromes in general practice. JAMA 164:732–738, 1957.

65. Levine DB: The painful back. Arthritis and Allied Conditions, 10th Ed. Edited by DJ McCarty. Philadelphia, Lea & Febiger, 1985.

66. Sternbach RA, Murphy RW, Akeson WH, Wolf SR: Chronic low-back pain: The "low-back loser." Postgrad Med 53:135–138, 1973.

67. Dillane JB, Fry J, Kalton G: Acute back syndrome—a study from general practice. Br Med J 2:82–84, 1966.

68. Nachemson A: Adult scoliosis and back pain. 1979: Spine 4:513–517. National Institute of Health: Biofeedback for Patients with Raynaud's Phenomenon. JAMA 242:509–510, 1979.

69. Wilberger JE: The silent danger of asymptomatic lumbar disk herniation. J Musculoskel Med 1:33–42, 1984.

70. Gelmers HJ: Entrapment of the sciatic nerve. Acta Neurochir 33:103–106, 1976.

71. Gold S: Unicyclist's Sciatica—A Case Report. N Engl J Med 305:231–232, 1981.

72. Breneman JC: The herniated disc syndrome. J Occup Med 11:475–479, 1969.

73. Retzlaff EW, Berry AB, Haight AS, et al: The piriformis muscle syndrome. J Am Osteopath Assoc 73:799–807, 1974.

74. Pace JB, Nagle D: Piriform syndrome. West J Med 124:435–439, 1976.

75. Brown BR: Diagnosis and therapy of common myofascial pain. JAMA 239:646–648, 1978.

76. Hallin RP: Sciatic pain and the piriformis muscle. Postgrad Med 74(2):69–72, 1983.

77. Simons DG, Travell JG: Myofascial origins of low back pain—1. Principles of diagnosis and treatment. Postgrad Med 73(2):66–108, 1983.

78. Banerjee T, Hall CD: Sciatic entrapment neuropathy. J Neurosurg 45:216–217, 1976.

79. Kestler OC: Posterior lumbar fusions, spinal stenosis, and arachnoiditis. An overview. Contemp Orthop 1:43–53, 1979.

80. Shenkin HA, Hash CJ: Spondylolisthesis after multiple bilateral laminectomies and facetectomies for lumbar spondylosis. J Neurosurg 50:45–47, 1979.

81. Choudhury AR, Taylor JC: Occult lumbar spinal stenosis. J Neurol Neurosurg Psychiatry 40:506–510, 1977.

82. Wiltse LL: Common problems of the lumbar spine: Degenerative spondylolisthesis and spinal stenosis. JCE Orthop 7:17–30, 1979.

83. Wilson ES, Brill RF: Spinal stenosis: The narrow lumbar spinal canal syndrome. Clin Orthop 122:244–248, 1977.

83a. Hall S, Bartoleson JD, Onofrio BM et al.: Lumbar spinal stenosis. Ann Intern Med 103:271–275, 1985.

84. Keim HA: Awareness that spinal nerve entrapment syndromes really exist is most important step in treatment. Orthop Rev 7:79–86, 1978.

85. Verbiest H: A radicular syndrome from developmental narrowing of the lumbar vertebral canal. J Bone Joint Surg 36:230–237, 1954.

86. Singewald ML: Sacroiliac lipomata—an often unrecognized cause of low back pain. Johns Hopkins Med J 118:492–498, 1966.

87. Bywaters EGL: Tendinitis and bursitis. Clin Rheum Dis 5:883–927, 1979.

88. Sarno J: An unorthodox approach to ending back pain. Therapaeia Feb:47–56, 1982.

89. Fowler WM, Taylor RG: Differential diagnosis of

muscle diseases. *In* Musculoskeletal Disorders: Regional Examination and Differential Diagnosis. 2nd Ed. Edited by RD D'Ambrosia. Philadelphia, JB Lippincott, 1984.

90. Fairbank JCT, Obrien JP: The Iliac Crest Syndrome—a treatable cause of low-back pain. Spine 8:220–224, 1983.

91. Martens G, Hoogmartens M, Vaniseghem J: Tight hamstrings syndrome. Acta Ortho Belgica 47:560–569, 1981.

92. Ries E: Episacroiliac lipoma. Am J Ob Gyn 34:490–494, 1937.

93. Pace JB, Henning C: Episacroiliac lipoma. Am Fam Phys 6:70–73, 1972.

94. Blumer D, Heilbronn M: Chronic pain as a variant of depressive disease, the pain-prone disorder. J Nerv & Ment Dis 170:381–431, 1982.

95. Leavitt F: Evaluation of psychological disturbance in low back pain using verbal pain measurement. IM 4:43–49, 1983.

96. Capra P, Mayer TG, Gatchel R: Adding psychological scales to your back pain assessment. J Musc Med 2:41–52, 1985.

97. Crown S: Psychological aspects of low back pain. Rheumatol Rehabil 17:114–122, 1978.

98. Forrest AJ, Wolkind SN: Masked depression in men with low back pain. Rheumatol Rehabil 13:148–153, 1974.

99. Pheasant HC: The problem back. Curr Pract Orthop Surg 7:89–115, 1977.

100. MacNab I: Backache. Baltimore, Williams & Wilkins, 1977.

101. Mooney V: Evaluating low back disorders in the primary care office. J Musculoskel Med. 1:16–26, 1984.

102. Hall H: Examination of the patient with low back pain. Bull Rheum Dis 33:1–8, 1983.

103. Chadwick PR: Examination, assessment and treatment of the lumbar spine. Physio Therapy 70:2–7, 1984.

104. Hochschuler SH: Diagnostic studies in clinical practice. Ortho Clin N Am 14:517–526, 1983.

105. Selby DK: Conservative care of nonspecific low back pain. Ortho Clin N Am 13:427–437, 1982.

106. Calin A, Kaye B, Sternberg M, et al: The prevalence and nature of back pain in an industrial complex. Spine 5:201–205, 1980.

107. Benson DR: The back: Thoracic anbd lumbar spine. *In* Musculoskeletal Disorders: Regional Examination and Differential Diagnosis. 2nd Ed. Edited by RD D'Ambrosia. Philadelphia, JB Lippincott, 1984.

108. Hadler NM: A rheumatologist's view of the back. J Occup Med 24:283–285, 1982.

109. Currey HLF, Greenwood RM, Lloyd GG, Murray RS: A prospective study of low back pain. Rheumatol Rehab 18:94–101, 1979.

110. Blower PW: Neurologic patterns in unilateral sciatica. Spine 6:175–179, 1981.

111. Nelson MA, Allen P, Clamp SE, et al: Reliability and reproducibility of clinical findings in low-back pain. Spine 4:97–101, 1979.

112. Brown MD: Diagnosis of pain syndromes of the spine. Orthop Clin N Am 6:233–248, 1975.

113. ARA Glossary Committee: Dictionary of Rheumatic Diseases. Vol I: Signs and Symptoms. American Rheumatism Assn, New York, Contact Associates, 1982.

114. McRae IF, Wright V: Measurement of back movement. Ann Rheum Dis 28:584–589, 1969.

114a. Merritt JL, McLean TJ, Erickson RP et al.: Measurement of trunk flexibility in normal subjects: Reproducibility of three clinical methods. Mayo Clin Proc 61:192–197, 1986.

115. Goto I. Nagasaka H, Kuroiwa Y: Rigid spine syndrome. J Neurol Neurosurg, Psych 42:276–279, 1979.

116. Felsenthal G, Reischer MA: Asymmetric hamstring reflexes indicative of L5 radicular lesions. Arch Phys Med Rehabil 63:377–378, 1982.

117. Kopp JR: Examining the patient with low back pain efficiently. J Musculoskel Med 1:11–17, 1984.

118. Biering-Sorensen F: Physical measurements as risk indicators for low-back trouble over a one-year period. Spine 9:107–116, 1984.

119. Hadler NM: Legal ramifications of the medical definition of back disease. Ann Intern Med 89:992–999, 1978.

120. Lehmann TR, Brand RA: Disability in the patient with low back pain. Ortho Clin N Am 13:559–568, 1982.

121. Waddell G, Main CJ: Assessment of severity in low-back disorders. Spine 9:204–208, 1984.

122. Pope MH, Rosen JC, Wilder DG, Frymoyer JW: The relation between biomechanical and psychological factors in patients with low-back pain. Spine 5:173–180, 1980.

123. Scavone JG, Latshaw RF, Rohrer GV: Use of lumbar spine films. JAMA 246:1105–1108, 1981.

124. Liang MW, Larson MG, Cullen KE, et al: Comparative measurement efficiency and sensitivity of five health status instruments for arthritis research. Arth Rheum 28:542–547, 1985.

125. Granda JL, Wertheimer TM, Salas JM, Karvonen RL, Lang EF, Nepjuk CAT: X-ray changes in the lumbar spine. (Abstract #248) Arth Rheum 25 (No. 4) [Supp], 1982.

126. Frymoyer JW, Newberg A, Pope MH, Wilder DG, Clements J, MacPherson B: Spine radiographs in patients with low back pain. J Bone Joint Surg 66A:1048–1055, 1984.

127. Pening L, Wilmink JT, van Woerden HH: Inability to prove instability; critical appraisal of clinical-radiological flexion-extension studies in lumbar disc degeneration. Diagn Imag Clin 53:186–192, 1984.

128. Dupuis PR, Young-Hing K, Cassidy JD, Kirkaldy-Willis WH: Radiologic diagnosis of degenerative lumbar spinal instability. Spine 10:262–279, 1985.

129. Lawrence JS, Bremner JM, Bier F: Osteoarthrosis: Prevalence in the population and relationship between symptoms and x-ray changes. Ann Rheum Dis 25:1–24, 1966.

130. Lawrence JS: Disc degeneration: Its frequency and relationship to symptoms. Ann Rheum Dis 28:121–138, 1969.

131. Raskin SP: Introduction to computed tomography of the lumbar spine. Orthopedics 3:1011–1023, 1980.

132. Jackson DW: Low back pain in young athletes: eval-

uation of stress reaction and discogenic problems. Am J Sports Med 7:364–366, 1979.

133. Alarcon GS, Ball GV, Blackburn WD, Vitek JJ, Barger BO, Acton RT: The value of CT scan in the evaluation of inflammatory back pain. (Abstract #52) Arth Rheum 28: (No. 4) [Supp], 1985.

134. Wiesel SW, Sourmas N, Feffer HL, Citrin CM, Patronas N: Non-specific back pain. Spine 9:549–552, 1984.

135. Bell GR, Rothman RH, Booth RE: A study of cat. II. Comparison of metrizamide myelography and CAT in diagnosis of herniated lumbar disc and spinal stenosis. Spine 9:552–7, 1984.

136. Modic MT, Pavlicek W, Weinstein MA, et al: Magnetic resonance imaging of intervertebral disk disease. Radiology 152:103–111, 1984.

136a. Lynch MC, Taylor JF: Facet joint injection for low back pain. J Bone Joint Surg 68B:138–141, 1986.

137. Dory MA: Arthrography of the lumbar facet joints. Radiology 140:23–27, 1981.

138. Murphy WA: The facet syndrome. Radiology 151:533, 1984.

139. Porter RW, Wicks M, Ottewell D: Measurement of the spinal canal by diagnostic ultrasound. J Bone Joint Surg 60B:481–484, 1978.

140. Abraham EA: Thermography: Uses and Abuses. Contemp Ortho 8:95–99, 1984.

141. Bywaters EGL: Viewpoint, mobility with rigiditis: a view of the spine. Ann Rheum Dis 41:210–214, 1982.

142. Terry AF, DeYoung R: Hip disease mimicking low back disorders. Ortho Review 8:95–104, 1979.

143. Beals RK, Hickman NW: Industrial injuries of the back and extremities. J Bone Joint Surg 54A:1593–1611, 1972.

144. Lane N, Bloch D, Jones H, Wood P, Fries JF: Running and osteoarthritis: a controlled study. (Abstract #46) Arth Rheum 28 (No. 4) [Supp], 1985.

145. Keegan JJ: Alterations of the lumbar curve related to posture and seating. J Bone Joint Surg 35A:586–603, 1953.

146. Wosk J, Voloshin AS: Low back pain: conservative treatment with artificial shock absorbers. Arch Phys Med Rehabil 66:145–148, 1985.

147. White AH, White LA, Maltmille WA: Back school and other conservative approaches to low back pain. St Louis; CV Mosby, 1983.

148. Zachrisson MF: The back school. Spine 6:104–106, 1981.

149. Simmons JW, Dennisz MD, Rath D: The back school, a total back management program. Orthopedics 7:1453–1456, 1984.

150. Berquist-Ullman M, Larsson UL: Acute low back pain in industry. A controlled prospective study with special reference to therapy and confounding factors. Acta Ortho Scand 170:1–117, 1977.

151. Kraus H: Clinical Treatment of Back and Neck Pain. New York, McGraw-Hill, 1970.

152. Pearce J, Moll JMH: Conservative treatment and natural history of acute lumbar disc lesions. J Neurol Neurosurg Psychiatry 30:13–17, 1967.

153. Swezey RL: The modern thrust of manipulation and traction therapy. Seminars Rheum Dis 12:321–331, 1983.

154. Mathews JA, Hickling J: Lumbar traction; A dou-

155. Mooney V, Cairns D: Management in the patient with chronic low back pain. Ortho Clin N Am 9:543–557, 1978.

156. Saunders HD: Use of spinal traction in the treatment of neck and back conditions. Clin Ortho Research 179:31–38, 1983.

157. Million R, Nilsen KH, Jayson MIV, et al: Evaluation of low back pain and assessment of lumbar corsets with and without back supports. Ann Rheum Dis 40:449–454, 1981.

158. Nachemson A: Physiotherapy for low back pain patients: A critical look. Scand J Rehabil Med 1:85–90, 1969.

159. Friberg TR, Weinrab RN: Ocular manifestations of gravity inversion. JAMA 253:1755–1757, 1985.

160. Kendall PH, Jenkins JM: Exercises for backache: A double-blind controlled trial. Physiotherapy 54:154–157, 1968.

161. Kendall PH, Jenkins JM: Lumbar isometric flexion exercises. Physiotherapy 54:158–163, 1968.

162. Ekholm J, Arborelius U, Fahlcrantz A, Larsson A-M, Mattsson G: Activation of abdominal muscles during some physiotherapeutic exercises. Scand J Rehab Med 11:75–84, 1979.

163. Blackburn SE, Portney LG: Electromyographic activity of back musculature during Williams' flexion exercises. Phys Ther 61:878–885, 1981.

164. McKenzie RA: Prophylaxis in recurrent low back pain. New Z Med J 89:22–23, 1979.

165. Kraus H, Nagler W: Evaluation of an exercise program for back pain. AFP 28:153–158, 1983.

166. Abraham EA, Leifer LJ: Study results of a group therapeutic exercise program. Contemp Orthop 5:47–53, 1982.

167. Davies JE, Gibson T, Tester L: The value of exercises in the treatment of low back pain. Rheumatol Rehab 18:243–247, 1979.

168. Overman SS, Rockey PH, Dickstein DA, Larson JW: Physical therapists as primary care providers for low back pain: a controlled trial. (Abstract #49) Arth Rheum 25 (No. 4) [Supp], 1982.

169. Coxhead CE, et al: Multicenter trial of physiotherapy in the management of sciatic symptoms. Lancet 1:1065–1068, 1981.

170. Woolbright JL: Exercise protocol for patients with chronic back pain. JAOA 82:919–932, 1983.

171. Hindle TH III: Comparison of carisoprodol, butabarbital, and placebo in treatment of the low back syndrome. Cal Med 117:7–11, 1972.

172. Beaumont G: The use of psychotropic drugs in other painful conditions. J Int Med Res 4:[Supp] (2)56–57, 1976.

173. deJong RH: Central pain mechanisms. JAMA 239:2784, 1978.

174. Pheasant H, Bursk A, Goldfarb J, Azen SP, Weiss JN, Borelli L: Amitriptyline and chronic low-back pain. Spine 8:552–557, 1983.

175. Berry H, Bloom B, Hamilton EBD, Swinson DR: Naproxen sodium, diflunisal, and placebo in the treatment of chronic back pain. Ann Rheum Dis 41:129–132, 1982.

176. Steindler A, Luck JV: Differential diagnosis of pain low in the back: Allocation of the source of pain by

the procaine hydrochloride method. JAMA
110:106–113, 1938.

177. Dilke TFW, Burry HC, Grahame R: Extradural
corticosteroid injection in management of lumbar
nerve root compression. Br Med J 2:635–637, 1973.

178. Bourne IHJ: Treatment of backache with local injections. Practitioner 222:708–711, 1979.

179. Hameroff SR, Crago BR, Blitt CD, Womble J,
Kanel J: Comparison of bupivacaine, etidocaine,
and saline for trigger-point therapy. Anesthesia Analgesia 60:752–755, 1981.

179a. Sonne M, Christensen K, Hansen SE, Jensen EM:
Injection of steroids and local anesthetics as therapy
for low-back pain. Scand J Rheum 14:343–345,
1985.

180. Cuckler JM, Bernini PA, Wiesel SW, Booth RE,
Rothman RH, Pickens GT: The use of epidural ste-
roids in the treatment of lumbar radicular pain. J
Bone Joint Surg 67A:63–66, 1985.

181. Hendler N, Fink H, Long D: Myofascial syndrome:
response to trigger-point injections. Psychosomatics 24:993–999, 1983.

182. Brown BR: Myofascial and musculoskeletal pain.
Int Anesthiol Clin 21:139–151, 1983.

183. Reed JW, Harvey JC: Rehabilitating the chronically
ill: A method for evaluating the functional capacity
of ambulatory patients. Geriatrics 19:87–103, 1964.

184. Matheson LN, Ogden LD, Violette K, Schultz:
Work hardening: Occupational therapy in industrial rehabilitation. Am J Occup Therapy
39:314–321, 1985.

185. Guten G: Herniated lumbar disk associated with
running. Am Ortho Soc Sports Med 9:155–159,
1981.

186. Richardson RR, et al: Transcutaneous electrical
neurostimulation in functional pain. Spine
6:185–188, 1981.

187. Murphy TM: Subjective and objective follow-up
assessment of acupuncture therapy without suggestion in 100 chronic pain patients. In Advances
in Pain Research and Therapy. Vol. I. Edited by JJ
Bonica, DG Albe-Fessard. New York, Raven Press,
1976.

188. Mendelson G, Selwood TS, Kranz H, Loh TS, Kid-
son MA, Scott DS: Acupuncture treatment of
chronic back pain: A double blind placebo controlled trial. Am J Med 74:49–55, 1983.

189. Maigne R: Orthopedic Medicine: A New Approach
to Vertebral Manipulations. Springfield, Charles C
Thomas, 1972.

190. Glover JR, Morris JG, Khosla T: Back pain: A randomized clinical trial of rotational manipulation of
the trunk. Br J Ind Med 31:59–64, 1974.

191. Doran DML, Newell DJ: Manipulation in treatment of low back pain: A multicentre study. Br Med
J 2:161–164, 1975.

192. Firman GJ, Goldstein MS: The future of chiropractic: A psychosocial view. N Engl J Med
293:639–642, 1975.

193. Kane RL, Leymaster C, Olsen D, et al: Manip-
ulating the patient: A comparison of the effectiveness of physician and chiropractic care. Lancet
1:1333–1336, 1974.

194. Godfrey CM, Morgan PP, Schatzker J: A random-

ized trial of manipulation for low-back pain in a
medical setting. Spine 9:301–304, 1984.

195. Jayson MIV, Sims-Williams H, Young S, Baddeley
H, Collins E: Mobilization and manipulation for
low-back pain. Spine 6:409–416, 1981.

196. Sims-Williams H, Jayson MIV, Young SMS, et al:
Controlled trial of mobilisation and manipulation
for patients with low back pain in general practice.
Br Med J 2:1338–1340, 1979.

197. Greenland S, et al: Controlled clinical trials of manipulation: A review and a proposal. J Occup Med
22:670–676, 1980.

198. Hoehler FK, Tobis JS, Buerger AA: Spinal manipulation for low back pain. JAMA 245:1835–1838,
1981.

199. Cox JM, Shreiner S: Chiropractic manipulation in
low back pain and sciatica: statistical data on diagnosis, treatment, response of 576 consecutive
cases. J Man Physio Therap 7:11, 1984.

200. Haldeman S: Spinal manipulative therapy. Clin
Orth Related Res 179:62–70, 1983.

201. Waring EM, Weisz GM, Bailey SI: Predictive factors in the treatment of low back pain by surgical
intervention. In Advances in Pain Research and
Therapy. Vol 1. Edited by JJ Bonica, DG Albe-
Fessard. New York, Raven Press, 1976.

202. Finneson BE: Modulating effect of secondary gain
on the low back pain syndrome. In Advances in
Pain Research and Therapy. Vol I. Edited by JJ
Bonica, DG Albe-Fessard. New York, Raven Press,
1976.

203. Stanton-Hicks M: Therapeutic caudal or epidural
block for lower back or sciatic pain. JAMA
243:369–370, 1980.

204. Tarlov E: Therapeutic caudal or epidural block for
lower back or sciatic pain. JAMA 243:369, 1980.

205. Oudenhoven RC: The role of laminectomy, facet
rhizotomy, and epidural steroids. Spine 2:145–147,
1979.

206. Wallace G, Solove GJ: Epidural steroid therapy for
low back pain. Postgrad Med 78:213–218, 1985.

207. McCulloch JA: Chemonucleolysis for relief of sciatica due to a herniated intervertebral disc. Can
Med Assoc J 124:879–882, 1981.

208. Javid MJ, et al: Safety and efficacy of Chymopapain
(Chymodiactic) in herniated nucleus pulposus with
sciatica. JAMA 249:2489–2494, 1983.

209. Crawshaw C, Frazer AM, Merriam WF, Mulholland RC, Webb JK: A comparison of surgery and
chemonucleolysis in the treatment of sciatica: a prospective randomized trial. Spine 9:195–199, 1984.

210. Gottlieb H, Strite LC, Koller R, et al: Comprehensive rehabilitation of patients having chronic
low back pain. Arch Phys Med Rehabil 58:101–108,
1977.

211. Hubbard JH: Chronic pain of spinal origin: ration-
ales for treatment. In The Back, edited by RH
Rothman and FA Simeone. Philadelphia, WB
Saunders, 1982.

212. Cairns D, Thomas L, Mooney V, Pace JB: A comprehensive treatment approach to chronic low back
pain. Pain 2:301–308, 1976.

213. Newman RI, Seres JL, Yospe LP, et al: Multidisciplinary treatment of chronic pain: Long-term fol-

low-up of low-back pain patients. Pain 4:283–292, 1978.

214. Blaschke JA: Clinical characteristics of osteitis condensans ilii. Abstract. Paper presented to VI Pan-American Congress on Rheumatic Diseases, June, 16–21, 1974.

215. Singal DP, deBosset P, Gordon DA, et al: HLA antigens in osteitis condensans ilii and ankylosing spondylitis. J Rheumatol [Supp (3)]4:105–108, 1977.

216. Arturi AS, Marcos JC, Maldonado-Cocca JA, et al: Osteitis condensans ilii in apatite crystal deposition disease. Arth Rheum 26:567–569, 1983.

217. Samellas W, Finkelstein P: Osteitis pubis: Its surgical treatment. J Urol 87:(4)553–555, 1962.

218. Scott DL, Eastmond CJ, Wright V: A comparative radiological study of the pubic symphysis in rheumatic disorders. Ann Rheum Dis 38:529–534, 1979.

219. Pinals RS: Traumatic arthritis and allied conditions. In Arthritis and Allied Conditions. 10th Ed. Edited by DJ McCarty. Philadelphia, Lea & Febiger, 1985.

220. O'Duffy JD: Increasing evidence suggests polymyalgia rheumatica is not a muscle disease. Wellcome Trends in Rheumatology 1:1–2, 1979.

221. Barnes WC, Malament M: Osteitis pubis. Surg Gynecol Obstet 117:277–284, 1963.

222. Wiley JJ: Traumatic osteitis pubis: the gracilis syndrome. Am J Sport Med 11:360–363, 1983.

223. Thiele GH: Coccygodynia and pain in the superior gluteal region and down the back of the thigh. Causation by tonic spasm of the levator ani, coccygeus, and piriformis muscles and relief by massage of these muscles. JAMA 109:1271–1275, 1941.

224. Sinaki M, Merritt, JL, Stillwell GK: Tension myalgia of the pelvic floor. Mayo Clin Proc 52:717–722, 1977.

225. Johnson PH: Coccygodynia. J Arkansas Med Soc 77:421–424, 1981.

226. Sohn N, Weinstein MA, Robbins RD: The levator syndrome and its treatment with high-voltage electrogalvanic stimulation. Am J Surg 144:580–582, 1982.

227. Nicosia JF, Abcarian H: Levator syndrome; a treatment that works. Dis Colon Rectum 28:406–408, 1985.

228. Swartout R, Compere EL: Ischio-gluteal bursitis. JAMA 227:551–552, 1974.

229. DeValera E, Raftery H: Lower abdominal and pelvic pain in women. In Advances in Pain Research and Therapy. Vol 1. Edited by JJ Bonica, D Albe-Fessard. New York, Raven Press, 1976.

230. Applegate WV: Abdominal cutaneous nerve entrapment syndrome. Am Fam Physician 8:132–133, 1973.

231. Kopell HP, Thompson WA; Peripheral Entrapment Neuropathies. Huntington, NY, RE Krieger, 1976.

232. Hameroff SR, Carlson GL, Brown BR: Ilioinguinal pain syndrome. Pain 10:253–257, 1981.

233. Sheon RP: A joint protection guide for nonarticular rheumatic disorders. Postgrad Med 77 (5):329–338, 1985.

9

The Hip and Thigh Region

Pain in this region may be referred from disorders arising in the low back, abdomen, peripheral nerves, retroperitoneal region (with irritation of the psoas muscle), within the hip joint, or may result from lesions in the soft tissue of the hip region. Patients often interpret low back or presacral pain, or ischiogluteal discomfort, as "hip pain." Always ask the patient to point to the area of greatest discomfort. True hip pain usually is groin pain or is referred to the medial aspect of the knee. Patients with intrinsic hip disease usually have the associated complaint of limitation of movement. For example, the most specific complaint is loss of the ability to rotate the leg into abduction when putting on a slipper or stocking in the morning. In essence, the patient is performing the Patrick or "Fabere test." The *Fabere test* is comprised of the abbreviations for four maneuvers: *F*lexion, *Ab*duction, *E*xternal *R*otation and *E*xtension.[1] As mentioned previously, night pain often is the result of inflammation of myofascial structures, bursitis, or tumor. If a patient with known hip disease does suffer night pain, the clinician should be alert to a coexisting extra-articular treatable soft tissue cause for the pain, although severe intra-articular disease can also cause night pain. Numbness, tingling, stabbing, and sciatica-like pain may be of myofascial origin rather than disc disease, or the symptoms may result from an entrapment neuropathy. Entrapment neuropathies are characterized by intermittency of symptoms, lancinating pain, and aggravation by a particular motion. (See Danger List, Table 9–1.)

The fascia lata and its component, the iliotibial tract, are important soft tissue structures, the involvement of which is capable of causing frustrating chronic leg pain (see An-

Table 9–1. Danger List for the Hip Region

1. Fever and chills
2. Weight loss
3. Lymphadenopathy
4. Hip claudication
5. Thigh atrophy
6. Reflex change
7. Painful gait

atomic Plates X and XI).[2] The fascia lata is a thickened deep fascia of the lateral thigh. Superiorly the fascia lata attaches to the anterior superior iliac spine, the inguinal ligament, the body of the pubic bone, the ischial tuberosity, the sacrotuberous ligament, the sacrum, and the iliac crest. The iliotibial tract is a conjoint aponeurosis of the fascia lata and the gluteus maximus muscle. The iliotibial tract inserts on the anterolateral aspect of the tibia.[1] If contracted, it exerts a pull upon the hip resulting in flexion and abduction; it can also cause the "snapping hip syndrome." Tendinitis of the gluteus medius and minimus at their insertion also causes lateral hip pain. Distinction from trochanteric bursitis is difficult and is probably unnecessary as treatment is the same for both. Knowledge of the location of the superficial and deep trochanteric bursae, the iliopectineal bursa, and the origin and points of potential injury or entrapment of the various superficial peripheral nerves of this region allow the examiner to palpate for trigger points and to reproduce the pain that results from disturbances of these soft tissue structures.

Physical Examination. The following degrees of hip movement are considered normal: Flexion—120 to 135 degrees; abduction in extension—35 to 40 degrees; abduction in flexion—70 to 75 degrees; adduction (crossing leg)—25 to 30 degrees; internal rotation in extension or flexion—45 degrees; external rotation in extension or flexion—45 degrees; and hip extension—20 to 30 degrees[3] (Fig. 9–1).

The examiner should measure leg lengths, after determining the patient's ability to fully straighten the knees. With the leg drawn straight and the patient lying flat on her back, the true leg length can be measured from the anterior-superior iliac spine to the medial malleolus of each ankle. Normal individuals may have as much as 1-cm discrepancy without symptoms. "Apparent" limb length disparity is determined by measuring the distance from the umbilicus to each medial malleolus.[3] An examination of the abdomen, back, and groin and a careful neurologic examination should be performed appropriate to the clinical presentation (Table 9–2: Decision Chart for the Hip Region).

Special Maneuvers or Other Tests. The *Trendelenburg* test is important for the detection of involvement of the hip stabilizers (gluteus medius, gluteus minimus). The examination consists of having the patient stand with her back to the examiner; two points are marked on each of the posterior iliac spines; then the patient stands on one foot and raises the other; the side supporting the body's weight is the side being tested. If the pelvis falls on the side *not* bearing weight the test is positive and suggests muscle disease affecting the abductors or the stabilizers of the hip, congenital dislocation of the hip, coxa vara, Legg-Calvé-Perthes disease, or abnormalities in the proximal femoral epiphysis.[3]

The *Fabere test* (also called Patrick's test) is a physical examination maneuver that requires placing the foot of the involved extremity on the opposite knee. The examiner then presses the knee and thigh downward and pain results if intrinsic hip disease is present (Fig. 9–2).

Erichsen's sign: The examiner provides compression across the iliac bones; if pain occurs, the test is suggestive for sacroiliac joint inflammation.

Ober's test (for contracture of the iliotibial band): The patient lies with the affected side up and the opposite side down; the uppermost leg (symptomatic side) is drawn backward at the hip (with hyperextension of the hip) and then bent at the knee (Fig. 9–3). The Ober test is positive if, after letting go of the involved thigh, the knee does not drop to the table. Failure of the leg to fall suggests a contracture of the iliotibial band. The Ober test (Fig. 9–3) also reproduces pain resulting from hip flexor muscle contractures.[3]

Differential Diagnosis. The conditions described in this chapter are regional local disorders. However, pain in the region can also arise from systemic or multifocal disease, such as herniation of a lumbar disc, Paget's disease, migratory osteolysis, inflammatory rheumatic diseases, panniculitis, occult sepsis, or neoplastic disorders.[4–7] Hip fracture in the elderly is not uncommon and can be missed; the patient often forgets the traumatic incident. Any elderly person with an abnormal gait should be examined for this as a cause of symptoms. The fracture may not be visible at first roentgenographic study, but will usually be evident at following roentgenographic examination.[8] Constant groin pain can result from other articular and non-articular causes. Recurrent groin strain is common among hockey and soccer players. Injury to the pubis with resultant osteitis pubis should be considered.[9] Other causes for groin pain include conditions of the femoral triangle such as abscesses, hernias, cellulitis, hematomas, lipomas, aneurysm, femoral vein thrombosis and tumors. Use of computed tomography[10,11] or ultrasound examination of this region can be helpful[12] (Table 9–1, Danger List). Patients with persistent pain in this region require appropriate laboratory and radiographic examinations. Radiographic examination should include the spine and both hips for appropriate evaluation. An erythrocyte sedimentation rate, a complete blood count, urinalysis, rectal examination, and stool examinations for occult blood are essential in patients with any persistent pelvic or hip region pain. A careful vaginal pelvic examination should be performed by the clinician experienced in this examination. The

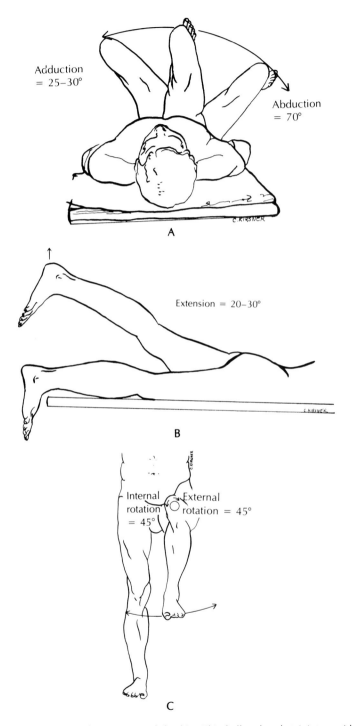

Fig. 9–1. Examination for range of movement of the hip. This ball-and-socket joint provides, *A*, adduction, abduction, and flexion: *B*, extension; *C*, internal and external rotation. These illustrations demonstrate some of the methods for the determination of these movements.

Table 9–2. Decision Chart, The Hip and Thigh

Feature	Action	Further Actions
A. Lateral Hip Pain Not acute, no limp Painful when lying on side Normal hip motion	CONSERVATIVE CARE Correct aggravating factors Prescribe exercises Provide pain relief with NSAID's Inject bursae if tender Analgesics, relaxants	Repeat Roentgenographic Examination CT Scan Repeat general physical examination Orthopedic/Rheumatologic Consultation Physiatric consultation
B. Lateral Hip Pain Limp, weakness Neurologic findings positive or suspicious	Roentgenographic examination in older patient → Physical therapy consult if needed Electrodiagnostic study as appropriate	
C. Anterior Hip Pain Morning stiffness Limited motion No neurologic findings	⟶ + Ultrasound or CT Scan	
D. Acute Hip Pain Older patient Limps, and limited motion	⟶ Immediate roentgenographic exam	
E. Danger List present Constitutional features Lymphadenopathy/Mass Claudication, limb discoloration Atrophy	⟶ Immediate Appropriate Action	

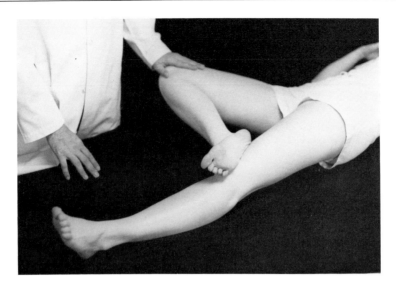

Fig. 9–2. The Patrick or Fabere test: If pain results when the examiner presses the knee and thigh downward, then intrinsic hip disease should be suspected.

pelvic ligaments are uncommon sites of origin for low pelvic pain in females, and the degree of tenderness is a subjective determination.

MYOFASCIAL PAIN SYNDROMES

Snapping Hip

An actual dislocation of the hip is painful, whereas the snapping hip is a painless an-noying noise.[13] The snapping hip often results from a taut iliotibial band slipping over the greater tuberosity.[1,3] Other causes for snapping hip include the iliopsoas tendon jumping across the iliopectineal eminence,[14] the gluteus maximus sliding across the greater trochanter, and generalized joint laxity. Arthrography, with special attention to the iliopsoas tendon during hip motion, under fluoroscopy

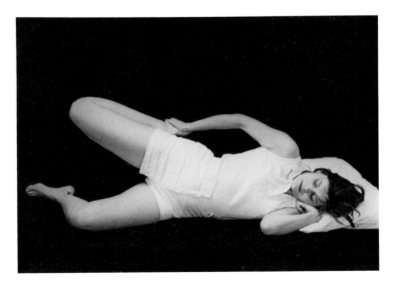

Fig. 9–3. The Ober test: This test is useful for determining the presence of a contracture of the iliotibial band or tightness in the hip flexor musculature.

may be necessary for diagnosis. In our experience the iliotibial band is most often the culprit, and treatment provides benefit thus alleviating the need for expensive diagnostic tests. Treatment consists of stretching the iliotibial band for a few moments twice daily (Fig. 9–4). Usually within a period of weeks the snapping diminishes.

Fascia Lata Fasciitis

Symptoms may result from inflammation or tightness of the fascia lata due to overuse or disuse. The patient may describe vague discomfort upon arising in the morning and after prolonged walking. Initially, symptoms may be relieved by walking, only to be aggravated by further prolonged walking. The discomfort is a dull ache over the low back and lateral hip and thigh region radiating down the lateral thigh to the lateral knee region. Physical examination requires positioning the patient on the examining table with the involved hip uppermost. The straight leg is then drawn over the edge of the table and pressure is placed upon the ankle (Fig. 9–4). The weighted straight leg is drawing the fascia lata taut. In a slender individual we have seen dimpling along the fascia resulting from adhesions (Fig. 9–5). The dimpling or tenderness to palpation may be detected in the region of

the trochanteric bursa, 2 inches below the trochanteric bursa, and then along the crevice palpable between the anterior and posterior muscle compartments of the lateral thigh. These areas should be marked for later injection. Tenderness should be sought as high as the gluteus medius and as low as 2 to 3 inches below the fibular head. Treatment consists of injecting local anesthetic-corticosteroid mixture into the involved symptomatic locations. The fascia should be stretched by having the patient assume the same position as described for the examination. The patient lies on the edge of a bed with a weight (ranging from 3 to 10 pounds depending on tolerance) applied to the ankle. The patient should flex the hip to a degree that allows a pulling sensation to be felt along the lateral compartment of the thigh[2] (Fig. 9–4). Persistent pain should lead to suspicion of an L-4–5 herniated disc with referred pain to the lateral hip area.

BURSITIS

Of the 18 or more bursae described in the hip region, the most important are the trochanteric, iliopectineal, and ischiogluteal bursae.

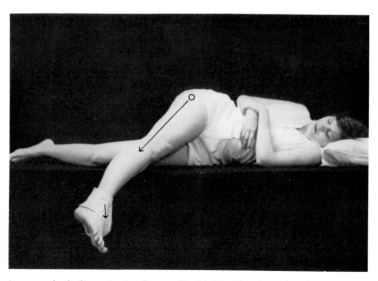

Fig. 9–4. Exercise or method of examination for taut iliotibial band or fascia lata fasciitis.

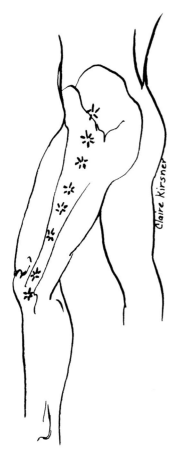

Fig. 9–5. Sites of tenderness or adhesions along the fascia lata.

Trochanteric Bursitis

The deep trochanteric bursa lies between the tendon of the gluteus maximus and the posterolateral prominence of the greater trochanter.[1,3,15] A more superficial bursa directly over the greater trochanter may also become inflamed and tender. Characteristic night pain of bursitis may be added to that secondary to osteoarthritis of the hip. Point tenderness over the trochanteric bursa with pain reproduction is strong evidence for the presence of bursitis. This point of tenderness usually lies approximately an inch posterior and superior to the greater trochanter, and is located about 3 inches deep to the skin. Obesity, compression injury, or other minor local trauma may be aggravating factors. The act of arising from a position of lumbar spine flex-

ion (back bent forward), while the knees are kept straight requires a lever action of the glutei and is perhaps the most common cause for gluteal strain, which in turn may predispose to trochanteric bursitis. Such patients must learn to bend their knees before bending their backs. Treatment consists of injecting the trochanteric bursa with a local anesthetic-corticosteroid agent (Fig. 9–6), sleeping with a small pillow under the involved buttock to keep the body weight shifted off of the bursa, and stretching the gluteal muscles utilizing knee chest exercises (Fig. 8–11). The need for repeated injections of the hip should lead to consideration for other diagnoses, aggravating factors, or additional consultation. Repeated injections can result in osteonecrosis.[16] Surgical excision is rarely necessary.[17]

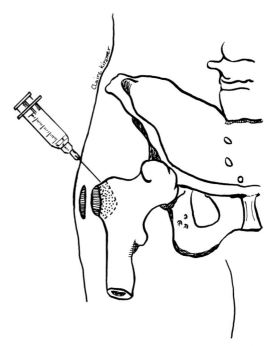

Fig. 9–6. Superficial (adventitial) and deep trochanteric bursitis: After localizing the points of maximum tenderness by deep palpation, a 1½- to 4-in. needle is used as a probe; the points of maximum tenderness are determined, and aliquots of a corticosteroid-local anesthetic are injected into each site.

Iliopectineal and Iliopsoas Bursitis

The iliopectineal bursa lies between the iliopsoas muscle and the iliopectineal eminence. Posteriorly it lies lateral to the femoral vessels and overlies the capsule of the hip. The iliopsoas bursa lies medially in Scarpa's triangle. Bursitis in the anterior hip region (rare in our experience) causes pain in the anterior pelvis, groin, and thigh region.[1,3] The iliopectineal bursa often communicates with the hip joint; bursitis may result from intrinsic joint disease.[1] Diagnosis can be confirmed by ultrasound or computed tomography. Careful injection of the bursa with a corticosteroid-local anesthetic mixture probably is best performed by a rheumatologist or orthopedist. Persistence may indicate surgical intervention and excision of the bursa.

ENTRAPMENT NEUROPATHIES

Symptoms of intermittent numbness, tingling, and a sensation of swelling suggest an entrapment neuropathy.

Obturator Nerve

Often following a pelvic fracture, osteitis pubis, or development of an obturator hernia, the patient notes pain and paresthesia in the groin that travels down the inner aspect of the thigh; these symptoms are aggravated during passive or active hip motion.[18] Local nerve block is necessary to establish the diagnosis.

Meralgia Paresthetica

Entrapment of the lateral femoral cutaneous nerve is a frequent entrapment neuropathy of the thigh region. Intermittent paresthesia, hypesthesia, or hyperesthesia over the upper anterolateral thigh occur (Fig. 9–7). The entrapment usually occurs at the anterior superior iliac spine where the nerve passes through the lateral end of the inguinal ligament or adjacent iliacus fascia.[18,19] The nerve also perforates the sartorius muscle and exits through a canal in the fascia lata.[20] Entrapment may also occur within the spinal

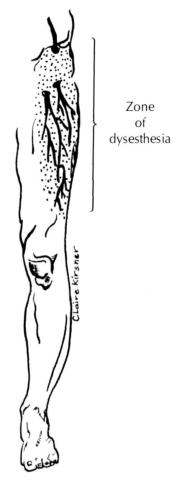

Zone of dysesthesia

Fig. 9–7. Entrapment of the lateral femoral cutaneous nerve (meralgia paresthetica): The nerve is frequently impinged at the anterosuperior iliac spine; dysesthesias are noted over the upper anterior lateral thigh.

canal, intervertebral foramina, or in the retroperitoneal region. Trauma, a pelvic tilt resulting from a short limb, prolonged sitting with crossed legs, or increased abdominal girth with bulging fat may be causative. Pregnancy, rapid weight gain, and constriction from a corset, belt, or seatbelt are other common causes.[21] Treatment includes local infiltration with anesthetic-corticosteroid agents into the site of nerve exit at the inguinal ligament and into the region of dysesthesia. Also helpful are avoiding contact pressure in the region of the inguinal ligament, loss of

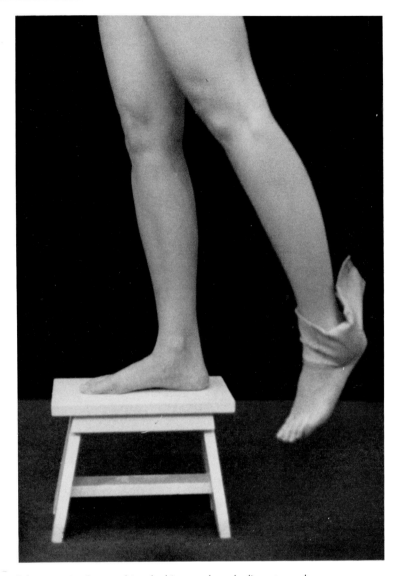

Fig. 9–8. Pendulum exercise for stretching the hip capsule and adjacent muscles.

weight, and if necessary, use of a heel-lift for a short limb.[18]

Sciatic Pseudoradiculopathy

A pseudoradiculopathy may result from trochanteric bursitis; relief of the sciatica-like pain occurs following injection of the trochanteric bursa.[22] Sometimes hip capsule stretching is of additional help (Fig. 9–8). In addition, the sciatic nerve may be involved in disease entities beyond the pelvis. Con-

stricting myofascial bands in the posterior thigh have been described.[23]

No single entity stands out as a cause for low pelvic, hip, and thigh region pain. We have presented a potpourri of disorders seen frequently as causes for treatable discomfort in the hip and thigh (Table 9–2 Decision Chart for the Hip Region). Management obviously depends on careful assessment. The relief provided by treatment often establishes the diagnosis. However, failure to recognize an aggravating factor often results in recurrence. The six points of management described previously apply to this body region as well.

REFERENCES

1. Turek SL: Orthopaedics: Principles and Their Application. 4th Ed. Philadelphia, JB Lippincott, 1984.
2. Lowman EW: Connective tissue diseases. *In* Handbook of Physical Medicine and Rehabilitation. 2nd Ed. Edited by FH Kruzen. Philadelphia, WB Saunders, 1971.
3. D'Ambrosia RD: The hip. *In* Musculoskeletal Disorders. Philadelphia, JB Lippincott, 1977.
4. Benson R, Fowler PD: Treatment of Weber-Christian disease. Br Med J 2:615–616, 1964.
5. Pinals RS: Traumatic arthritis and allied conditions. *In* Arthritis and Allied Conditions. 10th Ed. Edited by DJ McCarty. Philadelphia, Lea & Febiger, 1985.
6. Swezey RL. Transient osteoporosis of the hip, foot, and knee. Arthritis Rheum 13:858–868, 1970.
7. Duncan H, Frame B, Frost HM, Arnstein AR: Migratory osteolysis of the lower extremities. Ann Intern Med 66:1165–1173, 1967.
8. Aaron JE, Gallagher JC, Anderson J, et al: Frequency of osteomalacia and osteoporosis in fractures of the proximal femur. Lancet 1:229–233, 1974.
9. Muckle DS: Associated factors in recurrent groin and hamstring injuries. Br J Sports Med 15:37–39, 1982.
10. Kovarsky J, Davis R: Compression of obturator nerve by lipoma. Arth Rheum 23:871–872, 1980.
11. Penkava RR: Iliopsoas bursitis demonstrated by computed tomography. Am J Roentgen 135:175–176, 1980.
12. Gitschlag KF, Sandler MA, Madrazo BL, Hricak H, Eyler WR: Disease in the Femoral Triangle: Sonographic Appearance. AJR 139:515–519, 1982.
13. Carter C, Wilkinson J: Persistent joint laxity and congenital dislocation of the hip. J Bone Joint Surg 46B:40–45, 1964.
14. Lyons JC, Peterson LFA: The snapping iliopsoas tendon. Mayo Clin Proc 59:327–329, 1984.
15. Swezey RL, Spiegel TM: Evaluation and treatment of local musculoskeletal disorders in elderly patients. Geriatrics 34:56–75, 1979.
16. Roseff R, Canoso JJ: Femoral osteonecrosis following soft tissue corticosteroid infiltration. Am J Med 77:1119–1120, 1984.
17. Brooker AF Jr: The surgical approach to refractory trochanteric bursitis. Johns Hopkins Med J 145:98–100, 1979.
18. Kopell HP, Thompson WA: Peripheral Entrapment Neuropathies. Huntington, NY, RE Krieger, 1976.
19. Dan NG: Entrapment syndromes. Med J Aust 1:528–531, 1978.
20. Brown PW: Peripheral nerve lesions. *In* Musculoskeletal Disorders. Edited by RD D'Ambrosia. Philadelphia, JB Lippincott, 1977.
21. Hench PK: Nonarticular rheumatism. *In* Rheumatic Diseases: Diagnosis and Management. Edited by WA Katz. Philadelphia, JB Lippincott, 1977.
22. Swezey RL: Pseudo-radiculopathy in subacute trochanteric bursitis of the subgluteus maximus bursa. Arch Phys Med Rehabil 57:387–390, 1976.
23. Banerjee T, Hall CD: Sciatic entrapment neuropathy. J Neurosurg 45:216–217, 1976.

10

The Knee

The knee performs a complex series of gliding, sliding, rotating, and bending functions.[1] Knee movement includes the "screw home" mechanism; specifically, as the knee extends or straightens from the bent position, the tibia rotates externally and the femur rotates internally. This rotation mechanism requires joint stability, particularly while running. Although the functions of the menisci are not completely understood, they act both as shock absorbers and as stabilizers to help rotational stability.[1] At least a dozen bursae are situated in the knee region; several of them communicate with the joint itself (Fig. 10–1).

A diagnosis of osteoarthritis must not be taken for granted as the only cause for knee pain. When roentgenographic evidence of osteoarthritis has been noted, that change may have little to do with the patient's complaints. A primary or contributing soft tissue problem which may be present can be easily diagnosed and treated. In one study of 91 patients with osteoarthritis, the origin of pain was assessed by local anesthetic blocks with notation as to whether pain was relieved (>75% relief on a verbal analog scale). In this manner, Traycoff and Trapp noted that 26% of knee pain originated in soft tissue structures alone; in an additional 12% there were both soft tissue and intra-articular causes for symptoms.[2] Similarly, 60% of patients referred to a tertiary care center for osteoarthritis of the knee had signs and symptoms of anserine bursitis.[2a]

History. The physician who deals with disabling problems of knee pain must consider the age of the patient, any preceding injury, and the pain pattern. In addition, the mode of onset, the localization of pain, and any associated phenomena of locking, clicking, catching, buckling, swelling, or loss of motion should be noted.[3,4] Features suggesting the need for more detailed evaluation and consultation are detailed in Table 10–1, Caution Signs for Knee Evaluation. A careful history for improper use or resting positions is important (see Table 10–2, Joint Protection Guide for the Knee).

Intermittent "giving way" (buckling) or locking, followed by a period of recovery, may result from a torn meniscus, intra-articular loose bodies, plicae, cruciate ligament inadequacy, patellofemoral instability, hypertrophy of the infrapatellar fat pad, or intra-articular tumors of the knee. These disorders collectively are termed "internal derangements of the knee."[5] Early recognition of an internal derangement of the knee, followed by appropriate therapy, may relieve symptoms and prevent secondary osteoarthritis. Warmth and swelling in association with a persistent locked knee are signs of serious internal derangement; surgical consultation is often required (Table 10–1, Danger Signs for the Knee).

Asking the patient to point to the area of maximum pain, or having the patient indicate whether the pain is anterior, posterior, medial, or lateral assists the clinician in diagnosis. Pain at the medial joint line is seen with injury to the medial collateral ligament, disease of the medial joint compartment, anserine bursitis, or an internal derangement. Pain posterior to the knee joint may result from a shortened hamstring, a popliteal cyst, or tendinitis. Pain at the lateral aspect of the knee joint may represent bursitis adjacent to the head of the fibula, arthritis, or internal derangement of the lateral compartment of the knee. Pain anterior to the knee is strongly suggestive of patellofemoral disturbances or derangements of the quadriceps mechanism. Although pain location is helpful, referred

217

View of the medial aspect of the knee

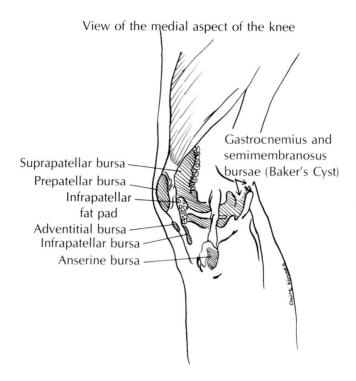

Suprapatellar bursa
Prepatellar bursa
Infrapatellar fat pad
Adventitial bursa
Infrapatellar bursa
Anserine bursa

Gastrocnemius and semimembranosus bursae (Baker's Cyst)

Fig. 10–1. Bursae of the knee region: The suprapatellar, prepatellar, infrapatellar, and adventitial bursae lie anteriorly; the anserine bursa and the sartorius bursa (not shown) are located on the medial aspect; posteriorly, the large popliteal (Baker's cyst) may originate from the gastrocnemius or semimembranosus bursa.

Table 10–1.   Caution Signs for Knee Evaluation

1. Warmth and redness
2. Constitutional symptoms such as weight loss, fever, night pain
3. Regional lymphadenopathy
4. Quadriceps atrophy
5. Positive stress tests
6. Lateral knee instability (excess motion)
7. Limb claudication
8. Limb discoloration
9. Increasing pain during weight bearing
10. Locking and buckling
11. Numbness, tingling, and weakness

pain may be present and confuse the diagnosis. Burning, throbbing, or other neuritic-like symptoms may result from reflex sympathetic dystrophy in the knee region,[6] or from a prepatellar neuralgia[7] (Table 10–3, Causes for Knee Pain).

Sport and industrial knee injuries are re-ceiving more study. Such injuries may result in part from underlying foot, ankle, leg, or hip problems. Overuse syndromes are particularly important and common. If not recognized, the aggravation will only be repeated, adding to physician and patient dissatisfaction. For example, middle-aged men might be advised to use stair climbing as exercise for cardiac conditioning and find themselves with patellofemoral pain. They often will not volunteer this information; it has to be questioned. Runners who overtrain with mileage in excess of 20 miles per week commonly get into trouble. Cycling, hockey, basketball, soccer, and downhill skiing may stress the collateral ligaments (Table 10–2, Joint Protection Guide for the Knee).

Physical Examination. A careful examination includes evaluation of the appearance of the extremity when the patient is lying, rising, standing, and walking. Some specific

Table 10–2.   Joint Protection for the Knee[61]

Harmful	Helpful
■ Pushing off from chairs with the hands wastes the quadriceps muscle.	■ Keep the hands in the lap when arising from a sitting position.
■ Repetitively twisting the knee while dancing or exercising can damage it.	■ Modify or avoid knee-twisting dance steps and exercises.
■ For some persons, bicycling can strain the knee.	■ Pace bicycling if it causes knee pain.
■ Engaging in sports activities on an occasional or weekend basis without proper conditioning or warm-up is potentially harmful to the knee.	■ Engage in sports activities regularly to stay in condition. Do warm-up exercises.
■ Climbing stairs repeatedly is irritating to the knee.	■ Limit stair climbing. If lack of a toilet on the first floor necessitates stair climbing, one solution is to place a portable commode somewhere on the first floor.
■ Sitting for prolonged periods allows the muscles behind the knee to tighten up.	■ Limit sitting to 30 minutes, then move around.
■ Having certain foot disorders can result in poor alignment of the leg bones, which in turn affects the knee.	■ Consult a physician.
■ Wearing shoes having worn-down heels can aggravate knee problems.	■ Buy shoes with proper heels and check them for signs of excessive wear.
■ Working on the hands and knees on a hard surface can result in bursitis in the front of the knee. Also known as water on the knee and housemaid's knee, this swelling is visible in front of the kneecap.	■ Instead of working on the hands and knees, use a mechanic's or milker's stool; either one sits low to the ground. Sit with the legs apart and reach forward to perform, with little effort, such tasks as gardening and washing floors.

physical examination maneuvers that assist in determining the integrity of the internal knee structures are described. A more comprehensive discussion and description of post-traumatic knee problems is beyond the scope of this book, and the interested reader may find the article by Hughston of value.[8]

While the patient is standing with feet slightly apart and parallel (pointing directly forward), the clinician may note congenital abnormalities, including genu recurvatum (excessive backward joint mobility), patella alta (a high-riding patella), or abnormal patellar alignment, when viewed in relation to the tibial tubercle. From the frontal view, the patellae each may point away from the midline, denoting lateral patellar subluxation ("grasshopper eye patellae"); this often occurs in association with chondromalacia patellae.[3,9]

Genu valgum* (knockknee) may also predispose to lateral patellar dislocation or displacement. Displacement may be observed as the seated patient straightens the knee and the patella moves outward instead of straight upward. Prepatellar bursitis, synovitis with suprapatellar fullness, or a Baker's cyst may be apparent by observation while the patient is standing. Pes planus (flatfootedness) may

---

*The terms varus, or valgus, through common usage, imply inward or outward deviation respectively. Recent discussions in the literature have emphasized that these commonly used terms are inaccurate.[10] Accordingly, it is usually best to add additional descriptions when defining changes related to these anatomic deviations.

Table 10–3. Causes for Knee Pain

I. Anterior Knee Symptoms:
    Patellofemoral pain syndrome (younger patient without significant disorder)
    Patellofemoral osteoarthritis (older patient)
    Overload syndromes (osteochondral injuries in runners, athletes)
    Malalignment (tracking) syndromes (with genu valgus or rotation abnormalities of
       the limb; quadriceps dysplasia; patellar dislocation; fracture)
    Other patellar disorders (patella alta, odd facet syndrome, chondromalacia, os-
       teochondritis)
    Cruciate ligament injury
    Synovial disorders (plicae, inflammatory arthritis, villonodular synovitis)
    Prepatellar neuritis, bursitis
    Reflex sympathetic dystrophy

II. Medial Knee Pain
    Ligamentous injuries (joint laxity, hypermobility syndrome, trauma)
    Anserine bursitis
    Meniscus lesions
    Medial plica syndrome
    Synovitis (arthritis)
    Referred pain from the hip
    Osteonecrosis

III. Lateral Knee Pain
    Fibular bursitis
    Meniscus injury
    Collateral ligament injury
    Iliotibial band friction syndrome
    Fascia lata fasciitis
    Pseudosciatica

IV. Posterior Knee Pain
    Tendinitis
    Capsulitis
    Bursitis
    Synovitis
    Peroneal nerve injury
    Vascular lesions
    Popliteal cyst

give rise to knee region discomfort and should be noted. The patient should be observed while rising from a seated position without the use of hands for assistance; this is a simple test for the integrity of the quadriceps extensor mechanism, but may also suggest knee disorders located in the patellofemoral region, or primary muscle disease. Inspection and palpation of the knee may reveal a relatively painless chronic granular cellulitis in the patellar region, as seen in coal miners (the beat knee).[11] Chronic prepatellar bursal thick-

ening occurs in relation to certain occupations, such as carpet laying (Fig. 10–2).

The joint capsule is supported on each side by complex medial and lateral collateral ligament systems,[8,12] and inadequacy of these structures may result in excessive sideway motion. Cruciate ligament insufficiency is associated with excessive anteroposterior motion. If there is any suggestion of instability, stress testing is important to help define the problem. Post-traumatic ligamentous instability that is not treated may lead to quadri-

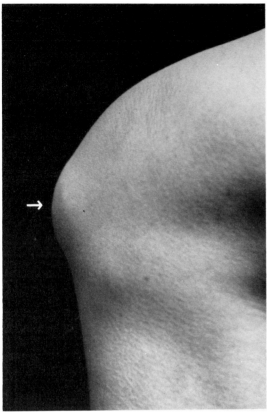

Fig. 10–2. Prepatellar bursitis: The bursitis is visible and palpable superficial to the patella.

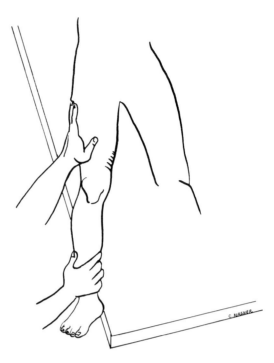

Fig. 10–3. The valgus stress test: When the examiner attempts to deviate the knee into a valgus position with the knee extended, the integrity of both the posterior cruciate and the medial collateral ligaments is tested; repeating the test with the knee bent tests the collateral ligament alone.

ceps atrophy, which complicates the clinical presentation.

Stress testing includes the collateral ligament stress test for excessive medial or lateral movement, and the "drawer tests" for anteroposterior instability. The collateral ligament stress tests are performed by the examiner first grasping the involved leg with the knee in full extension (Fig. 10–3); the test is then repeated with the knee flexed 30 degrees. The examiner attempts to deviate the foreleg away from the midline inwardly and outwardly (varus, valgus respectively). Performing the maneuver with the knee extended tests the integrity of both the posterior cruciate and collateral ligaments; repeating the stress test with the knee bent tests the collateral ligaments alone. The examiner observes for opening or widening of the medial or lateral joint compartment. Stress tests may

be misleading if reflex spasm from pain prevents relaxation during the examination.

The anterior drawer sign is performed with the patient supine, the hip flexed 45 degrees, and the patient's head supported on a pillow; otherwise, should the patient arise to look forward, the hamstring muscles may become tense. The involved knee is flexed approximately 80 to 90 degrees, and the foot is stabilized by the examiner sitting on it. The hamstrings should be relaxed. The tibia is gently pulled and pushed straight in and out, anterior and posterior, back and forth. The maneuver should be performed separately with the foot in the straight-forward or neutral position, then with the foot rotated internally, and lastly with the foot rotated externally. Both legs should be compared. Excessive anterior motion supports a diagnosis of insufficiency of the anterior cruciate ligament or of the medial portion of the joint capsule. Instability may be graded from 1 to 3+; greater than 5 mm of excess motion equals 1+ instability; greater than 10 mm equals 3+ instability.[8]

The posterior drawer sign is determined passively by observing whether the tibia is displaced posteriorly while the patient is resting in the same position as described for the anterior drawer sign. The examiner then grasps the tibia and attempts to displace it further posteriorly. A positive posterior drawer sign detects insufficiency of the posterior cruciate ligament.[13]

The McMurray sign and the Apley grinding maneuver may help distinguish a torn meniscus from other causes of internal knee derangement. The McMurray test is performed by acutely flexing the symptomatic knee, so that the heel of the involved extremity approximates the buttock. The examiner then grasps the ankle and straightens the tibia, while rotating the tibia medially and then laterally. A palpable or auditory click represents a positive test.[3,12,14] The Apley grinding maneuver is performed with the patient prone (on the stomach); the knee is flexed 80 to 90 degrees. The examiner than presses down upon the foot and foreleg while rotating them. Pain, clicking, or locking are noted if the Apley grinding maneuver is positive.[3] This usually indicates a derangement of the meniscus or articular surface rather than the ligament complex.

Sometimes a patient provides a history of the knee "giving way" but stress tests reveal only slight or no abnormal motion. In such patients a diagnosis of hypermobility syndrome with disuse quadriceps weakness should be considered; signs of joint laxity elsewhere in the musculoskeletal system should be sought.[2,12,15,16] Similar symptoms may result from patellofemoral disturbances (see "Disturbances of the Patella," this chapter).

Loose bodies (joint mice) may cause symptoms similar to that of a torn meniscus with sensations of locking, grating, giving way, and swelling of the knee. The loose body may represent a chondral or osteochondral fragment, meniscus material,[5] or a sequestered fragment from an osteochondritis dissecans lesion.[17] Radiographic evidence may not be apparent if the fragment is of cartilaginous origin or is hidden in the posterior compartment. Occasionally, a loose body may be the first sign of synovial chondromatosis. Periodic giving way or locking, without apparent injury, strongly suggests the presence of a loose body.

ARTHROSCOPIC EXAMINATION

Arthroscopic examination is indicated for patients with locking, buckling or other weight-bearing symptoms. This innovative high technology tool has provided a greater awareness of a wide variety of causes for such symptoms. The arthroscope can be used both for diagnosis and treatment. The instrument consists of a rigid tube about a half-centimeter in diameter, a light source, a TV setup for recording, and motorized instruments which may be used through the scope, such as a patellar shaver, meniscal "muncher", scissors, basket forceps, and a chondral edger. Conditions which may be evaluated by arthroscopy include meniscus tears, patellar problems, synovial lesions, condylar problems, extrasynovial lesions, loose bodies, plicae and various types of arthritis. Normal findings may be helpful in the management of the patient. Many abnormal conditions are treatable with this instrument, however, results are in direct relation to the experience of the operator. Arthroscopy should not be the first diagnostic study of a painful knee. Complications of arthroscopy include damage to the articular cartilage, hemarthrosis, infection, herniation of a fat pad, thrombophlebitis, granuloma formation, instrument breakage, neurovascular injury, and development of a fistula.[18,19] Often a therapeutic trial of conservative care will result in benefit and obviate the need for elaborate studies. If symptoms persist after a reasonable trial of conservative treatment, then further diagnostic studies are justified (see Decision Chart, Table 10–4).

Table 10–4. Decision Chart, The Knee

Feature	Action	Further Action

A. Anterior Knee Pain
  Diffuse pain, not acute
  Gait normal
  Interferes with sleep
  Normal motion
	CONSERVATIVE CARE
	Eliminate aggravating factors.
	Provide pain relief: NSAID's, local intralesional steroid injection
	Physical therapy
	Roentgenographic exam when appropriate
		Orthopedic Consultation

B. Patellofemoral pain		Arthroscopy/Arthrography Bracing Rest/Crutches ↓ Scintigraphy Systemic workup for inflammation
C. Medial or lateral pain and locking or buckling		

D. Swelling and stiffness
  Painful weightbearing
  Or Prepatellar Bursitis
	+ → + Synovial fluid analysis for crystals, gram stain, sugar	

E. Posterior knee pain	+ → + Aspirate Baker's Cyst	

F. DANGER LIST
  Warmth, discoloration
  Regional lymphadenopathy
  Constitutional symptoms
  Claudication
  Neurologic findings
  Positive stress tests
	→ Immediate Appropriate Action	→ Consultation:
		Orthopedist
		Rheumatologist
		Vascular studies

Often, in cases of suspected meniscus tear, the clinical diagnosis is found to be in error. For example, of 229 patients thought to have a torn medial meniscus, Lanny Johnson reports that with arthroscopy a different diagnosis was found in 56% of patients.[20]

Meniscus tears are particularly amenable to this treatment. Arthroscopic surgery has the advantages of outpatient care, lower risk, decreased morbidity, and less cost.[21,22] Many have suspected that meniscectomy leads to osteoarthritis and some investigations support the concept.[23] Arthroscopy may result in more accurate diagnoses, and earlier treatment. Certainly, untreated severe meniscus lesions are bad for the joint.

Plicae may be mistaken for arthritis, or may simulate meniscus tears, with locking, buckling or swelling after severe effort. These embryologic synovial folds, found in 20 to 60% of normal knees, are often delineated as the cause of symptoms during arthroscopy. Suprapatellar, mediopatellar, and an infrapatellar plicae may occur. Arthroscopic excision of the plica provides prompt relief of symptoms[24-26] (see the Plica Syndrome).

Partial tears of the cruciate ligaments may also result in locking. These can be also diagnosed by arthroscopy.[27]

Magnetic resonance imaging may be a valuable noninvasive technique in problems of internal knee derangement and patellofemoral pain syndromes. Menisci, ligamentous structures, patellar cartilage, and popliteal cysts can be delineated.[27a,27b]

QUADRICEPS MECHANISM DERANGEMENT

Quadriceps Muscle and Tendon Disruption

In young athletes the extensor quadriceps mechanism consists of strong tendons so that rupture generally involves the muscle mass. In older persons rupture usually occurs at the tendinous portion.[12] The injury generally occurs during forced knee joint flexion with a contracted quadriceps. Swelling occurs above the patella and the patient notes various de-

grees of loss of extension activity of the knee joint. With complete rupture at any age, immediate surgical repair is recommended. Occasionally a partial muscle rupture occurs with less severe trauma. In such patients, acute pain, swelling, and hemorrhage occur, but knee extension is possible. These patients are treated by immobilization in extension, followed by gentle physical therapy and exercise.[12]

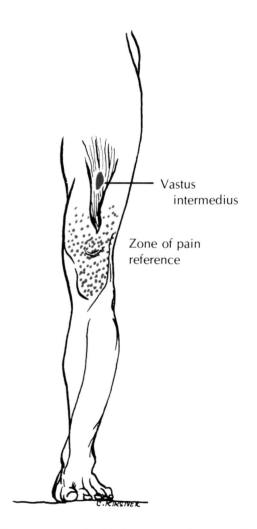

Vastus intermedius

Zone of pain reference

Fig. 10–4. A myofascial trigger point in the region of the insertion of the vastus intermedius may cause pain in the anterior lower leg and knee region.

Disuse Atrophy

This is one of the most common disorders leading to knee joint instability. It occurs secondary to other knee joint disturbances, including rheumatoid arthritis and osteoarthritis. Often disuse quadriceps atrophy results from the chronic use of hands to assist in the act of rising from the seated position. Middle-aged and elderly persons should be advised to use their thighs, not their hands when rising from a chair. This prophylactic advice may prevent a significant number of chronic painful joint disabilities. Often a trivial self-limited knee joint disturbance becomes a major disability because of disuse quadriceps atrophy or myofascial pain (Fig. 10–4). Resistant quadriceps exercise may be performed by patients at any age in the comfort of their home, and does not require frequent physical therapy supervision (Fig. 10–5) (see Exercises 1–4, Table 10–5). Hip stretching is helpful in patients with a taut vastus intermedius (Fig. 10–6).

Acute Calcific Quadriceps Tendinitis

Pain in the region of the suprapatellar pouch may be associated with calcification in the region of the quadriceps tendon, particularly at the superior pole of the patella (anterosuperior patellar whiskers). These radiographic findings may be seen in patients without symptoms; when associated with chronic knee pain, such patients frequently have evidence of degenerative joint disease.[28] Accordingly, the calcification may be an asymptomatic coincidental finding. The possibility that calcific quadriceps tendinitis is related to calcific tendinitis in other joint areas as a general metabolic disturbance has been suggested.[28]

DISTURBANCES OF THE PATELLA

Patellar region pain results from a number of complex problems; most of them respond well to nonsurgical treatment. These disorders include the patellofemoral pain syndrome, infrapatellar fat pad disturbances, infrapatellar tendinitis and bursitis, prepatellar bursitis, patellofemoral osteoarthritis, and prepatellar neuralgia. Patellar dysfunction may also result from contracture or insufficiency of the quadriceps mechanism, the hypermobility syndrome, or contracture of the iliotibial band (see Table 10–3, Differential Diagnosis). The disorders described often are symptomatic only because of injury or misuse, and although mild structural disturbances may coexist, symptoms respond to treatment with restoration of stability to the limb.

The Patellofemoral Pain Syndrome. This syndrome is characterized by pain and crepitation in the region of the patella during activities that require knee flexion under load conditions, such as stair climbing. Joint swelling may be seen; symptoms are often intermittent.[29] Primary idiopathic adolescent chondromalacia, post-traumatic adolescent chondromalacia, "patellofemoral syndrome of adolescents and young adults," and "adult chondromalacia with secondary degenerative joint disease" are various terms for a group of disorders with similar symptoms. Underlying etiologic disturbances include malalignment of the quadriceps with lateral patellar subluxation,[5] an abnormal medial patellar facet,[30] the patella alta, and the hypermobility syndrome. Findings of joint mobility, Q angle measurement, genu valgum and anteversion were not different among athletes with and without anterior knee pain.[31] Chondromalacia of the patella is a prominent associated finding in patellofemoral pain. The exact relationship of patellofemoral crepitation to the presence of pain is debatable.[5,28,29,32,33]

In one study of "normal" students, more than half had patellofemoral crepitation unrelated to the presence or absence of patellar pain.[29] The "cinema sign" describes patellofemoral pain following prolonged sitting with knees in flexion, relieved by subsequent knee extension.[12]

Physical findings suggestive of the patellofemoral pain syndrome include reproduction of pain when the examiner presses the patella against the femur during knee motion,

Table 10–5. Knee Exercises

1. Isometric quadriceps strengthening: Sit on a chair, knees bent, and feet resting about 2 feet out from the chair; cross good leg over bad, at the ankle. Now attempt to raise the bad leg against the good one. But resist the upward thrusting leg with the other leg. No actual motion takes place. Hold for 10 seconds and repeat for 5 minutes. If both legs are bad then later in the day, repeat the exercise reversing the legs.

2. Bed exercise for debilitated or recently injured patients: Place a rolled towel beneath the knee and press straight leg downward against towel using a maximum quadriceps contraction. Hold for 5 seconds, repeat 10 to 100 times. Do one leg at a time.

3. Isotonic quadriceps strengthening: Sit on a hard chair or edge of a firm bed with knees just over the edge and a firm towel rolled under lower thigh. If long legged, place two telephone books (4") under heel so the foot begins up about 4" from the floor. Lift foot slowly but not fully out straight. Hold for count of 5. Repeat for 5 minutes.

4. Add 3 to 25 pounds to the ankle and perform as above. If pain is minimal, this exercise can be done by starting with the most weight that can be lifted, from 2 to 25 pounds and hold for the count of 5. Do this until painful or fatigued, then take off 5 pounds and continue to lift. Keep removing the weights as needed. Do the lifting for a total of 5 minutes. Do one leg in the morning and the other leg in the evening (Fig. 10–5).

5. Hamstring and leg stretch: Lie with one leg bent at knee and lift other leg. Place 4 foot long rope over ball of foot. Pull rope and lift leg high, knee straight, ankle at 90 degrees. Gradually increase tension on hamstring muscles. Hold 1 minute. Repeat with other leg (Fig. 10–10).

6. Hamstring strengthening: Strap 3 to 10 pound weights to ankles, lie face down with feet hanging off end of bed, lift leg bending the knee. Keep thigh in contact with the bed. Draw foreleg back toward 90 degrees and return to straight position slowly. Repeat 30 times, then do other leg.

7. Isometric adduction: Place a plastic wastebasket between ankles while lying out straight. Squeeze legs together trying to crush the wastebasket. Hold for 20 seconds, repeat 10 times.

8. Isometric abduction: Make a loop out of a 4-inch ACE elastic bandage (looped around ankles, about 6 inches apart, then safety-pinned to make it permanent). Slip loop over both ankles then while lying flat, draw both legs apart against the loop for 20 seconds, 10 repeats.

9. Hip flexor and quadriceps stretch: Lie along side of edge of bed (Fig. 10–6), apply 2 pound weights just above knee and at ankle. Draw opposite knee toward chest, hang weighted leg off side of bed with knee straight. Allow weights to stretch leg for 3 minutes. Repeat twice daily.

or detecting tenderness over the medial articulating surface of the patella. Patellofemoral crepitation during knee flexion and extension is usually palpable.[30] Pain may be reproduced by patellofemoral compression with the knee flexed or straight as the patella is pushed from side to side (Perkin's test).[3,12] The examiner must avoid squeezing the synovium during the examination. The young adult or teenager with patellofemoral pain should be observed for lateral patellar displacement (dislocation or subluxation) during knee flexion and extension.

Lateral patellar subluxation can be detected by having the patient seated, and the examiner's index finger and thumb positioned upon the lateral and medial upper borders of the patient's patella. The examiner observes and palpates for lateral patellar displacement as the flexed knee is extended; this finding is commonly seen in patients with hypermobility syndrome. "Grasshopper eye patellae" is a term in which the patellae point outward from the midline, suggesting the appearance of grasshopper's eyes when viewed from the

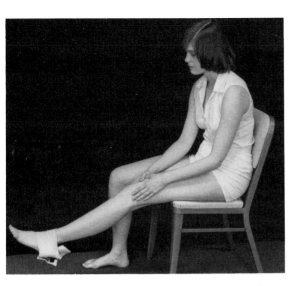

Fig. 10–5. Resistance quadriceps exercise: Utilizing weights ranging from 10 to 30 or more pounds, the arc of movement must be determined for each patient depending on comfort and tolerance. Often the patient notes an arc that achieves maximum results.

front.[3] This correlates with lateral patellar subluxation and chondromalacia.

Hoffa's Disease. This syndrome refers to hypertrophy of the infrapatellar fat pad in young persons after mild injury. The infrapatellar fat pad may then become impinged between the femur and tibia when the flexed knee is suddenly extended. Pain is localized and occurs during weight-bearing knee activity. Symptoms simulate internal knee de-

rangements, but locking does not occur. Physical examination reveals swelling on either side of the infrapatellar ligament, and quadriceps atrophy may be seen.[14] Hypertrophy of the infrapatellar fat pad may be recurrent as a premenstrual syndrome.

Infrapatellar Tendinitis. This disorder is common in persons with lateral patellar displacement or malrotations of the tibia or fibula.[1] Infrapatellar pain or crepitation may result from jumping in athletic endeavors (Jumper's knee).[3] Other sports that can result in patellar tendinitis include volleyball, soccer, and bicycling. Most respond to conservative measures[34] (see Management). Infrapatellar bursitis causes similar discomfort in the infrapatellar region.

Traumatic Prepatellar Neuralgia.[7] This type of neuralgia follows trauma to the anterior patella and may be preceded by transient prepatellar swelling. After a few weeks, exquisite tenderness occurs over the medial outer border of the patella at the site of emergence of the neurovascular bundle; even slight stroking is exquisitely painful. Treatment with a local anesthetic or corticosteroid injection into the point of maximum tenderness is usually helpful.[7,12]

Etiology. These patellofemoral disturbances are often associated with conditions that result in a change in the angle of pull of the patellar tendon. Such disturbances include malrotation of the tibia or femur, alteration

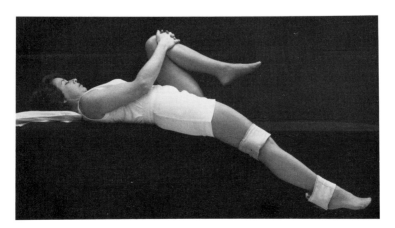

Fig. 10–6. Stretching the hip flexors and quadriceps mechanism for patients with myofascial knee region pain.

of the quadriceps muscle, abnormal position of the iliotibial band, or malformation in the posterior surface of the patellae or femoral condyles. Also, patellofemoral compression syndrome with tightness of the lateral capsule and patellofemoral ligament can occur.[30a] Symptoms may also result from chronic trauma, such as repeated scrubbing of floors on hands and knees. Hypermobility syndrome has been noted as a predisposing disorder. Degenerative pathologic findings of cartilage softening and fissuring are frequently noted; there is often a lack of correlation between pathologic findings and symptoms.

Laboratory and Radiographic Findings. Inflammatory connective tissue disease is rarely associated with these patellar disturbances. Therefore, tests of inflammation are normal. Radiographic examination should include the tangential patellofemoral roentgenographic techniques (skyline, Hughston views) that best demonstrate the patellar facets and lateral patellar deviation.[5] Radiographic findings unfortunately may add little to the diagnosis. When 71 patients operated upon for patellofemoral disturbances were compared with 97 others operated upon for meniscectomy, radiographic findings were poorly correlated with operative findings.[35] Nevertheless, in the older patient, osteoarthritis, osteonecrosis, fracture, tumor, or rheumatoid arthritis may be seen and defined. Athletes may develop osteochondritis of the patella or femur. Patella alta can be measured on lateral roentgenogram; the lengths of the patella and patellar tendon should be equal. If the tendon length exceeds the patella length by 10%, patella alta can be diagnosed.[36] Others feel that patella alta is a rare finding and not relevant to the young athlete.[37] Bone scan for stress fractures, osteonecrosis, or reflex dystrophy is sometimes indicated depending upon clinical presentation. Arthroscopy for more definitive diagnosis is indicated if conservative measures fail to provide symptomatic relief in 3 to 6 months.[33] Thermography suggested quadriceps muscle imbalance in one study of 30 athletes with patellofemoral pain; all responded to physical therapy and exercise.[33a]

Differential Diagnosis. In addition to syndromes already presented (Table 10–2), anterior knee pain may be referred from other soft tissue structures. Anterior knee pain in the absence of locking strongly suggests the patellofemoral pain syndromes, but may also occur from a tight hamstring. In the latter instance, straight leg raising to the point of maximum tolerance may reproduce the anterior knee distress.

Management. Conservative measures that are helpful include aspirin or other nonsteroidal anti-inflammatory agents for pain, restriction of competitive activities or overuse, weight reduction for obese patients, and resistance quadriceps strengthening exercises. Bracing with an elastic support and a lateral felt pad may also be tried. A trial of isometric quadriceps strengthening exercises with maximum resistance is essential. The leg should be almost in full extension as the quadriceps exercise is performed. The short arc of leg lift against resistance should not be painful. If painful then the patient can lie flat and hold the limb straight while lifting the entire limb for 500 repetitions[32] (see Exercise 2, Table 10–5). In a series of 100 patients graded according to arthroscopic findings and followed for 2 years, conservative measures of rest and traction followed by isometric exercises resulted in complete recovery in 100% of those with no demonstrable intraarticular abnormality and in 75% of those with only patellar cartilage fibrillation. However, in the small group with fibrillation of both the patella and femur, conservative measures often failed and surgical care was required.[38]

Disturbances of the infrapatellar fat pad, infrapatellar ligament, and the infrapatellar bursa usually respond to rest followed by graded resistance quadriceps exercise; relief usually requires many weeks of therapy. Injecting the infrapatellar fat pad with a local anesthetic-corticosteroid is rarely needed. If necessary, the injection is administered from a lateral approach; the needle should rest well beneath the tendon (Fig. 10–7). One ml 1%

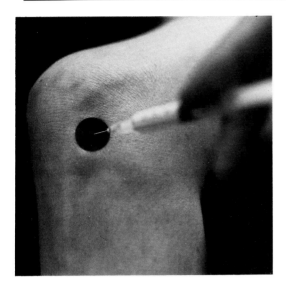

Fig. 10–7. Injection for disturbances of the infrapatellar region must be performed with the needle well beneath the infrapatellar tendon. Furthermore, patients receiving such an injection must be warned to limit stressful activities for several weeks in order to avoid tendon disruption.

procaine mixed with 20 mg triamcinolone may be injected with a 1 inch #23 needle, ½ injected into the medial and lateral borders of the fat pad. The tendon must not be penetrated as future tendon rupture may occur. These patients rarely require more than one injection. *Athletes or persons who must kneel repeatedly should not be given a local corticosteroid injection.*[39] Management also requires recognition and prevention of aggravating factors, such as improper kneeling, working on the hands and knees excessively, and prolonged sitting (see Table 10–2).

Outcome and Additional Suggestions. Adolescents with patellofemoral pain syndrome (chondromalacia patellae) frequently have spontaneous improvement without residual disturbance.[2,12,29,30] As mentioned, the key to managing patellar disturbances is to maintain a strong quadriceps mechanism with normal alignment. Special braces are available and include the patellar stabilization brace for lateral patellar dislocation; and bracing for patellar tendinitis, knee hyperextension, rotation abnormalities, and joint laxity.[40] Orthopedic consultation would be wise be-

fore assuming the responsibility for ordering special braces for young athletes.

In patients in whom symptoms are resistant to conservative programs, surgical intervention may be indicated. Surgery may have to be directed toward the underlying basic abnormality, such as patella alta or recurrent subluxation with hypermobility. Other corrections may have to be directed toward more general problems, such as genu valgum or tibial torsion. Surgery may have to be directed as well toward any chondromalacia present. Therapeutic procedures for the latter include patellar shaving, drilling, and rarely, patellectomy. The former may be accomplished with arthroscopy. When chondromalacia patellae is associated with lateral patellar displacement or dislocation, the future development of osteoarthritis may be prevented or retarded by surgical repair.[13,41]

Although surgery may be indicated at times, quadriceps setting exercises and associated conservative management measures often result in pain relief in patients with patellofemoral pain syndrome. We strongly encourage an intensive trial of conservative therapeutic modalities for all patients with this entity.

BURSITIS ABOUT THE KNEE

At least 12 bursae regularly occur in the knee region: the suprapatellar, prepatellar, infrapatellar, and an adventitious cutaneous bursa lie in the anterior knee region; the gastrocnemius and semimembranosus bursae are located in the posterior region and often give rise to a popliteal (Baker's) cyst; the sartorius and anserine bursae lie medially; three bursae lie adjacent to the fibular collateral ligament,[42] and the popliteus tendon in the lateral region of the knee.[12,14,43–45] Not to be forgotten is the "no name-no fame" bursa of Stuttle,[46] located at the front edge of the anterior fibers of the medial (tibial) collateral ligament.

Bursitis is characterized by pain, which is aggravated by motion and which at times is worse at night. Point tenderness is present over the involved bursa; active motion may or may not be limited. Inspection may immediately reveal a swollen prepatellar bursa. *Prepatellar* bursitis may be a chronic condition secondary to certain occupations, such as coal mining, farming, or activities performed by overconscientious housewives.[45] The "no name-no fame" bursa may be palpable during knee flexion when the examiner feels a small tender rounded nodule jumping onto the leading edge of the medial collateral ligament.[46] Another bursa, the adventitious cutaneous bursa, may be palpable as a swelling over the tibial tuberosity.[14] Popliteal bursitis is discussed under the commonly used term "Baker's cyst" in this chapter.

Anserine bursitis should be suspected when pain occurs in the medial knee region. It is often bilateral, and may accompany panniculitis in obese postmenopausal females.[44] Osteoarthritis often is present and may predispose to bursitis. Pain originating in the medial collateral ligament may also coexist. Pain of both anserine bursitis and medial collateral ligament disease is worse with activity. Pain at night is more characteristic of anserine bursitis.

Etiology. Bursitis about the knee often occurs in females. Pes planus may be a predisposing cause for bursitis in the medial knee region.[46] The suprapatellar bursa and the posterior bursae often communicate with the knee joint. Swelling of these "pouches" often reflects synovial swelling due to inflammatory arthritis or internal derangement of the true knee joint; the most common cause is rheumatoid arthritis.[14] None of the bursae in the medial or lateral knee regions communicate with the synovial cavity; therefore, inflammatory joint disease rarely is related to inflammation of these bursae.[44] Women with large fat panniculi overlying the medial knee joint may present with pain that is worse at night; this nocturnal pain should alert the physician to the presence of an anserine bursitis deep to the panniculus. Whether pressure from the panniculus is significant in the cause of anserine bursitis is unknown. Following treatment, the bursitis seldom recurs despite the continued presence of the panniculus.

Laboratory and Radiographic Examination. Prepatellar bursitis, though usually secondary to pressure phenomenon, may also result from infection. Aspiration of prepatellar bursa fluid for white cell count and differential, gram stain, sugar, culture and sensitivity determination, and crystal identification are diagnostically indicated. In acute knee bursitis of local origin, tests for systemic inflammation are normal. Radiographic examination is seldom abnormal but may reveal osteoarthritis consistent with age. Calcific tendinitis and bursal calcification may rarely be seen. Chondrocalcinosis with pseudogout syndrome may occur in elderly patients with bursitis, but the findings are likely coincidental. Contrast arthrography (pneumoarthrogram) for the diagnosis of some types of knee pain may be required, but the procedure is probably best considered only after orthopedic consultation when diagnosis is difficult. The choice between arthroscopy and arthrography requires further clinical assessment and experience. Subtle disorders of the popliteus bursa evident on arthrography may be observed and can suggest tears of the lateral meniscus, discoid menisci, adhesive capsulitis, and anatomic variants.[47] Arthroscopy is not without risk, as has been mentioned.

Differential Diagnosis. Diagnosing acute bursitis is seldom a problem. Swelling in the region of the bursa may also result from tumors of the bursae, including osteochondromatosis, villonodular synovitis, xanthomatosis, and synovioma.[12]

A patient with osteonecrosis of the femur may present with medial compartment knee pain that is constant (day and night). Radiographic features may be normal. Radionuclide imaging with strontium 85 or technetium 99 reveals a localized increased area of uptake in the involved femoral condyle.[48]

Management. Nonseptic bursitis about the knee responds readily to reduction in local pressure and local corticosteroid-anesthetic injections[44] (Fig. 10–8). Patients with bursitis

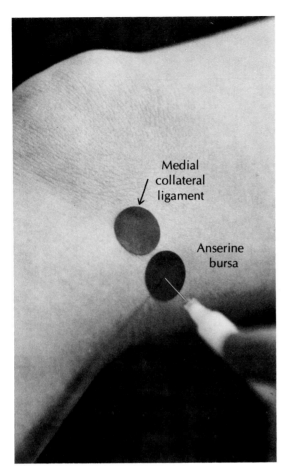

Medial collateral ligament

Anserine bursa

Fig. 10–8. Injection of the medial collateral ligament or the anserine bursa: Tenderness in the medial region of the knee may result from one or both structures, and with the needle used as a probe, points of maximum tenderness should be injected. A 1½-inch No. 22 or No. 23 needle is appropriate.

in the medial aspect of the knee should sleep with a small cushion placed between the thighs so that the opposite knee does not rest upon the medial aspect of the involved knee. Use of kneeling pads is important for miners and other persons whose occupations expose them to prepatellar bursitis. Septic bursitis requires the use of parenteral antibiotics and immobilization. Aspiration and open drainage may be required. Ho and Su report the advantage of using antibiotic therapy for 5 days after documented sterile cultures. Although they report oral antibiotic use for some cases of olecranon bursitis, their series of patellar

bursitis were treated with intravenous antibiotics, with cure in all cases.[49] Recurrence of infection should lead to consideration of total bursal excision during the quiescent phase of the disease.

Outcome and Additional Suggestions. Chronic bursitis about the knee is rarely encountered; it is limited mostly to the prepatellar bursa.[45] Gout, rheumatoid arthritis, and villonodular synovitis are differential diagnostic entities that should be considered in patients with bursitis. As noted, surgical excision may be indicated in chronic bursitis.[45]

POPLITEAL CYST (BAKER'S CYST)

Swelling in the posterior aspect of the knee (in the popliteal fossa) may occur in children and adults. In children, the cyst is usually congenital and usually disappears spontaneously after a prolonged period of observation; surgery is rarely indicated.[50,51] In adults, a Baker's cyst is usually secondary to underlying disease of the knee joint, such as internal derangement, osteoarthritis, or rheumatoid arthritis. The patient frequently presents with aching discomfort in the popliteal region, leg, and calf. The discomfort is aggravated by walking, and often relieved by rest. Frequently the patient reports the presence of an egg-shaped mass behind the knee (Fig. 10–9).

When a Baker's cyst is suspected but not certain after physical examination, have the patient perform the hamstring stretching exercise using a 4-foot length of rope to pull the leg up in the air (Fig. 10–10); this results in a more readily palpable cyst. Needle aspiration of the Baker's cyst reveals fluid ranging from jelly-like consistency or cholesterol-laden fluid to acute inflammatory fluid, depending on the presence of underlying inflammatory disease in the knee joint. A large-bore (15 gauge) needle may be needed for aspiration.

Occasionally a Baker's cyst ruptures acutely before the physician has been consulted. This may occur with any activity, but is especially common during repetitive squat-

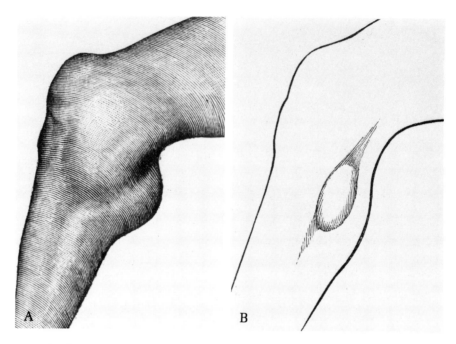

Fig. 10–9. Popliteal (Baker's cyst) bursitis. Reprinted from the original report by W.M. Baker. Saint Bartholomew's Hospital Reports, London, 1877.

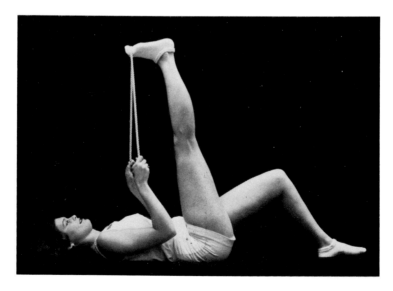

Fig. 10–10. Hamstring and posterior leg muscle stretching may be helpful by providing a more readily palpable popliteal bursa. Hamstring stretching exercise is useful for treatment of posterior myofascial pain disorders of the posterior knee region.

ting movements, such as taking inventory or redoing the stock in a store. Patients with a *ruptured Baker's cyst* present with features suggestive of thrombophlebitis. They may have minimal or no synovitis in the knee, the cyst is often no longer palpable, and swelling, heat, and diffuse tenderness of the calf and posterior foreleg is evident.

A Homan's sign, suggestive of phlebitis, may be positive. At this point it is apparent that the diagnosis may be uncertain, and the differential between a ruptured popliteal cyst and acute phlebitis is an important consideration. In those patients in whom the diagnosis is unclear, studies should be performed to exclude phlebitis to clarify this important question. Ultrasound or CT scan may be warranted if diagnosis is unclear.[52] Contrast pneumoarthrograms reveal evidence of rupture with extravasation of dye into the calf. Although this study is diagnostically confirmatory, it is not always essential if clinical findings are characteristic. Gompels and Darlington compared ultrasonography with arthrography in 48 knees. The ultrasound technique missed 3 cysts and gave 3 false positive results in these 48 cases.[52] The non-invasiveness of the procedure is a distinct advantage, but we would prefer arthrography when a ruptured cyst is suspected. Nuclear magnetic resonance tomography may be the most sensitive diagnostic test.[27b]

In patients in whom the diagnosis of ruptured cyst has been made, management consists of treatment with bed rest, heat, and elevation. Introduction of local steroids into the joint that has an effusion may be helpful. Nonsteroidal anti-inflammatory agents may also be of assistance. After symptoms have begun to show significant improvement, ambulation can slowly be increased. Patients sometimes demonstrate evidence of both popliteal cyst formation, with or without rupture, and thrombophlebitis. This combined process results when prolonged pressure from the cyst has led to venous stasis.

Management of an uncomplicated Baker's cyst includes aspiration of the contents of the cyst (and of the knee if synovitis is present), and instillation of a corticosteroid-anesthetic mixture into the cyst and joint cavity. A mild pressure bandage applied to the posterior popliteal region is helpful, as are isometric quadriceps exercises (see Exercise 1, Table 10–5). Weightbearing should be minimized for several days or weeks.

The need for surgical excision of the cyst depends on recurrences and the presence of primary disease within the knee joint. Cyst excision without therapy directed to the primary knee disease is usually associated with cyst recurrence. This results from fluid transmission through the one-way valve, which exists in the communication between the knee and cyst. The fluid accumulates in the bursa and is unable to go back into the knee. The bursa gradually descends into the calf; it may rupture and produce further local inflammation. Proper care of the underlying knee joint arthritis or internal derangement is essential.

MISCELLANEOUS DISORDERS OF THE KNEE

Popliteal Region Tendinitis

Tenosynovitis of the popliteal tendon or hamstring may cause pain in the posterior or posterolateral aspects of the knee. Tenderness to palpation with the knee at 90 degrees may be found,[3] and straight leg raising to maximum tolerance can accentuate the tenderness. Palpation during straight leg raising reveals marked tightness in the involved muscles.[53] Corticosteroid-anesthetic injections into points of tenderness often provide prompt relief. Hamstring stretching exercises performed twice daily are helpful.[54] Hamstring injuries are common in runners. The "pulled hamstring" injury is aggravated during the runner's long stride. Tenderness can be detected at the origin or insertion of the muscle; rest, ice followed by stretching, is helpful.[55]

Pellegrini Stieda Syndrome

Following knee strain, an occasional patient notes progressively worsening symptoms, and knee joint *flexion* becomes restricted. Presumably a soft tissue injury in the region of the medial tibial collateral ligament is followed by *calcification* in this area with permanent obstruction to knee joint motion.[12] Similar medial joint calcification has been reported in the ankle and elbow joint regions.[14] If present, synovitis is usually transient. Palpable indurated swelling in the soft tissues about the femoral condyle, restriction of knee joint flexion, and evidence of calcification on roentgenographic films of the knee joint are noted. Adult males are most commonly affected. The calcification appears 3 to 4 weeks following injury, and has the appearance of a narrow elongated amorphous shadow adjacent to the medial aspect of the femoral condyle (Fig. 10–11). Similar calcification may be seen without symptoms.[12] Pain gradually disappears over a period of months or years. Surgical excision of the bony mass may be considered if symptoms persist.

Iliotibial Band Friction Syndrome

The iliotibial band is a thickened part of the fascia lata that inserts over the lateral tibial condyle. Patients with this syndrome present with pain in the region of the lateral knee joint following vigorous running or hiking. These patients develop a painful limp and experience point tenderness over the lateral femoral condyle. Friction is thought to provoke the inflammation. Pain is accentuated by having the patient support all of his weight on the affected leg with the knee bent 30 to 40 degrees. Furthermore, a palpable "creak" during flexion and extension of the knee is noted; this has the consistency of rubbing over a wet balloon.[56] Synovial effusion or excessive lateral joint motion does *not* occur. Nonsteroidal anti-inflammatory drugs and joint rest are helpful. Local corticosteroid injection into the point of insertion may be attempted, if necessary. In a series of 100 long distance runners with this affliction, rest and reduction of the training program, and a single steroid injection resulted in relief in 30 patients; 21 others required 2 injections; and 8 required 3 injections. Five patients re-

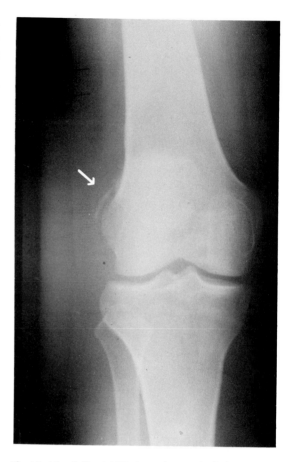

Fig. 10–11. Pellegrini Stieda syndrome of calcification in the region of the medial or lateral tibial collateral ligament. This narrow elongated amorphous shadow adjacent to the femoral condyle may occur in patients with or without symptoms. (Courtesy of Toledo Hospital.)

quired surgery. Others required total rest from running for 4 to 6 weeks.[57]

Knee problems in runners are often secondary to abnormal foot positions, flatfeet, or high arches. Stretching exercises, proper shoes, and if necessary, an orthotic insert consisting of leather with a molded plastic insert is usually beneficial.[58]

The Plica Syndrome

Folds, pleats, bands, or shelves of synovium are normally present in the knee joint; the term "plica" is used to describe these synovial remnants.[59] The most common remnant is the medial suprapatellar plica originating beneath the quadriceps tendon and extending to the medial wall of the joint. Also common is the infrapatellar plica, which is attached to the intercondylar notch and runs distally to the infrapatellar fat pad. Knee joint pain and effusion often follow a blunt or twisting trauma. Many cases arise from overuse. Additional features, similar to internal derangement, include a sensation of giving way. During physical examination a palpable snap may occur. Definitive diagnosis is based on demonstrating the plica(e) by arthroscopy or pneumoarthrography. Conservative treatment with hamstring stretching, rest, heat, and anti-inflammatory agents is helpful in some patients;[60] in others the plica can be released during arthroscopy, but some patients require arthrotomy and partial synovectomy.

BOWLEG AND KNOCK KNEE

When a patient under age 30 has significant genu varum (bowleg) or genu valgum (knock knee) deformity, careful assessment should be performed regarding the potential benefit of surgical intervention. Tibial osteotomy may prevent serious osteoarthritis in well selected cases. In the older patient, or those with mild deformity, exercises aimed at improving alignment should be tried. For bowleg or knock knee deformity, the isometric adduction exercise (Exercise 7, Table 10–5), the isometric abduction exercise (Exercise 8, Table 10–5) and a quadriceps exercise have provided symptomatic relief as well as measurably improved alignment in some cases, in our experience. Joint protection measures are also helpful.

REFERENCES

1. Grossman RB, Nicholas JA: Common disorders of the knee. Orthop Clin N Am 8:619–640, 1977.
2. Trayoff R, Trapp R: Extra-articular pain syndrome: Frequency of osteoarthritis of the knees and effect on responsiveness to intra-articular corticosteroids. (Abstract #246) Arth Rheum 25 (No. 4) [Supp], 1982.
2a. Larsson L, Baum J: The syndrome of anserine bursitis. An overlooked diagnosis. Arth Rheum 28:1062–1065, 1985.
3. James SL: The knee. In Musculoskeletal Disorders. Edited by RD D'Ambrosia. Philadelphia, JB Lippincott, 1977.
4. Burry HC: The painful knee. Practitioner 215:46–54, 1975.
5. Johnson RP, Brewer BJ: Mechanical disorders of the knee. In Arthritis and Allied Conditions. 10th Ed. Edited by DJ McCarty. Philadelphia, Lea & Febiger, 1985.
6. Kim HJ, Kozin F, Johnson RP, Hines R: Reflex sympathetic dystrophy syndrome of the knee following meniscectomy. Arth Rheum 22:177–181, 1979.
7. Gordon GC: Traumatic prepatellar neuralgia. J Bone Joint Surg 34B:41–44, 1952.
8. Hughston JC, Andrews JR, Cross MJ, Moschi A: Classification of knee ligament instabilities. J Bone Joint Surg 58A:159–172, 1976.
9. Dehaven KE, Dolan WA, Mayer PJ: Chondromalacia patellae and the painful knee. Am Fam Physician 21:117–124, 1980.
10. Houston CS, Swischuk LE: Varus and valgus—no wonder they are confused. N Engl J Med 302:471–472, 1980.
11. Sharrard WJ: Aetiology and pathology of beat knee. Br J Ind Med 20:24–31, 1963.
12. Turek SL: Orthopaedics: Principles and Their Application. 4th Ed. Philadelphia, JB Lippincott, 1984.
13. Kennedy JC, Roth JH, Walker DM: Posterior cruciate ligament injuries. Orthop Digest 7:19–31, 1979.
14. Duthie RB, Ferguson AB: Mercer's Orthopedic Surgery. 8th Ed. Baltimore, Williams & Wilkins, 1983.
15. Kirk JA, Ansell BM, Bywaters EGL: The hypermobility syndrome; Musculoskeletal complaints associated with generalized joint hypermobility. Ann Rheum Dis 26:419–425, 1967.
16. Howorth MB: General relaxation of the ligaments. Clin Orthop 30:133–143, 1963.
17. Zeman SC, Nielsen MW: Osteochondritis dissecans of the knee. Orthop Rev 7:101–112, 1978.
18. Hadied AM: An unusual complication of arthroscopy: a fistula between the knee and the prepatellar bursa. J Bone Joint Surg 66A:624, 1984.
19. Lindenbaum BL: Complications of knee joint arthroscopy. Clin Ortho 160:158, 1981.
20. Johnson LL: Impact of diagnostic arthroscopy on the clinical judgement of an experienced arthroscopist. Clin Ortho 167:75–83, 1982.
21. Sprague NF III: Arthroscopic surgery: degenerative and traumatic flap tears of the meniscus. Contemp Ortho 9:23–46, 1984.
22. Pettrone FA: Meniscectomy: arthrotomy versus arthroscopy. Am J Sport Med 10:355–359, 1982.
23. Seale KS, Haynes DW, Nelson CL: The effect of meniscectomy on knee stability. (Abstract # 42) Arth Rheum 25 (4) [Supp], 1982.
24. Reid GD, Glasgow M, Gordon DA, Wright TA: Pathological plicae of the knee mistaken for arthritis. J Rheum 7:573–576, 1980.
25. Munsinger U, Ruckstuhl J, Scherrer H, Gschwend N: Internal derangement of the knee joint due to pathologic synovial folds: the mediopatellar plica syndrome. Clin Orth 155:59–64, 1981.
26. Blatz DJ, Fleming R, McCarroll J: Suprapatellar plica: A study of their occurrence and role in internal

derangement of the knee in active duty personnel. Orthopaedics 4:181–184, 1981.

27. Monaco BR, Noble HB, Bachman DC: Incomplete tears of the anterior cruciate ligament and knee locking. JAMA 247:1582–1584, 1982.

27a. Soudry M, Lanir A, Angel D, et al: Anatomy of the normal knee as seen by magnetic resonance imaging. J Bone Joint Surg 68:117–120, 1986.

27b. Hull RG, Rennie JN, Eastmond CJ, et al: Nuclear magnetic resonance (NMR) tomographic imaging for popliteal cysts in rheumatoid arthritis. Ann Rheum Dis 43:56–59, 1984.

28. Trujeque L, Spohn P, Bankhurst A, et al: Patellar whiskers and acute calcific quadriceps tendinitis in a general hospital population. Arth Rheum 20:1409–1412, 1977.

29. Abernethy PJ, Townsend PR, Rose RM, Radin EL: Is chondromalacia patellae a separate clinical entity? J Bone Joint Surg 608:205–210, 1978.

30. Goodfellow J, Hungerford DS, Woods C: Patellofemoral joint mechanics and pathology. J Bone Joint Surg 58B:291–299, 1976.

30a. Yates C, Grana WA: Patellofemoral pain—a prospective study. Orthopedics 9:663–666, 1986.

31. Fairbank JCT, Pynsent PB, van Poortvliet JA, Phillips H: Mechanical factors in the incidence of knee pain in adolescents and young adults. J Bone Joint Surg 66B:685–693, 1984.

32. Insall J: Current concepts review patella pain. J Bone Joint Surg 64:147–152, 1982.

33. Radin EL: Chondromalacia of the patella. Bull Rheum Dis 34:1–6, 1984.

33a. Devereaux MD, Lachmann SM, Thomas DP, et al: Thermographic diagnosis in athletes with patellofemoral arthralgia. J Bone Joint Surg 68B:42–44, 1986.

34. Martens M, Wouters P, Burssens A, Mulier JC: Patellar tendinitis: pathology and results of treatment. Acta Orthop Scand 53:445–450, 1982.

35. Perrild C, Hejgaard N, Rosenklint A: Chondromalacia patellae. Acta Orthop Scand 53:131–134, 1982.

36. Worrell RV: The diagnosis of disorders of the patellofemoral joint. Ortho Review 10:73–76, 1981.

37. Radin EL: Anterior knee pain, the need for a specific diagnosis, stop calling it chondromalacia! Ortho Review 14:33–39, 1985.

38. Wissinger HA: Chondromalacia patella: A nonoperative treatment program. Orthopedics 5:315–316, 1982.

39. Ismail AM, Balakrishnan R, Rajakumar MK: Rupture of patellar ligament after steroid infiltration: Report of a case. J Bone Joint Surg 51B:503–505, 1969.

40. Malone T, Blackburn TA, Wallace LA: Knee rehabilitation. Phys Therapy 60:1602–1610, 1980.

41. Grana WA, O'Donoghue DH: Patellar-tendon trans-

fer by the slot-block method for recurrent subluxation and dislocation of the patella. J Bone Joint Surg 59A:736–741, 1977.

42. Hendryson IE: Bursitis in the region of the fibular collateral ligament. J Bone Joint Surg 28:446–450, 1946.

43. Moschcowitz E: Bursitis of sartorius bursa: an undescribed malady simulating chronic arthritis. JAMA 109:1362–1364, 1937.

44. Brookler MI, Mongan WS: Relief for the pain of anserina bursitis in the arthritic knee. Cal Med 119:8–10, 1973.

45. Quale JB, Robinson MP: An operation for chronic prepatellar bursitis. J Bone Joint Surg 58B:504–506, 1976.

46. Stuttle FL: The no-name and no-fame bursa. Clin Orthop 15:197–199, 1959.

47. Pavlov H, Goldman AB: The popliteus bursa: An indicator of subtle pathology. Am J Rheum 134:313–321, 1980.

48. Lotke PA, Ecker ML, Alavi A: Painful knees in older patients. J Bone Joint Surg 59A:617–621, 1977.

49. Ho G Jr., Su EY: Antibiotic therapy of septic bursitis: Its implication in the treatment of septic arthritis. Arth Rheum 24:905–911, 1981.

50. Dinham JM: Popliteal cysts in children: The case against surgery. J Bone Joint Surg 57B:69–71, 1975.

51. Wigley RD: Popliteal cysts: variations on a theme of Baker. Sem Arth Rheum 12:1–10, 1982.

52. Gompels BM, Darlington LG: Evaluation of popliteal cysts and painful calves with ultrasonography: comparison with arthrography. Ann Rheum Dis 41:355–359, 1982.

53. Halperin N, Axer A: Semimembranous tenosynovitis. Orthop Rev 9:72–75, 1980.

54. Weiser HI: Semimembranosus insertion syndrome: a treatable and frequent cause of persistent knee pain. Arch Phys Med Rehabil 60:317–319, 1979.

55. Leach RE: Running injuries of the knee. Orthopedics 5:1358–1378, 1982.

56. Renne JW Lt Cdr: The iliotibial band friction syndrome. J Bone Joint Surg 57A:1110–1111, 1975.

57. Noble CA: Iliotibial band friction syndrome in runners. Am J Sports Med 8:232–234, 1980.

58. Lutter LD: Foot related knee problems, presented to Am Orthopaedic Foot Society. San Francisco. Orthop Rev 8:123–126, 1979.

59. Hardaker WT, Whipple TL, Bassett FH: Diagnosis and treatment of the plica syndrome of the knee. J Bone Joint Surg 62A:221–225, 1980.

60. Whipple TL, Hardaker WT: Symptomatic plica and shelf syndromes in knee. Ortho Review 14:61–64, 1985.

61. Sheon RP: A joint protection guide for nonarticular rheumatic disorders. Postgrad Med 77(5):329–338, 1985.

11

The Foreleg Region

Overuse from running, jogging, or other conditioning activities often results in pain syndromes of the lower extremities. The potential damage that may result from "cumulative impact loading" during jogging is the subject of much speculation in the current literature. Little hard data are presently available but we currently would advise that the runner limit mileage to about 15 or 20 miles per week. Other disorders of diverse or unknown etiology are presented in this chapter with suggestions for safe and empiric therapy.

SHIN SPLINTS

"Shin splints syndrome" is loosely used jargon that has been applied to a symptom complex of pain and discomfort in the lower leg after repetitive overuse, such as in running, jogging, or walking. Discomfort emanates from the lower half of the posteromedial border of the tibia, the anterior tibial compartment, the tibia itself, or the interosseous membrane region of the foreleg. The symptoms are a dull ache followed by a gradually worsening pain, which is at first relieved by rest, and later becomes continuous. Accompanying foreleg pain, numbness or loss of sensation over the fourth toe may be noted. The pain and discomfort in the leg are associated with repetitive running, particularly on a hard surface, or with forcible, excessive use of foot flexors. Usually the pain is confined to the anterior portion of the leg, but the site of involvement may be more diffuse. Tenderness can usually be elicited over symptomatic sites.[1] Stress fractures, periostitis, tears of musculotendinous structures, or definite ischemic compartment syndromes are important alternate diagnostic considerations,[2,3]

Etiology. Shin splints syndrome often is related to overuse of underdeveloped, untrained muscles, particularly the posterior tibial muscle.[1,2] Small tears at the origin of the muscle or herniation of the muscle through fascia are thought to occur.[3] The lesion may be located at the origin, belly, or musculotendinous junction of the involved muscles;[2] or may be a periostitis. Normal intramuscular pressure in the posterior compartment of the leg in cases with the shin splints syndrome has been reported.[4] When tenderness is localized to the medial border of the tibia and the patient has pronated feet, a periostitis may be present. This in turn may result from biomechanical stress on the soleus muscle.[5]

Differential Diagnosis. If pain is out of proportion to the clinical findings, an intermittent or complete ischemic compartment syndrome should be excluded. A compartment syndrome results from any increased tissue pressure within an anatomic space that compromises the circulation to the compartment.[6–8] It requires a constricting envelope (a constricting fascia or cast) and an increased volume (blood, swelling). Ischemic compartment syndromes that must be distinguished from shin splints include those due to involvement in the anterior tibial compartment.[9] Symptoms related to these ischemic syndromes often begin 10 to 12 hours after unaccustomed exercise, or in association with serious trauma; aching pain in the compartment region is noted. Increased pain in the anterior compartment following passive flexion of the toes is an early sign. Pain, pallor, and pulseless paralysis are late hallmarks of the serious ischemic post-traumatic compartment syndromes. Elevated compartment pressure is a confirmatory diagnostic finding. In addition to ischemic compartment syndrome, fracture and vascular claudication must also be considered in the differential diagnosis of severe shin splints syndrome.[6,9,10,11]

Stress fractures resulting from athletic competition or jogging must be recognized early in order to prevent more serious injury. Radionuclide bone scan is more reliable than conventional roentgenograms for diagnosis.[12] Such fractures may occur in the spine, femur, tibia, fibula, calcaneus, or metatarsal bones. Pain may be referred to sites distant from the fracture. The etiology is thought to be bone "fatigue". Female runners over the age of 30 tend to fracture the inferior ramus of the pubis; high school track or cross country runners tend to fracture the distal fibula.[13] Tenderness and pain is well localized, usually persists several weeks, and swelling without redness may be present. Treatment measures include rest, substitution of sports such as swimming, strengthening exercises, gentler training, and monitored return to running. Orthotics are of uncertain value.

Management. Application of ice packs for 15 minutes at a time and leg elevation are initial treatment measures. Local subfascial injection of a corticosteroid agent may be helpful. Stretching followed by strengthening exercises directed to the musculature of the involved site of the leg are helpful. Use of proper footgear is important; runners should avoid running on hard surfaces.

Outcome and Additional Suggestions. Brief rest usually allows the pain to subside, at which time activity may be resumed. Local tenderness should no longer be palpable. Recurrent or persistent pain requires exclusion of a true compartment syndrome or a stress fracture.[9] The latter may be difficult to distinguish from shin splints; bone scans, positive in the presence of stress fracture, are diagnostically helpful.[1,12,14]

OTHER LEG PAIN AND DYSFUNCTION

Patients may suffer from a partial rupture of one of the calf muscles. Symptoms commonly are due to a tear of the plantaris muscle, but may also result from a partial rupture of any of the other muscles of the popliteal and calf region. The term "tennis leg" has been given to this symptom complex. The patient often perceives a "snap" followed by a sudden burning in the calf; the leg gives way and the patient finds himself on the ground. Examination reveals pain aggravated by passive dorsiflexion of the ankle. Treatment of the partial tear is protective with the use of adhesive strapping to immobilize the ankle in plantarflexion and to limit weight bearing; the use of heat, massage, and gentle exercise are helpful. Limited activity for 3 to 4 weeks is usually needed.[15]

Spontaneous *rupture* of the *posterior tibial tendon* results in pain, tenderness, and swelling behind and below the medial malleolus with loss of foot stability. Often a tenosynovitis characterized by slight swelling behind and beneath the medial malleolus has been present for some time. Lower leg pain after walking is noted.[15]

Osgood Schlatter Disease

Usually seen in boys during periods of rapid growth, patients with this disease have pain, tenderness, and soft tissue swelling about the tibial tubercle just below the patella. Pain occurs when climbing stairs, kneeling, or kicking in association with quadriceps muscle contraction. The discomfort and swelling usually cease before or by age 18.

The etiology is thought to be traumatic and may result from avulsion of the tibial tubercle during adolescence.[10] Radiographic findings may include swelling of the patellar ligament, fragmentation of the tibial tubercle, soft tissue swelling, avulsion of an ossification center,[10] or avascular necrosis.

Treatment includes the use of a cylinder cast for several weeks, avoidance of contact sports, and maintenance of quadriceps strength with cautious use of isometric exercise (10 to 20 pounds, depending on age and size of the patient). The end result is a prominent tubercle that is usually painless. In one study, 116 of 142 patients recovered within 1 year with conservative measures. In the others, surgical intervention consisted of excision of a portion of the surface of the tibial tuberosity and multiple perforation with a thin drill point.[16]

Growing Pains

The term "growing pains" attributed to Deschamp in the early 19th century[17] is in fact a misnomer, because the most common age of occurrence is *not* at the time of rapid growth. These pains usually occur around age 8 and disappear by age 12.[18] The discomfort is described as an intermittent annoying pain or ache usually localized to the muscles of the legs and thighs, associated with a feeling of restlessness. These pains do not occur in joint areas and are often bilateral;[17] they often awaken the child from sleep and may be relieved by movement such as walking about the room. A hot tub bath, leg elevation, and leg massage are additional helpful measures. The discomfort is accentuated by running or other strenuous play activities.

Naish and Apley, in a study of British school children, noted leg pain in 5% of the children.[18] Patients identified in the study had a history of nonarticular pain of at least 3 months' duration, and severe enough to cause some limitation of activity. The sexes were equally involved. Except for two children who were found to have tuberculosis, and one child who developed osteochondritis of the knee, the remainder had a confirmed diagnosis of benign leg pain after 1 to 3 years of observation. A family history of rheumatic pain was found in over half the children with growing pains, compared to 10% in a control group. A child with only nocturnal pain often had relatives with only nocturnal pain, whereas children with diurnal pain had a strong family history of diurnal pain. Although no acceptable cause for these pain disturbances has been recognized,[17] a relation to exertion, fatigue, mechanical factors, and structural deficits such as pes planus or scoliosis has been noted.[18]

The differential diagnosis of recurrent pain in the lower limbs in children and adolescents includes trauma, occult infection, avascular necrosis of bone, vascular disturbances, con-genital structural disorders, tumors, connective tissue diseases, and the soft tissue rheumatic pain disorders. Workup might include an erythrocyte sedimentation rate complete blood count, and roentgenogram of the limb and chest if clinically indicated.[17,18] Benign causes of leg pain are usually bilateral, whereas most of the serious disorders with leg pain are unilateral.

Treatment for children with these benign leg pains is empiric. If the leg muscles are tight, gentle hamstring muscle stretching exercises may be beneficial. These should also be done as a warmup before competitive sports. When myofascial trigger points have been found, a vapocoolant spray has been found to be helpful. Improvement with these measures aids in diagnosis of a soft tissue rheumatic pain disorder.[19] Most children seem to improve by age 12.

Infrequently the clinician sees a child or adolescent with leg pain without any distinguishing features; psychogenic factors may have to be considered.[18,20] The clinician should then look for the following:

1. Death of a parent or separation from a significant other person.
2. Marital discord between parents.
3. Family history or similar complaints of pain in parents or siblings.
4. Difficulty in school with academic subjects, teachers, or peers.

When an emotionally charged situation has been discovered, therapeutic intervention must focus on the psychosocial disorder as well as on its resulting symptoms. With removal of the emotionally charged situation, the pain or dysfunction state often improves.[20]

Night Cramps

Cramps that involve the legs and feet are probably more common than physicians realize. Effective treatment may be a problem. Patients often do not mention the complaint unless asked. Inappropriate use of folk medicines and snake venom for this and other pain syndromes serves only to emphasize our failure to understand and treat this syndrome adequately.

Benign nocturnal leg and foot aches and cramps may be related to exertion, and often awaken the patient. These patients usually have normal peripheral pulses on examination and no evidence of significant vascular disease. Symptoms have to be differentiated from pain of intermittent claudication, which occurs during limb use and is relieved by rest. Although common in childhood and in the elderly, night cramps occur in all decades of life. Patients with the complaint of nocturnal leg and foot pain and cramp should be carefully examined for structural disorders, including flat feet, genu recurvatum, hypermobility syndrome, and inappropriate leg position during sedentary activity. Patients who sit for prolonged periods or who tuck a leg up under themselves may be predisposed to night cramp. Diuretics, excessive sweating without salt replacement, hypocalcemia, low serum magnesium, and motor neuron disease are additional causes of cramp.[21]

A history of working on a concrete floor, or having moved to a home built on a cement slab foundation (even with floor coverings) may correlate with the occurrence of leg cramps. Wearing thick crepe-soled shoes is often helpful in such situations. Symptoms frequently recur in clusters. Quinine given at bedtime may be helpful in preventing recurrences. This agent is administered daily at bedtime until the patient has been free of night cramps for several days. Therapy is then discontinued and reinstituted when a new cluster of cramps recurs. In patients allergic to this agent, or who fail to respond, a trial of diphenhydramine (Benadryl) may be of value. Other medications recommended for night cramps include vitamin E,[22] meprobamate, and other simple muscle relaxants.[22–24] Chloroquine phosphate, 250 mg daily for 2 or 3 weeks was reported to be effective within 1 to 3 weeks. Thereafter, 250 to 500 mg given once a week provided preventive benefit.[25] This has been helpful in our experience.

If a structural disorder or muscle contraction is found, muscle stretching or strengthening exercises, and use of long-countered shoes and other proper footgear may be of value. If a cramp occurs, walking or leg "jiggling" followed by leg elevation may be helpful. Leg stretching, by standing 2 to 3 feet out from a wall, placing hands on the wall, then climbing hands up the wall, keeping the heels on the floor;[23] hold 20 seconds, repeat 3 times in succession, 4 times a day for 1 week; then twice a day thereafter (see Exercise #1, Table 12–3 and Fig. 11–1). In most cases, these stretching exercises may prevent leg cramps. Use of a warm tub bath may be prophylactic. Judicious use of brandy is a time-honored remedy.

The *postphlebitic syndrome* presentation of gradual onset of aching calf pain and dependent edema, a sensation of fullness in the calf, and worsening with prolonged standing and walking, and relieved by rest and elevation should be considered. The presentation may mimic deep vein thrombosis. The pathogen-

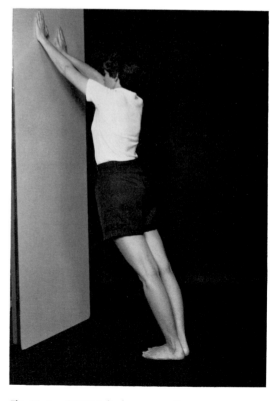

Fig. 11–1.   Exercise for leg cramps.[23]

esis is unknown but probably reflects venous hypertension.[25a]

Restless Leg Syndrome

Painless, spontaneous, continuous leg movements are often of psychogenic origin,[26] but may also accompany organic disease states. Hypoglycemia, hyperglycemia, hypothyroidism, neuropathies, uremia, anemia, and caffeinism have been associated with the syndrome.[21,27] If accompanied by expressions of exquisite pain, they may be of hysterical origin. The use of low-dose tricyclic antidepressant medication and leg stretching exercises have been helpful.[24] Other recommended treatment includes propranolol;[28] carbamazine 100 mg hs or more gradually increased;[29] or clonazepam.[30] Stretching exercises for the posterior leg muscles should be performed before retiring (see Fig. 10–10, p. 232).

Night Starts

Although not limited to the leg, sudden jerking contractures of the limbs that occur shortly after falling asleep are common. They awaken the patient, and the severity of the jerky movements is frightening. Upon falling back to sleep, they seldom recur. No definite cause is known. The condition is self-limited, and treatment is reassurance of the benign temporary nature of the disturbance.

Anterior leg pain and a sensation of swelling, which is lateral and inferior to the tibial tubercle, can result from a contracted or tight hamstring muscle. In any event, the pain is *not* articular. The anterior leg pain is reproduced during straight-leg-raising examination, as the leg is forced straight upward. Pain is relieved by exercises that stretch the hamstring muscles (Fig. 10–10, p. 232).

Reflex Sympathetic Dystrophy

As described previously in Chapter 3, throbbing, burning, aching pain following trauma suggests this disorder. The lower limb is less commonly involved, but when it occurs, diagnosis may be difficult. The pain quality is suggestive of the diagnosis if throb-

bing and burning occur. The limb is often discolored with dependent rubor or cyanotic mottling noted about the entire foot and lower foreleg. The skin is cool, and hyperhidrosis may be present. Diffuse swelling throughout the ankle and forefoot is noted. Radiographic evidence of spotty osteoporosis is suggestive but not diagnostic. Bone scans reveal either decreased or increased uptake. A short course of prednisone, beginning with doses of 20 to 30 mg daily, may be beneficial. Patients in whom steroids are contraindicated or ineffective may benefit from a series of lumbar sympathetic blocks. Sympathetic drugs such as guanethedine, 10 mg tid or phenoxybenzamine, 10 mg tid are less consistently effective. Use of a transcutaneous nerve stimulator (TENS) unit may provide symptomatic benefit.

NODULES

Pseudorheumatoid nodules have already been mentioned in the discussion of the upper extremity regions; they also occur in the pretibial region in infants and children. No articular abnormalities are seen, and the nodule is painless. Recently, a "hidden" 19 S IgM rheumatoid factor that is complement-fixing has been detected in the sera of such patients.[31] No treatment is necessary. *Surfer's nodules* also may occur in the pretibial foreleg region. They result from activities in which the foreleg and the hyperextended ankle are brought in contact with a hard surface. Recurrent bumping from a surf board is a known cause. The lesions may resemble rheumatoid nodules. Avoiding surface contact is curative. Similar nodules can occur on children's forefeet if they repeatedly sit on their legs with their feet plantarflexed and in contact with hardwood floors. Similarly, painter's bosses are nodules where the foreleg strikes the rungs of a ladder.[32] Other etiologies include panniculitis due to infectious agents (tuberculosis, histoplasmosis);[33] erythema nodosum; sarcoidosis; streptococcal infections; peripheral manifestations of inflammatory bowel disease, occult neoplasm; and primary bone tumors of the foreleg.

REFERENCES

1. Baugher WH, Balady GJ, Warren RF, Marshall JL: Injuries of the musculoskeletal system in runners. Contemp Orthop 1:46–54, 1979.
2. Slocum DB: The shin splint syndrome. Am J Surg 114:875–881, 1967.
3. Garfin S, Mubarak SJ, Owen CA: Exertional anter-olateral-compartment syndrome. J Bone Joint Surg 59A:404–405, 1977.
4. Mubarak SJ, Gould RN, Lee YF, Schmidt DA, Hargens AR: The medial tibial stress syndrome. Am J Sport Med 10:201–205, 1982.
5. Michael RH, Holder LE: The soleus syndrome, a cause of medial tibial stress. Am J Sports Med 13:87–94, 1985.
6. Matsen FA: Compartmental syndromes. N Engl J Med 300:1210–1211, 1979.
7. Mubarak SJ, Hargens AR, Owen CA, et al: The wick catheter technique for measurement of intramuscular pressure. J Bone Joint Surg. 58:1016–1019, 1976.
8. Mubarak, SJ, Owen CA: Double-incision fasciotomy of the leg for decompression in compartment syndromes. J Bone Joint Surg 59:184–187, 1977.
9. Matsen FA: Compartmental syndromes. Hosp Pract 15:113–117, 1980.
10. Turek SL: Orthopaedics; Principles and Their Application. 4th Ed. Philadelphia, JB Lippincott, 1984.
11. Detmer DE, Sharpe K, Sufit RL, Girdley FM: Chronic compartment syndrome: diagnosis, management, and outcomes. Am Ortho Soc Sport Med 13:162–170, 1985.
12. Norfray JF, Schlachter L, Kernahan WT Jr, et al: Early confirmation of stress fractures in joggers. JAMA 243:1647–1649, 1980.
13. Warren RF, Sullivan D: Stress fractures in athletes: recognizing the subtle signs. J Musculoskel Med 1 (March):33–35, 1984.
14. Brady DM: Running injuries. Clin Symp 32 4:2–36, 1980.
15. Pinals RS: Traumatic arthritis and allied conditions. In Arthritis and Allied Conditions. 10th Ed. Edited by DJ McCarty. Philadelphia, Lea & Febiger, 1985.
16. Soren A, Fetto JF: Pathology, clinic, and treatment of Osgood-Schlatter Disease. Ortho 7:230–234, 1984.
17. Peterson HA: Leg aches. Ped Clin N Am 24:731–736, 1977.
18. Naish JM, Apley J: "Growing pains": A clinical study of non-arthritic limb pains in children. Arch Dis Child 26:134–140, 1951.
19. Bates T, Grunwaldt E: Myofascial pain in childhood. J Pediatr 53:198–209, 1958.
20. Caghan SB, McGrath MM, Morrow MG, Pittman LD: When adolescents complain of pain. Nurse Practit 3:19–22, 1978.
21. Whiteley AM: Cramps, stiffness and restless legs. Practitioner 226:1085–1087, 1982.
22. Ayres S Jr, Mihan R: Nocturnal leg cramps (systremma). Southern Med J 67:1308–1312, 1974.
23. Daniell HW: Simple cure for nocturnal leg cramps. N Engl J Med 301:216, 1979.
24. Lee HB: Cramp in the elderly. Br Med J 2:1259, 1976.
25. More on muscle cramps. Drug Therapeutics Bulletin 21:83–84, 1983.
25a.Leclerc JR, Jay RM, Hull RD, et al: Recurrent leg symptoms following deep vein thrombosis. Arch Intern Med 145:1867–1869, 1985.
26. Smythe HA: Nonarticular rheumatism and psychogenic musculoskeletal syndromes. In Arthritis and Allied Conditions. 10th Ed. Edited by DJ McCarty. Philadelphia, Lea & Febiger, 1985.
27. Lutz EG: Restless legs, anxiety and caffeinism. J Clin Psych 39:11–16, 1978.
28. Derom E, Elinck W, Buylaret W, Van Der Straeten N: Which beta-blocker for the restless leg? Lancet 1:857, 1984.
29. Telstad W, Sorensen O, Larsen, S, Lillevold PE, et al: Treatment of the restless legs syndrome with carbamazepine: double blind study. Br Med J 288:444–447, 1984.
30. Montplasir J, Godbout R, Boghen D, DeChamplain J, Young SN, Lapierre G: Familial restless legs with periodic movements in sleep: electrophysiologic, biochemical, and pharmacologic study. Neuro 35:130–134, 1985.
31. Moore TL, Doner RW, Zuckner J: Complement-fixing hidden rheumatoid factor in children with benign rheumatoid nodules. Arth Rheum 21:930–934, 1978.
32. Ehrlich GE: Painter's bosses. Arch Intern Med 116:776–777, 1965.
33. Pottage JC, Trenholme GM, Aronson IK, Harris AA: Panniculitis associated with histoplasmosis and alpha 1-antitrypsin deficiency. Am J Med 75:150–153, 1983.

12

The Ankle and Foot

From the Madison Avenue slogan "clothes make the man," one should conclude "shoes make the foot." However, although improper shoes may produce a multitude of forefoot and toe problems, they should not be incriminated in all painful soft tissue disorders of the foot. Improper shoes can cause or exacerbate hallux valgus, hammer-toes, hard corns, and plantar keratoses. Proper shoes should provide comfort (proper fit) for the weightbearing foot, room for the toes to fully extend, and lack of crowding of the foot.[1] "First and foremost one should remember that the shoe should protect the foot, not disturb it."[2]

Every physician is familiar with problems created by the narrow-toed, high-heeled contemporary female dress shoe, In the last 20 years, greater strides have been made by shoe manufacturers to provide reasonable covering for the foot: a cushion or crepe sole for walking on concrete floors, a toe box with adequate space, and lacing or straps that hold the foot in the shoe.[3] The "earth shoe" relieves metatarsal weightbearing and returns the weightbearing line of vertical force to the more normal position just anterior to the ankle joint (Fig. 12–1). This has been reported to be helpful for a number of painful disturbances of the *forefoot*.[3] The running or jogging shoe is particularly comfortable for walking or working on concrete, and it may prevent metatarsalgia. This shoe differs from a tennis shoe in having a layer of microcellular foam in the sole; the arch is soft but elevated; and the forefoot is rigid. It has a neutral heel; the heel and sole are at the same level. The shoe makes the wearer use the entire foot more evenly when walking or running (Fig. 12–2). Adapting shoes to the patient can be a valuable contribution to the comprehensive treatment of rheumatic diseases of the foot.[4]

Because weight should be borne evenly between the heel and the toe and more toward the first metatarsal, shoes may require modification to correct minor structural disorders that change this weightbearing distribution.[5] Some basic features of "specialized" shoes include a heavier rib steel shank that provides rigidity to the forefoot, a long counter to within ⅜ inch of the first metatarsophalangeal joint for support of the longitudinal arch, and a Thomas heel that projects forward on the medial side. These features maintain the arch and prevent the heel from turning out (valgus heel).[6] A combination last represents a shoe three widths smaller in the heel than in the forefoot area.[6] Shoe modifications, including extra depth to provide insoles or inlays, are discussed throughout this chapter.

The diagnosis of most foot and ankle disorders is aided by the fact that the bones are palpable, the soft tissues can be tested for their supporting functions, and vascular changes are readily apparent.[7] The foot consists of 28 bones and 57 articulations that provide the ability to walk on any surface, to run, or to jump. The intrinsic muscles of the foot provide all the means necessary for grasping. The articulating bones and joints provide the longitudinal arch.[8] (See Anatomic Plates XII and XIII.)

The Examination. Foot complaints must be assessed in a logical sequence in order to determine local versus systemic causes, or traumatic, genetic, or acquired disturbances (Table 12–1, Danger Signs for the Leg and Foot). The quality of pain should help distinguish neuropathic types of discomfort (burning, tingling) from the more common deep-aching symptoms of tissue strain or injury. When symptoms are intermittent rather than persistent, further inquiry should include the

243

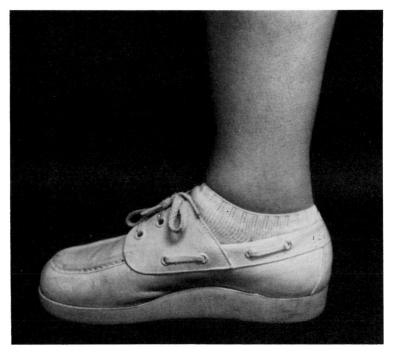

Fig. 12–1. The neutral shoe: Originally the earth shoe distributed weight back upon the heel. Modification of the principle resulted in the neutral shoe, which shifts weight off the metatarsophalangeal joint region toward the ankle. A slightly rounded sole may also act as a rocker bar. The neutral shoe may be helpful for patients with metatarsalgia or rheumatoid arthritis of the forefoot.

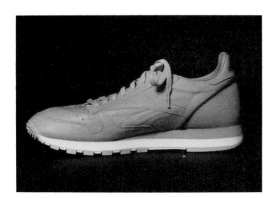

Fig. 12–2. A running shoe has microcellular foam and a rigid forefoot. These are important differences from other sport shoes.

Table 12–1. Danger Signs for the Foot and Ankle Region

1. Discoloration of the leg and foot
2. Swelling, warmth, erythema of limb
3. Regional lymphadenopathy
4. Intermittent claudication
5. Weight-bearing pain of increasing intensity
6. Night pain
7. Paresthesias aggravated by coughing
8. Neurologic deficits
9. Compartment symptoms: Pain, paresthesia, pulselessness.

type of flooring in the home or job, any recent change in occupation that might require prolonged standing, or whether recent recovery from a protracted illness has occurred. New activities such as jogging, racquetball, or other impact foot activities should be discussed (Table 12–2, Aggravating Factors).

Inspection of the foot while the patient is seated includes noting skin color, hair distribution on the foot and foreleg, presence of a normal arch, forefoot width, and the presence of calluses and other dermatologic features. Next, with the patient standing, the physician

Table 12–2. Joint Protection (From Sheon[78])

Harmful	Helpful
■ Being loose-jointed may provoke repeated ankle injury, with the ligaments at the outside of the ankle giving way and tearing	■ Wear low-heeled shoes that tie up close to the ankle; high-necked shoes that tie above the ankle may give less support to the ankle. Good walking shoes have rubber soles and stiff heel counters.
■ Having flat arches, a condition common in loose-jointed persons, may cause joint and muscle fatigue. Working on a hard surface, standing in one position for prolonged periods, or being overweight compounds the problem.	■ Use arch supports if deemed necessary by a physician. Many loose-jointed, flat-footed persons have no ankle problems and thus do not need to wear arch-preserving shoes.
■ Wearing shoes with crepe soles, many of which are too flexible to support the metatarsal area, can be injurious.	■ Invest in a pair of running shoes. One of the best-designed types of shoes available, they are cushioned, have a moderate arch, and shift body weight back toward the ankle and away from the metatarsal arch, or ball of the foot.
■ Wearing slippers or moccasins or going barefoot aggravates metatarsal and toe pain.	■ Try running shoes for everyday use. Always wear shoes that shift body weight behind the metatarsal arch and that tie or buckle to keep the feet from slipping forward.
■ Walking and/or standing on concrete (which we all are doing increasingly) promotes joint and muscle fatigue. This is true even when the concrete is covered with carpeting.	■ Select shoes with rubber soles, which act as shock absorbers.
■ Squeezing the forefoot, which tends to widen with age, into too narrow a shoe may cause nerves to be pinched between the bones of the toes. Having bunions can also be problematic. Neuralgia, with a burning sensation and aching pain in the forefoot radiating to the toes (usually the third and fourth), is symptomatic of improper shoe fit.	■ Ensure that shoes fit properly. Sometimes, use of an external metatarsal bar helps to spread the toe bones. Wear shoes with enlarged toe boxes to accommodate troublesome bunions. Fortunately, today's specialty stores usually stock shoes having extra depth and enlarged toe boxes.
■ Having burning pain in the feet at night suggests a pinched nerve at the ankle or neuritis caused by diabetes or a nutritional deficiency.	■ Consult a physician.

looks for spinal curvatures, pelvic tilt, femoral or tibial torsion, patellae rotating away from the midline, and the direction of the weight-bearing foot. The flatfoot is accompanied by pronation, a tilting outward of the foot, and valgus deviation of the heel. This can be seen best by inspecting the foot from behind the standing patient. From the frontal view, a line carried from the midpoint of the patella down the anterior spine of the lower tibia should project forward through the web between the second and third toes.

While the patient is standing, the physician should look for toe deformities, particularly hallux valgus, metatarsus primus varus of the first toe (the first metatarsus is shortened and deviated to the midline, and the toe is rotated slightly medially as noted by the slant of the toe nail), and for evidence of toe crowding. With the patient lying supine the examiner should next determine the rigidity or softness of the plantar fascia. This is performed by grasping the toes and dorsiflexing them with one hand while palpating the plantar aspect of the foot, particularly the bands compressing the plantar fascia. Only by examining many normal feet can the physician become familiar with the pathologic tightly bound plantar fascia (Fig. 12–3). The assessment of the circulation and neurologic status of the foot should complete the examination.

SOFT TISSUE INJURY OF THE ANKLE

Sprains

The most common problems of the soft tissue-supporting structures of the ankle joint are sprains. The ligamentous structures of the

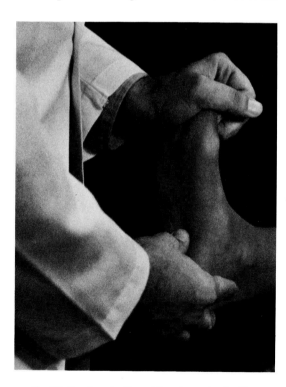

Fig. 12–3. Examination of the plantar fascia: The toes are drawn into extension, thus tensing the bands of the plantar fascia. Palpation reveals points of induration and tenderness. The two feet should be compared.

medial side of the ankle are less commonly injured than those of the lateral side. Sprains may be subclassified into 3 types: type 1 is a mild stretching of the ligament with the fibers still intact; type 2 is a more severe injury with partial disruption of the fibers of the ligaments; and type 3 is a complete disruption of the ligament. The more severe sprains should be referred to an orthopedic surgeon.

The lateral-collateral ligaments, composed of the anterior talofibular ligament, the posterior talofibular ligament, and the calcaneofibular ligament are most commonly involved in ankle sprains.[9] Usually the patient notes pain associated with an inverted ankle, and has a sensation of "giving way" of the ankle. Pain is increased upon forced-ankle inversion. The examiner can palpate for tenderness and often determines which portion of the ligament is involved. The medial collateral ligament (the deltoid ligament) can also suffer sprain; gentle eversion accentuates this pain. Swelling, local tenderness, and ecchymosis may occur and weightbearing becomes painful.

Management of type 1 sprain includes immediate application of cold with compression, elevation, and rest for the first 24 to 48 hours. In most cases, radiographic examination to exclude bony injury should be carried out. Special radiographic procedures including arthrography and stress roentgenographs may be needed to define the extent of injury.[10,11] In mild injury when the edema subsides, adhesive strapping or elastic support should be accomplished and continued until symptoms subside. A corticosteroid-anesthetic mixture may be injected into the region of the injury if symptoms persist.[9,12] *Chronic instability of the ankle joint* often results from the additive damage of multiple "turned ankles;" therefore, proper care of the acute injury is essential.[9,12]

Athletic injuries to the ankle may appear to be trivial, but are important in the context of the athlete's future endeavors.[13] Prevention of further injury includes ankle strapping to limit inversion or eversion, use of elastic ankle supports, and shoes with rigid-toe boxes and firm soles. Inflatable ankle supports, laced supports with malleable metal stays, and light-weight plastic posterior leg splints have been advocated for some ankle problems (see Decision Chart, Table 12–5). Following recovery from injury, the athlete should progress from walking to jogging, and then to running in figure eights, with gradually tighter circles in order to test the stability of the ankle before competitive activity is resumed. The patient should be referred to physicians who are expert in this area if the injured joint has not improved within 2 to 3 weeks,[13] or if there is any question about the degree of sprain.

Tendinitis

Inflammation of a tendon sheath about the ankle may result from repetitive activity or unaccustomed extraordinary work.[13,14] Other causes include improper footwear resulting in injury, particularly to the extensor hallucis longus or to the Achilles tendon. The shoe vamp may impinge upon the tendons of the dorsum of the ankle and forefoot, and local heat, redness, and tenderness may occur. Severe or repeated traumatic tenosynovitis may result in scarification and require surgical excision of the tendon sheath.

A chronic nonspecific tendinitis may affect several tendons at the ankle, similar to that seen in DeQuervain's tenosynovitis at the wrist.[9,12,15,16] Tenosynovitis involving the tibialis anterior, tibialis posterior, extensor digitorium longus, or peroneal tendons at the ankle may occur where the tendons become angulated at the ankle; friction can then cause inflammation of the tendon sheath. A bulbous swelling that occurs distally to areas of constriction is helpful in demonstrating points of constriction.[15] Histologic examination of the tendon sheath demonstrates nonspecific inflammation. Occasionally rheumatoid arthritis, spondylarthritis and rarely oxalosis, xanthomas, or giant cell tumors are found,[9,17] Tuberculosis is uncommon in this region.[15] Radiographic abnormalities are usually absent although new bone formation over the posterior aspect of the medial malleolus has

rarely been described.[18] Treatment of tendinitis includes partial immobilization of the ankle with bandaging or an elastic ankle support, and physical therapy to maintain range of motion. Sometimes complete immobilization in a cast is helpful. Tendon sheath injection with a corticosteroid-anesthetic mixture may be tried. Excision of the tendon sheath for diagnosis and treatment is rarely necessary. Persistent symptoms in a 20 to 30 year old should raise suspicion for a tarsal coalition. This fusion of 2 or more tarsal bones may give rise to vague foot pain after use or prolonged standing, and peroneal muscle spasm. Roentgenographic examination with attention to this possible etiology should be considered.[19]

Tendon Dislocation

The peroneal tendon is the most commonly dislocated leg tendon. It may become taut and dislocate, and the patient may experience an audible painless snapping sensation in this tendon. Such dislocation occurs in older children, and because walking is not affected, may go unrecognized.[12] The dislocated tendon may be seen lying over the lateral malleolus.[9,12] The patient notes the leg or ankle giving way if the peroneus longus muscle goes into spasm with abduction and plantarflexion of the foot.[21] Occasionally the dislocation may result from trauma; more often it results from a congenital shallowness of the tendon groove located on the posterior surface of the lateral malleolus.[9,12] Usually spontaneous reduction occurs; if not, active reduction may be required. After reducing the dislocation, treatment includes immobilization with a cast for 5 to 8 weeks, which usually results in permanent benefit. Occasionally, surgical intervention to reconstruct the sheath or to deepen the groove is necessary.[12,20]

Disorders of the Achilles Tendon Region

A tight Achilles tendon may result from disuse, from complex factors associated with growth, or more often as a problem occurring in women who wear high-heeled shoes. The patient presents with pain over the heel;[12]

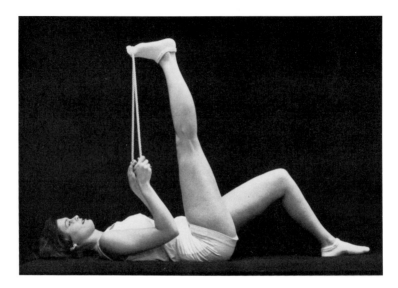

Fig. 12–4. Stretching and mobilizing exercise performed with this non-weightbearing technique is helpful for myofascial disturbances of the lower extremity and foot.

dorsiflexion of the ankle increases the pain and tenderness. Gentle progressive heel cord stretching exercise is helpful (see Exercise 1 to 3, Table 12–3, and Decision Chart, Table 12–5. Also, see Fig. 11–1 and Fig. 12–4). Achilles tendinitis in runners may respond to use of visco-elastic or other heel inserts to cushion and raise up the heel.[21]

Calcific tendinitis of the Achilles tendon produces swelling and often redness along the lower 5 cm of the tendon. Calcification may be evident in the tendon sheath on roentgenogram. A history of previous episodes of bursitis at the shoulder, hip or wrist may indicate more general calcium apatite deposition disease. Gout rarely strikes the posterior heel region but rheumatoid arthritis will involve the Achilles tendon on occasion. Treatment with nonsteroidal anti-inflammatory drugs is helpful. The condition may require several weeks of medication.

Bursitis may involve bursae that lie superficial and deep to the tendon near its insertion onto the calcaneus. Neither the deep bursa nor the tendon sheath should be injected because of the possibility of tendon rupture as a result of steroid-induced atrophy. Oral non-

steroidal anti-inflammatory agents are helpful.

Rupture of the Achilles Tendon. Rupture may occur after abrupt calf-muscle contraction. Usually the patient is a male over 30 years of age who sporadically engages in sports. The patient may note an audible snap, followed by pain in the calf as if struck with a baseball. The patient may then be unable to stand up on his toes. The Thompson test may be performed for further evidence of rupture of the Achilles tendon. The patient kneels on a chair with the feet hanging over the edge; when the examiner squeezes the calf muscle on the normal side, the foot responds with plantar flexion. When performing this examination on the suspected side, there is no foot response. Orthopedic consultation for immobilization or surgical repair is necessary.[2]

Adhesive Capsulitis of the Ankle

An adhesive capsulitis may follow an interarticular fracture or other severe injury. Persistent pain and limitation of motion develop. Arthrography is a useful diagnostic test. During arthrography a decreased capacity of the joint is evident. Instillation of a corticosteroid into the ankle and aggressive physical therapy may restore ankle motion.[22]

HEEL PAIN

The following conditions cause heel disturbance or pain: pump bumps, tendinitis, periostitis of the calcaneus, piezogenic papules, apophysitis, retrocalcaneal bursitis, neoplasms, calcaneal spurs, and plantar fasciitis.[9,12,23-26] Referred pain to the heel may result from disease of the subtalar joint or from sciatic nerve impingement.

"Pump bumps" are visible, firm, nodular lesions at the lower end of the tendo Achillis. They are commonly associated with wearing high-heeled pumps or loafers.[9] The bump may be an exostosis of the superior tuberosity of the calcaneus,[2] or may appear as a hatchet-shaped calcaneus with a prominent postero-superior margin.[25,27] They often are bilateral and asymptomatic.[2] Occasionally an overlying bursa becomes inflamed.[2] Symptomatic pump bumps are often the result of wearing closely contoured heel counters.[25] The pump bump may also be associated with an adventitial bursitis located at the posterior surface of the calcaneus lateral or medial to the Achilles tendon. Ill-fitting shoes may cause another adventitial bursitis, "last bursitis" located lateral to the heel.[28]

Rheumatoid nodules in this region can be distinguished from pump bumps: the former occur 1 or 2 in. *above* the point of attachment of the tendon to the calcaneus. Conversely, pump bumps are lower down at the superior border of the calcaneus. Treatment includes use of sandals or laced shoes, protective padding or a plastic heel cup, a heel lift, and rarely a corticosteroid injection into the adventitial superficial bursa.[2,9,29] Conservative therapy is helpful; if not, resection of the posterior prominence of the calcaneus may be necessary[25] (Table 12-4).

Pain accompanied by exquisite tenderness at the posterior point of the heel may also result from a *bursitis* secondary to calcific tendinitis.[26] Treatment with systemic nonsteroidal anti-inflammatory agents is helpful.

Tenosynovitis or bursitis near the heel are usually acute self-limited disorders. However, if chronic and accompanied by the wearing of boots, the condition is known as "Winter's heel" or "Haglund's disease."[12] Heel pads or molded heel cups are helpful.[30]

A bursitis at the insertion of the tendo Achillis may also occur in athletes, and requires a change in the heel counter of the athlete's shoe.[9] When an Achilles tendinitis coexists, the heel should be elevated $\frac{1}{4}$ to $\frac{1}{2}$ inch with heel padding.[1]

Calcaneal periostitis may result from trauma, Reiter's disease, ankylosing spondylitis, psoriatic arthritis, or rheumatoid arthritis.[26] The resulting painful heel may have to be raised 1 to 2 cm with a heel lift for relief.[12] *Calcaneal spurs* develop on the plantar tuberosity, and extend across the entire width of the calcaneum. The apex is imbedded in the plantar fascia. Pain occurs if the apex is angled downward by depression of the long arch.

In the past, an acutely painful heel spur was thought to be a manifestation of gonorrhea. More recent studies have demonstrated the cause to be due to other diseases, such as ankylosing spondylitis, Reiter's syndrome, or rheumatoid arthritis. Heel spurs are more often asymptomatic or innocent bystanders that rarely cause pain themselves. When symptomatic, another mechanical etiology is usually responsible. Plantar fasciitis is a likely cause of heel pain with or without spur formation. Use of shoes with cushion- or crepe soles, cut-out heels, heel inversion, or arch supports that reduce the forces acting upon the plantar aponeurosis are helpful. A local corticosteroid injection into the point of maximum tenderness is usually helpful.[31,32]

Painful heel pad syndrome in marathon runners and others is thought to result from disruption of the fibrous septa that compartmentalize the fat. The pain is localized to the heel pad; the plantar fascia is not tender and pain is not accentuated as the examiner dorsiflexes the toes. Insertion of heel cups is helpful.[33] Recently, Plastizote (trademark) that is individually molded to the patient's heel has proved very helpful.[34] Rarely, an osteocartilaginous nodule may be detected within the heel pad. Surgical excision may be necessary.[35]

Herniations of fat that occur as painful papules at the medial inferior border of the heel (piezogenic papules) may be noted only upon weightbearing, and are an uncommon cause of painful heels. Weight reduction, use of felt padding, and cushion- or crepe-soled shoes may provide relief.[24] We have noted these in asymptomatic patients.

In children, heel pain may result from an apophysitis, which often follows a change of shoe or increased sports activity. Tenderness at the posterior aspect of the heel and radiographic features of a fluffy, motheaten, flattened, and fragmented apophysis are seen. Treatment includes using a sponge-heel elevation, elastic strapping, avoiding vigorous running, and if necessary, injecting a local corticosteroid.[23]

"Black heel" is a black or bluish-black plaque that usually develops on the heel of the foot. The lesion is oval or circular and may develop on the posterior or posterolateral plantar surfaces of one or both heels. It results from a shearing force during sports that causes intracutaneous bleeding. The lesion is painless, most common in adolescents or young adults, and requires no treatment.[36]

PLANTAR FASCIITIS

Plantar fasciitis is one of the most common causes of foot pain.[37] Heel spurs often coexist and may represent a secondary response to an inflammatory reaction. The deep plantar fascia (plantar aponeurosis) is a thick, pearly white tissue with longitudinal fibers intimately attached to the skin. The central portion is thickest and attaches to the medial process of the tuberosity of the calcaneus; distally it divides into five slips, one for each toe.[15] Symptoms include pain in the plantar region of the foot, made worse when initiating walking. A hallmark for diagnosis is local tenderness. Point tenderness along the longitudinal bands of the plantar fascia is best determined by bimanual examination. The examiner dorsiflexes the patient's toes with one hand, pulling the plantar fascia taut. The examiner, with an index finger, palpates along the plantar fascia from the heel to the forefoot (Fig. 12–3). Points of discrete tenderness can be elicited, and may be marked for possible later local corticosteroid injection. The patient should be examined for inflammatory arthritis, the hypermobility syndrome, or pes planus with valgus heel deformity. The condition may be indistinguishable from anterior calcaneal bursitis, tenosynovitis of the flexor hallucis longus, and medial calcaneal nerve injury.[5]

Etiology. Strain of the plantar fascia often follows jumping, prolonged standing, or occurs in association with obesity and flatfeet;[4,31] a relation to heel spurs has been noted by most clinicians.[31] In one sizable study of plantar fasciitis,[31] rheumatoid arthritis, gout, and ankylosing spondylitis were diagnosed at the time of the initial examination in 10% of the patients. Subsequently, another 5% developed rheumatoid arthritis or gout. Thus, systemic rheumatic diseases occurred in 15% of the patients. Plantar fasciitis in association with obesity and pes planus was more common. Over half the patients had plantar spurs, but the presence or absence of plantar spurs had no relationship to the outcome. Plantar fasciitis is common among ballet dancers and those performing dance aerobic exercise. Plantar fascia strain and minute avulsions are more common in dancers with an inelastic arch. Fatigue fracture of the metatarsals must be ruled out in these patients.[39] Heel spurs probably are just a further development associated with plantar fasciitis.[38] Plantar pain may also result from use of fluoride for treatment of osteoporosis.[40]

Laboratory and Roentgenographic Examination. Unless systemic disease is also present, tests for inflammation are normal. Radiographic examination will delineate pressure spurs that are usually unrelated to symptoms or outcome. Tumors, fractures, periostitis, and the fluffy-bone change characterstic of Reiter's syndrome and other spondyloarthropathies, Lofgren's syndrome, and sarcoidosis are to be considered in differential diagnosis, and are further reasons for obtaining roentgenographs.

Management. Treatment of obesity, flatfeet, and systemic inflammation is undertaken when the respective conditions are present. Arch-supporting shoes, particularly with a long counter, or shoes with inserted foam-rubber raised arches and rubber or tub heels, rigid shanks, and cushion- or crepesoles are helpful. Initially the patient may not tolerate wearing the arch-supporting shoes all day. The patient can carry along an older pair of shoes when leaving the house, and after several hours may switch from the new shoes to the old ones. Within a short time the patient can usually tolerate the arch-supporting shoes and is grateful for the benefit received. In resistant cases, before considering molded shoe inserts, the points of tenderness along the plantar fascia may be injected with a corticosteroid-anesthetic mixture. A No. 23 or 25 needle inserted $\frac{1}{4}$- to $\frac{1}{2}$-inch deep into the plantar fascia for deposition of the steroid (not more than 40 mg for each foot) is utilized (Fig. 12–5).

Outcome and Additional Suggestions. If patients adhere to the program by wearing proper shoes for correction of associated structural foot disorders, benefit often occurs after several weeks in the majority of patients. Wearing slippers or going barefoot may result in recurrence. Patients who work or reside in buildings with concrete floors should use cushion- or crepe-soled shoes. Rigid inserts are of little value,[1] but heel cups may be helpful. Leather or rubber longitudinal arches may be added in $\frac{3}{16}$- to $\frac{1}{4}$-inch thicknesses. On occasion, patients respond to oral nonsteroidal anti-inflammatory agents. Local strapping of the plantar arch and midfoot may also be helpful.[1] A soft, moldable flexible insert that can be shaped to the foot while it is held in position of correction may be helpful, if structural deformities are also present.[1] In our experience, surgical intervention is rarely needed. Furey reported that only 2% of patients with plantar fasciitis required a Stein-dler stripping procedure (stripping of the plantar fascia).[31] Surgical intervention in massively obese patients with persistent symptoms may be justified if all other efforts fail.[41] Runners and dancers with persistent symptoms and a demonstrable exostosis on roentgenographic examination will usually benefit from excision of a portion of the plantar fascia and removal of the spur[42] (see Decision Chart, Table 12–5).

MIDFOOT AND METATARSAL PAIN

Following an inversion injury, a *ligamentous sprain* of the calcaneocuboid joint often occurs. Pain, swelling, and tenderness over the lateral border of the foot are noted. For treatment, the midfoot should be taped or wrapped with an elastic bandage or gelocast; following 24 to 48 hours of rest, recovery is the rule.

Tendinitis of the superficial extensor tendons of the foot commonly results from tight lacing, or from ridges on the tongue of the shoe. Frequently, point tenderness and pain follow the use of a new pair of work shoes; swelling is uncommon. To relieve the pressure, a lipstick mark is applied to the point of maximum tenderness, the shoe is replaced and laced; after removing the shoe, the lipstick mark will appear on the undersurface of the tongue of the shoe. A strip of adhesive-backed foam rubber $\frac{3}{8}$ to $\frac{1}{2}$ inches wide should be positioned on the undersurface of the tongue at each side of the lipstick mark, thus providing a gap over the point of tenderness. Use of elastic shoe laces may also be helpful.

A painful hard *spur* or *fibroma* on the dorsal aspect of the first tarsometatarsal joint in adults or children may result from tightfitting shoes.[9] Occasionally children suffer a painful disturbance beneath the first metatarsophalangeal joint. In the past this entity was thought to be due to sesamoiditis, but probably represents a *bursitis* associated with physical trauma.[7]

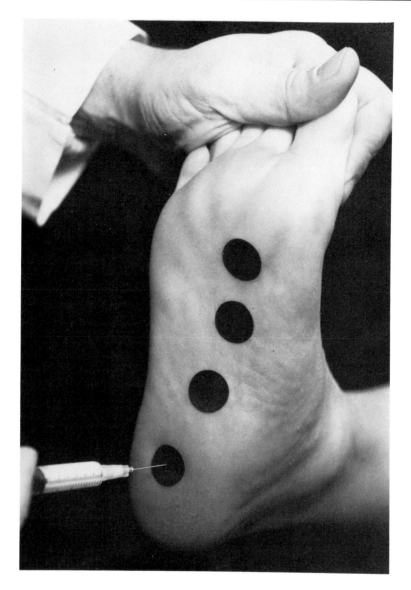

Fig. 12–5. Injection technique for the painful heel and plantar fasciitis. Using a 1-in. No. 23 or No. 25 needle, aliquots of a corticosteroid-local anesthetic mixture are introduced into the painful tissue. Alternatively these sites are approached from a lateral direction.

Metatarsalgia

Although Morton's neuroma is a common cause for forefoot pain, many other conditions occur in this region and must be distinguished. The disorders described here are *not* acute in onset, and although they may suggest mild gouty symptoms, they are not as abruptly painful as acute gout.

Disturbances of the metatarsal region may result from congenital structural abnormalities of the foot, weakness of intrinsic foot muscles, arthritis, or trauma.[2,12,15] Upon weight-bearing the "metatarsal arch" normally flattens and is therefore not a functioning arch.[2,12] The metatarsal arch created by the transverse metatarsal ligament and the abductor hallucis longus is further supported during push-off by the intrinsic toe flexors, which help to elevate the three central metatarsals.[15]

If a deformity of the first metatarsal is present, the axis of weightbearing may shift to the second metatarsal, with resultant strain upon the normal function of the metatarsal ligaments and musculature.[15] The most common of these deformities is probably metatarsus primus varus, in which the great toe is rotated on its longitudinal axis so that the toenail points medially. Metatarsal pain in the plantar region of the first metatarsal joint may result from a hallux valgus deformity, hallux rigidus (degenerative joint disease), or arthritis of a sesamoid articulation.[43] The second metatarsal bone is tightly fixed between the three cuneiforms and is therefore relatively immobile. The region under the second metatarsal head is easily aggravated by wearing high-heeled shoes, by weakness of the intrinsic foot muscles, or by contracture of the flexor tendons.[44] Congenital ligamentous laxity, particularly if associated with obesity, also may result in metatarsalgia during prolonged standing, and may result in a splay foot[11] with the development of plantar calluses under the second metatarsal head.[15]

A properly fitted shoe with a broad toe box, a metatarsal pad, or a metatarsal bar placed behind the metatarsal heads is helpful.[37] Calluses can be softened with 20% salicylic acid and collodion;[15] the application is removed after 2 or 3 days with warm soaking. Toe flexion exercises, such as crinkling newspaper with the toes, or curling the toes downward while standing on the edge of a phone book should be prescribed (see Exercise 5, Table 12–3). Weight reduction is essential in obese patients. The use of an anterior heel, "earth shoe," running shoe, soft insoles such as Spenco, Plastizote,[3] or comma-shaped inserts[2] are additional methods for relieving weightbearing from the metatarsal region (see Table 12–4).

Metatarsal bars may be straight or curved along the inferior surface. The short rocker bar, the most commonly prescribed type, $\frac{1}{4}$ inch thick, is placed externally behind the

metatarsal heads[45] (Fig. 12–6). The metatarsal bar may have a forward curve if the patient has this configuration of the metatarsal heads. A "horseshoe" bar may be used if there is a painful plantar callus. If the metatarsal bar is malpositioned it may aggravate pain and require revision.[1] When positioned properly, symptoms are usually promptly improved.

Plastizote insoles are self-molding but may require an extra-depth shoe with an enlarged toe box[1] (Fig. 12–7). The simple metatarsal foam rubber pad, approximately $\frac{3}{16}$ inch thick, is widely available. The patient can mark the painful area of the foot with lipstick, stand in the shoe, and then place the pad just behind the lipstick mark. Occasionally the pad requires a concave forward edge to accommodate a particularly painful metatarsophalangeal joint. Obviously, the shoe must hold the foot securely and prevent forward

Metatarsal bar   Thomas heel

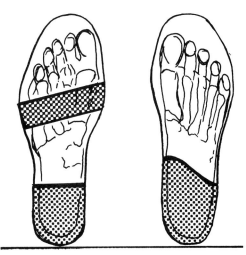

Fig. 12–6. *Left,* An external metatarsal bar distributes weight posterior to the metatarsal region. When standing, the patient should be certain the bar has been placed behind the metatarsophalangeal joints, or the bar should be removed and reattached in the proper location. The bar should be placed on both shoes to allow normal balance. A bar may also be inserted into the sole of a running shoe. *Right,* The Thomas heel provides support for patients with symptomatic pes planus, valgus heel deformity, or plantar fascia strain.

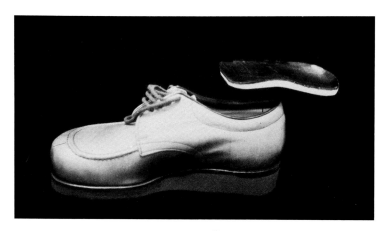

Fig. 12–7. The extra-depth shoe: Often prescribed with the additional feature of the enlarged toe box, this shoe is helpful for patients with metatarsal and metatarsophalangeal joint difficulties, hammertoe, rheumatoid or other inflammatory arthritides with forefoot deformity. If required, the molded soft plastic insert may be provided additionally. Occupational therapists, orthopedists, or podiatrists are skilled in making the mold.

slipping. This requires a strap or lacing. The sole should be firm but not rigid, and cushion or crepe soles are helpful.[3]

Metatarsalgia of traumatic origin may result from prolonged walking or jumping that results in a sprain of the intermetatarsal ligaments. Dancers may suffer a stress fracture of a sesamoid.[46] Swelling may or may not be present. An intermetatarsal bursitis from tight narrow shoes may also occur.[12,15,47] With aging, the metatarsal arch flattens, the metatarsal heads become broader, and the metatarsal heads often impinge upon the bursa. The resulting bursitis gives rise to symptoms similar to a Morton's neuroma.[47] Treatment of the bursitis with anti-inflammatory agents or local intralesional corticosteroid injection, and better fitting shoes will usually provide relief. Surgical intervention is not often necessary.[48] Sprain of the first metatarsophalangeal joint can incapacitate an athlete; tenderness in the great toe region is aggravated by running when compared to walking; roentgenograms are normal.[9] The adolescent, when engaged in sports, may suffer a stress fracture at the base of the fifth metatarsal, presenting with a painful prominence on the lateral side of the foot.[49] Treatment of the stress fracture includes relief from weight-bearing, and if symptoms persist a cast may be necessary.[49]

Fatigue (March) Fracture

A nondisplaced fracture that occurs just proximal to the metatarsal head is often a fatigue fracture. Although frequently seen in military personnel, particularly in new recruits after their first long march, this condition is also seen frequently in women after prolonged shopping, in joggers, in other overuse syndromes, and in persons with a short first metatarsal.[15,46,49,50] The second or third metatarsal shaft is most commonly fractured. These stress fractures rarely occur before age 12.[49] The patient notes tenderness and diffuse forefoot pain accompanied by swelling on the dorsal surface of the metatarsal region. Slight erythema may be present. The onset is subacute and never reaches the intensity of gout. Radiographic evidence of a fracture may be present only after several weeks (Fig. 12–8). A bone callus appears by 3 to 4 weeks and confirms the diagnosis.[51] A molded arch support, snug elastoplast wrapping, or support with a simple external short metatarsal rocker bar provides good results. Sometimes a walking cast is necessary.

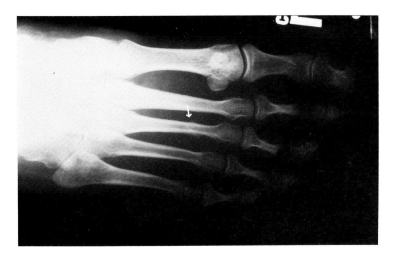

Fig. 12–8. Fatigue (march) fracture: Pain and swelling in the mid-metatarsal region on the dorsal aspect of the foot in a middle-aged patient is suggestive of a fatigue fracture. Roentgenographic examination 2 weeks following the pain should be scrutinized carefully for evidence of fracture and callus (see arrow).

Running Injuries

Long-distance runners may have complaints that result from the accumulated impact loading of long-distance running.[52-54] Often these problems relate to biomechanical overuse in patients with minor structural disorders. Malalignments with mechanical disadvantages, muscle contractures, and use of untrained muscles may lead to biomechanical failure.[53] Physical examination of the runner should include examination of the alignment of the entire lower extremities. The physician should note limb length, range of movement, configuration of the weightbearing foot and heel, and forefoot alignment. The vertical axis of the heel should be parallel to the longitudinal axis of the distal tibia when viewed posteriorly. The plane of the metatarsal head should be perpendicular to the heel.[52]

In a study of 180 injured runners, 232 abnormal structural conditions were noted on careful examination.[52] Of these injuries, 60% were the result of training errors, and of these, 29% were due to the accumulation of excessive mileage not tolerated by the subtle anatomic deformities found in these individuals. Shin splints and knee problems such as chondromalacia patellae and iliotibial tract tendinitis were also common (see Chapts. 10 and 11). Treating running injuries of the foot includes decreasing the runner's mileage, avoiding hard-surface running, changing the runner's stride, stretching the hamstring and calf muscles, and using shoes with waffle soles or orthotics when indicated, with alteration of the heel counter.[52,54]

FLEXIBLE FLATFEET

There are nearly as many terms for flatfeet as there are orthopedists writing about flatfeet. The flexible type is the most common and important type.[5,12,15] Blacks and American Indians normally have flatfeet yet they are not necessarily a precursor of painful feet.[13] Asymptomatic persons with flatfeet should be left alone. Flatfeet, however, do require more intrinsic foot muscle contraction with each step of walking;[55] nevertheless, the degree of flatness or pronation bears no correlation to future foot pain.[2] The flexible flatfoot, by definition, appears normal before it strikes the ground and bears weight; the arch flattens upon weightbearing. Symptoms, when present, include excessive muscular fatigue and aching, and intolerance to prolonged walking or standing. In some patients walking improves symptoms.[12] Symptoms often develop following a change in work habits that require prolonged standing. In addition, symptoms may follow other foot injuries that result in an abnormal gait. In some individuals, symptoms result from prolonged illness with resultant muscular atrophy.[13]

Physical examination reveals loss of the longitudinal arch upon weightbearing, increased prominence of the navicular bone and the head of the talus, or an exostosis on the medial aspect of the foot.[2] The calcaneus is everted (valgus position) as shown in Figure 12–9. The anterior and posterior tibial tendons and plantar muscles become stretched, and the tendo Achillis may become shortened.[15] The forefoot swings outward and the foot becomes rotated externally in relation to the leg. Occasionally, edema of the dorsum of the foot and tenderness over the medial aspect of the foot occur.[15]

The determination that the foot (subtalar joint) can be inverted is essential, in order to demonstrate the presence of a flexible rather than a rigid flatfoot.[2] Tenderness may also be noted over the navicular bone, the inferior calcaneonavicular ligament, or the sole of the foot.[12] While walking, the flatfooted patient raises the heel and toe together rather than using a heel-to-toe gait and demonstrates a splay foot with the toes turned outward. This results from an attempt to prevent strain on the tarsal or metatarsal ligaments.[12] The patient's gait has no "spring" to it. The shoe wears down more on the medial side of the sole than on the lateral sides. A corn on the fifth toe is further evidence of altered weightbearing. If the flatfoot is not evident from the frontal view, then it should become evident from a posterior view.

Etiology. The infant is born flatfooted and acquires an arch after a year or so of ambulation. The symptomatic flexible flatfoot may result from general hypermobility and a failure of postural muscle function to maintain the arch.[12] In any event, it is probably not a result of improper footwear. Of patients with flatfeet, 70% have an inherited predisposition to flatfeet.[12]

Laboratory and Radiographic Examination. Flatfeet may be a late manifestation of any inflammatory rheumatic disease, and other features of that disease should be manifest at the time of examination. When confronted with a *rigid* flatfoot, special roentgenographic techniques are required to demonstrate bony bridging due to inflammatory or congenital defects of the tarsal region.

Differential Diagnosis. The rigid flatfoot also results from congenital or acquired infection, or from inflammatory or traumatic

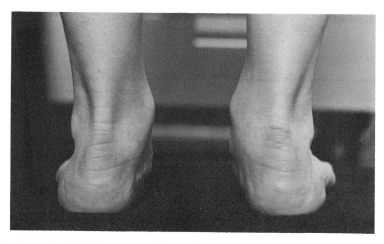

Fig. 12–9.   Pes planus (flatfeet) with eversion of the heels is best viewed posteriorly. Examination for pes planus should be part of the examination of any patient with a rheumatologic complaint in the lower extremity.

disturbances of the tarsal region.[15] Painful reflex spasm of the peroneal muscle[15] can result from a rigid flatfoot.[55]

Management. The most important rule in this chapter is not to treat asymptomatic flatfeet with a rigid arch support. Basic to the treatment of the symptomatic flatfoot is to move the center of gravity of the foot more to the outside of the foot and to remove points of pressure that are causing symptoms.[12] This can be accomplished by the use of a firm heel counter and a tight well-fitted instep with a low heel.[15] The physician may recommend a Thomas heel and a gradual shoe correction, and should not hastily order an expensive plastic rigid molded insert.[1] The Thomas heel for the symptomatic flatfoot should provide a varus tilt to the heel in order to put the ankle in a more vertical alignment. The Thomas heel can extend to the mid-part of the navicular so that it intersects the longitudinal axis of the fibula.[1] The shank of the shoe should remain flexible unless an appliance is being added to the shoe, or if a hallux rigidus coexists. Most patients require only a firm long-countered oxford shoe, and only a few require an insert. The examiner must determine whether the foot can be inverted, and if so an arch support can be tried. Such a support should not be rigid and should seldom exceed $\frac{1}{8}$ of an inch rise in the longitudinal arch.[2] Felt-type padding is not a permanent insert as it packs down. However, it is inexpensive and can be used to determine whether an insert will provide relief. If so, a permanent type should be prescribed for relief of pressure.[1] Only after failure of proper shoes without inserts, followed by a trial of flexible leather inserts, should moldable soft plastic inserts be considered. More often the latter inserts are used to treat structural foot disorders, such as forefoot or hindfoot varus, or valgus deformities. In general, the molded insert is not necessary in patients suffering from flexible flatfeet.

Recognition of aggravating symptomatic factors such as work on concrete floors, prolonged standing, obesity, or coexisting plantar fasciitis is essential for effective management. Grasping exercises for intrinsic foot muscles and mobilizing exercises that plantarflex the foot and invert the ankle are helpful. Crinkling newspaper with the feet on the floor, and ankle rotation performed with the foot constantly cupped, first clockwise, then counterclockwise, may help maintain mobility in the involved soft tissues (see Exercises 4 and 5, Table 12–3 and Fig. 12–10).

Outcome and Additional Suggestions. In our experience, patients with flexible flatfeet have self-limited episodes of pain brought about by prolonged weightbearing in improper shoes, excessive weight gain, carrying heavy objects, or moving to a home or job with a concrete floor. Often such episodes of pain are due to plantar fasciitis rather than flatfeet per se. Patients with chronic foot pain must be examined for systemic disorders mentioned in association with plantar fasci-

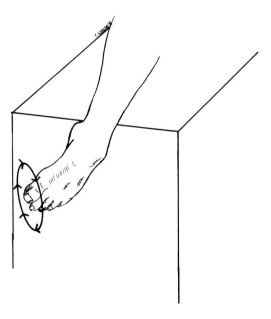

Fig. 12–10. Mobilizing exercise for the foot and ankle: While the toes are kept in downward flexion, the ankle is drawn to 90 degrees, and then a circular motion of the entire foot and ankle in one direction and then another is accomplished.

Table 12–3. Lower Leg and Foot Exercises

1. Face a wall in bare feet; stand about arm's length away. Reach palms to wall and "walk" palms up wall slowly until maximum stretch is felt at heel but do not let heel raise up from floor. Now push pelvis forward to increase the stretch, hold for 10 seconds and repeat 3 times. Perform the three stretches each time, 4 times a day. Continue for at least a week (Fig. 11–1).

2. Leg stretch: Lie on back. Place 4 foot rope across ball of one foot, draw this leg straight in the air while other leg is bent. Pull gently and with increasing force stretch muscles behind thigh, knee, and calf. Hold one minute, then stretch other leg. Repeat exercise twice daily (Fig. 12–4).

3. Stand with both foot on a step, hold on to bannister. Keep heels hanging off step; just the ball of foot is on the step. Raise up onto toes; then drop down letting heels drop below forefoot. The return to starting neutral position. Repeat; and gradually shift weight to involved leg. Repeat exercise twice daily.

4. Ankle mobilizing exercise: Barefoot, curl toes and keep foot in cupped position and rotate the forefoot in a circle with the great toe making a circle clockwise for a minute, then counterclockwise. Repeat exercise twice daily (Fig. 12–10).

5. Toe exercise: Stand on a telephone book and curl toes over edge for 1 minute. Place towel on floor in front of a chair. While sitting, repeatedly try to gather towel with toes. Place newspaper on floor and crinkle with toes. Repeat exercise twice daily.

itis. If symptoms have persisted despite conscientious use of proper foot gear, and no other underlying cause has been found, the clinician should carefully reexamine the entire lower extremity and lumbar spine for evidence of other disorders, such as peripheral neuropathy, gout, and lumbar disc disease.

TOE DISORDERS

The term "bunion" refers to soft tissue swelling over the first metatarsophalangeal joint. It is often mistakenly used to describe all disorders that enlarge the first metatarsophalangeal joint.[13] Several of the more common disorders of this joint region as well as disorders affecting the other toes are discussed.

Hallux Valgus Deformity

The patient with this common foot deformity presents with medial deviation of the head of the first metatarsal and lateral deviation of the great toe, often accompanied by a painful soft adventitial bursa. Because of this disorder, the second toe is forced dorsally and may develop into a hammertoe.[15] Displacement of

a sesamoid bone is often associated with this deformity. The condition occurs more commonly in cultures where shoes are worn and in females. Generally the large toe is rotated so that the nail faces medially. The bursa overlying the medial bony prominence may become secondarily infected or acutely inflamed from the pressure of ill-fitting shoes.[2,9,15] The patient often sees the physician not because of pain, but rather because of the inability to wear "dress shoes." (See Table 12–4.)

Hallux Rigidus

Progressive loss of motion of the great toe joint is associated with arthritis of the first metatarsophalangeal joint. This condition may follow hallux valgus deformity[15] or trauma, or may be associated with pes planus, the pronated foot, or metatarsus varus primus deformity.[56] Hallux rigidus is usually more disabling than hallux valgus deformity.[43]

Treatment of hallux valgus without rigidus includes the use of shoes with an enlarged toe portion, the use of a felt ring, or the use of a plastic cap.[15] Occasionally we have had a shoemaker remove the dorsal portion of the shoe and replace it with a wide roomy vinyl covering. Additional measures include pads of felt or rubber behind the first metatarsophalangeal joint, or arch supports with lateral and medial flanges to fit over medial and lateral bunions.[2] High-heeled or soft flexible shoes are not well-tolerated. Surgical intervention should be performed only for symptoms and not for cosmetic reasons.[15] Bunion surgery is 85% effective, yet 12,000 unsatisfactory operations are estimated to occur each year.[2] Use of joint replacement is still in the experimental stage.

If the bursa over a hallux valgus deformity is swollen and tender, measures to keep the shoe covering from rubbing against it are imperative. In summer months the use of an open sandal may be helpful. When a shoe must be worn, the vamp should be cut with a linear slit through the lining just above the sole and over the bunion.[57] We have found it advantageous for patients to cut a wide half-circle throughout the medial portion of an old laced shoe. This allows support for the hind foot, provides a rigid sole for the forefoot, and reduces friction across the medial surface of the first metatarsophalangeal joint.

In addition to the measures previously mentioned, treatment of hallux rigidus requires the use of a thick and rigid shoe sole.[12,14] The clinician may also try a long rocker bar to add rigidity to the sole.[45] On occasion, a local corticosteroid-anesthetic injection into the region of a dorsal exostosis at the first metatarsal joint line is helpful.[2,13] Stretching the toe downward for a moment or so, morning and evening, has also been helpful.[2] Joint fusion, debridement arthroplasty, or other surgical procedures may be necessary.[12]

HAMMERTOE DEFORMITY

This disorder is usually acquired as a result of pressure from hallux valgus,[15] from tight shoes,[1,15] or it may be congenital in origin. It is usually a bilateral deformity with the second toe nearly always involved. The toe is flexed at the proximal interphalangeal (PIP) joint and the tip of the toe points downward.[15]

Thus the middle and distal phalanges of the second toe are flexed on the proximal phalanges.[1] A painful bursa and callus often form over the dorsal aspect of the flexed proximal interphalangeal joint. The toe tip becomes broadened and thick.[15] In children with congenital hammertoe, treatment is best handled with adhesive strapping and use of shoes with an adequate depth of toe box.[15] An "X" incision in the shoe vamp over the pressure point is helpful.[57] When keratoses are also present, surgical correction is often necessary.[13]

None of these toe disorders result in soft tissue swelling of the toe. When swelling occurs, sepsis (felon or whitlow), systemic rheumatic disease (e.g., rheumatoid arthritis, psoriatic arthritis), and other disease entities (e.g., gout, tumors) are considerations.

Table 12–4 provides possible shoe modifications for various foot problems. Combinations of these modifications may be indicated depending upon careful assessment of the individual problem.

Information for moldable plastics or extra depth shoes may be obtained from the following sources:

AliMed, 138 Prince St., Boston, Mass. 02113; P.W. Minor & Son Inc., Batavia, New York 14020; and Alden Shoe Company, Taunton St., Middleborough, Mass. 02346.

ENTRAPMENT NEUROPATHIES

With the increased use of high boots with high heels and with the popularity of activities such as jogging, entrapment neuropathies of the foot and ankle are being seen more often. When the patient complains of burning paresthesia day and night, this disorder should be suspected. However, that history is often not volunteered and must be sought. Any nocturnal foot symptoms and foot pain that radiates out to the toes should suggest an entrapment neuropathy.[60,61]

Occupational entrapment neuropathies are not uncommon. Peroneal palsy, or foot drop syndrome, may result from occupations re-

Table 12–4.   Common Shoe Modifications[53,54]

Problem Area	Possible Shoe Modification
Great Toe	Broad toe box, shoe cutout around bunion, vinyl patch to enlarge toe box, thicker or more rigid sole, broad external rocker bar, felt ring, and plastic cap.
Other Toes	"X" incision above toe, wider shoe size, metartarsal pads, and extra-depth shoes.
Metatarsal Area	Pads, excavation of innersole beneath lesion, "closed cell" foam pad (Spenco), molded flexible insert with "open cell" foam (Plastizote), short external metatarsal bar (1 inch wide), longer external rocker bar, vinyl covering to widen toe box, and anterior placed heel.
Plantar region of midfoot, flexible flatfoot, plantar fasciitis	Long-counter shoe, Thomas heel, scaphoid pad, flexible arch support, cutout under heel spur, scaphoid pad, 3/16-inch foam medial arch insert, and wedging of the medial sole.
Dorsal Midfoot	Strips of foam rubber cemented to inner tongue to lift tongue off of lesion, and elastic shoe laces.
Heel	Heel lift, heel pad, cutout heel pad, excavation of innersole beneath heel spur or lesion, plastic heel cup and "V" incision into rim of counter.

quiring crouching, squatting or kneeling in such jobs as agriculturists, miners, and shoe salesmen. Peroneal palsy has been reported in a baseball catcher![62] Increased pressure at the popliteal fossa may occur in persons who tilt back in chairs; this may result in a posterior tibial nerve injury. Symptoms similar to that of the tarsal tunnel syndrome may occur. The tarsal tunnel syndrome itself may result from use of shoes with improper arch support. On the other hand, arch supports may induce the syndrome when arch supports were unnecessary![62] Kneeling with toes flexed inside tight shoes may cause interdigital nerve injury during work as might be seen in electricians or carpetlayers.

The Tarsal Tunnel Syndrome

This syndrome refers to an entrapment neuropathy of the posterior tibial nerve as it passes through the tunnel beneath the flexor retinaculum on the medial side of the ankle.[37,63,64] Beneath this retinaculum (or lancinate ligament)[65,66] lies a tunnel containing the tendons of the flexor digitorum longus and flexor hallucis longus, the vascular bundle, the posterior tibial nerve, and the medial and lateral plantar nerves[15] (Fig. 12–11). Most

commonly the patient presents with aching, burning, numbness, and tingling involving the plantar surface of the foot, the distal foot, the toes, and occasionally the heel. The pain may also radiate up to the calf or higher.[15,67] The discomfort is often nocturnal, and may be worse after standing; the discomfort sometimes leads to removal of the shoe even while driving. Physical examination seldom reveals swelling or atrophy. Sensory nerve loss is variable and often is not found.[15] The Tinel test, in which the nerve is tapped with the finger or reflex hammer, is often positive at the flexor retinaculum located posterior and inferior to the medial malleolus. To be complete, tapping must be performed over the entire course of the posterior tibial nerve or one of its branches.[68] Occasionally, firm-rolling pressure across the nerve may be required to reproduce the symptoms. A tourniquet applied just above the ankle may reproduce these symptoms by creating venous engorgement of the tarsal tunnel.[15]

Most often the tarsal tunnel syndrome results from a compression neuropathy in which the tarsal tunnel has been compromised by a tenosynovitis of one or more of the tendons passing through the region. This may result

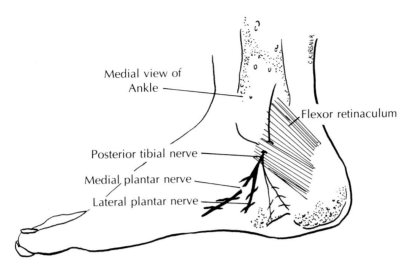

Fig. 12–11. Tarsal tunnel: Posterior tibial nerve is often trapped beneath the flexor retinaculum on the medial side of the ankle. Entrapment may also include the two branches, the medial and lateral plantar nerves.

from injury, from rheumatoid arthritis, or from other sources of inflammation.[15] or tumors.[69] Perhaps the most common cause for a tarsal tunnel syndrome is a fracture or dislocation involving the talus, calcaneus, or medial malleolus.[65,66] Previous involvement of a *carpal* tunnel has been described in patients who later develop a *tarsal* tunnel syndrome.[1,70] Most often the tarsal tunnel syndrome occurs in the absence of inflammatory rheumatic disease, but if other features are suggestive, the erythrocyte sedimentation rate and tests for rheumatic disease, including rheumatoid factor and antinuclear factor should be performed. Diabetic neuropathy may cause similar symptoms unrelated to tarsal tunnel involvement. Histopathologic study reveals preferential loss of large axons in fascicles at the periphery in comparison to fascicles in the center of the posterior tibial nerve. The changes differ from those associated with ischemia of the lower limb.[71]

Diagnosis of tarsal tunnel syndrome may be confirmed by electrodiagnostic tests. Tibial nerve conduction velocity normally is 49.9 ± 5.1 msec, and latency from the malleolus to the abductor hallucis normally is 4.4 ± 0.9 msec. Prolonged latency in excess of 6.1 msec for the medial plantar nerve and 6.7 msec for the lateral plantar nerve is indicative of dis-

ease;[15,66,72,73] however, normal values do not exclude the syndrome.[73] Perhaps the best diagnostic test is response to a local corticosteroid-anesthetic injection into the region of the tarsal tunnel, with relief confirming the presence of the syndrome.

In most cases a local corticosteroid-anesthetic mixture injected once or twice into the region inferior and posterior to the medial malleolus and injected in a fan-like manner provides relief (Fig. 12–12). We inject 20 mg methylprednisolone mixed with 1% procaine, taking care not to inject the nerve. Others report only a 30% response and recommend decompression surgery.[15,67,68] It may be that surgical intervention is most often required when the tarsal tunnel syndrome follows fracture or dislocation. If symptoms persist, local or systemic underlying disorders causing a tarsal tunnel or similar symptomatic syndromes must be considered. These include vascular disease with venous stasis, diabetes mellitus with neuropathy, rheumatoid arthritis, myxedema, pregnancy, and amyloidosis.[72] Children may develop the tarsal tunnel syndrome but symptoms differ from adults in that night pain is less common; the involvement is unilateral rather than bilateral; the symptoms more likely are burning pain in the sole while walking, or recurrent

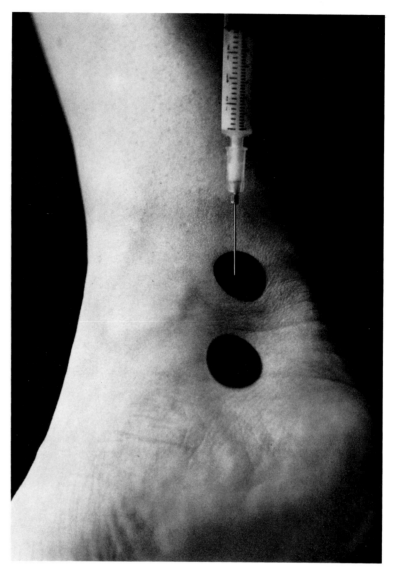

Fig. 12–12.   Sites for injection of the tarsal tunnel or posterior tibialis tendinitis on the medial aspect of the ankle. A 1-in. No. 23 needle should be used, and the medication instilled in a fan-like manner.

spontaneous sudden sharp pain in the foot. Paresthesias in the sole of the foot results when the nerve is percussed behind the medial malleolus. In one series, all patients involved were girls between the ages of 9 and 15. Trauma was unlikely as a cause. Often the child walked with the affected foot in supination, allowing only the lateral border of the sole to contact the ground.[74]

The Anterior Tarsal Tunnel Syndrome in which the deep peroneal nerve is entrapped beneath the inferior extensor retinaculum at the anterior aspect of the tarsal tunnel gives rise to paresthesias on the dorsum of the foot and often in the great toe. The discomfort is increased at night. Relief following local infiltration with corticosteroids, and an avoid-

Table 12–5. Decision Chart, Ankle and Foot Region

Problem	Action	Further Action
1. Posterior Heel Pain	Examine back and lower limb alignment Provide joint protection advice	Bone scan for fatigue fracture Tests for systemic inflammatory disease Stress roentgenograms of the ankle Weight bearing foot roentgenograms Rheumatology, orthopedic, podiatry, or other consultation
2. Plantar Heel Pain	Test for tight Achilles tendon Provide stretching exercises Prescribe proper shoes	
3. Ankle Pain and/or Instability	Prescribe rest, ankle support, exercise	
4. Midfoot Pain	Test for tendinitis, ligament laxity Provide arch or long counter shoe Protect foot from tight laces	
5. Metatarsalgia without Paresthesia	Provide broad toe shoe + / – metatarsal bars Prescribe NSAID's Intralesional steroid injection Foot Exercises	
6. Metatarsalgia with Paresthesia	Test for diabetes, vascular insufficiency; nerve entrapment Empiric steroid injection of intermetatarsal bursa	
7. Plantar Pain without Paresthesia	Examine for joint laxity, flat foot, tight and tender plantar fascia Prescribe proper shoe with long counter Provide mobilizing exercises, weight control program Inject plantar fascia	
8. Plantar Pain and Paresthesia Nocturnal aggravation	Test for Tarsal Tunnel Syndrome Inject Tarsal Tunnel	
9. Danger Signs: Color change or warmth Swelling Lymphadenopathy Paresthesia Increasing pain with weightbearing Claudication	Comprehensive examination and treatment Vascular, neurologic, endocrine studies or consultation.	

ance of boots, high-heeled shoes, or tight lacing is helpful and confirms the diagnosis.[75]

Compression Neuropathy of the Common Peroneal Nerve

Footdrop (inability to dorsiflex the foot) often results from peroneal nerve compression due to crossing the leg, hanging the leg over a constricting rigid object, or from direct trauma. A tight boot or cast may also result in sensory or motor peroneal nerve loss, and a partial or complete footdrop. A footdrop brace with a spring action that returns the foot to a 90-degree angle may be required for many months following injury.[64,65] Sometimes a simple plastic posterior splint will suffice.

Plantar Nerve Entrapment

Forced overpronation or pressure associated with a hallux rigidus, tenosynovitis, or venous engorgement of the posterior tibial veins may compress the plantar nerve on the medial aspect of the foot below the calcaneonavicular ligament.[64] The patient may present with a painful heel as well as numbness or tingling across the sole of the foot. A local corticosteroid injection at the site of compression and correction of abnormal foot mechanics with a medial shoe wedge, a scaphoid pad, or molded soft flexible inserts should provide relief.[65]

Interdigital Plantar Neuroma (Morton's Neuroma)

Entrapment neuropathy with or without an associated plantar neuroma often develops between the third and fourth toes on the plantar surface. This involves the anastomoses of the medial and lateral plantar nerves. Pain radiates forward from the metatarsal heads to the third and fourth toes. Similar involvement of other interdigital plantar nerves may occur. This entity, commonly called Morton's neuroma, has neuropathic features of hyperesthesia of the toes, numbness and tingling, and aching and burning in the distal forefoot. It is aggravated by walking on hard surfaces and wearing tight or high-heeled shoes.[15,64,65,68]

Physical examination reveals tenderness in the plantar aspect of the distal foot over the third and fourth metatarsals; compressing the forefoot reproduces the symptoms. The tenderness is occasionally aggravated by direct pressure to the plantar aspect of the third and fourth metatarsophalangeal joints. There should be a concomitant sensation of burning distally. Possible causes include excessive mobility of the fourth metatarsal,[68] nerve impingement between flattened metatarsal heads,[64,65] or compression of the nerve as it is angulated over the transverse tarsal ligament.[15,64,65,76] Chronic compression leads to neuroma formation. The signs and symptoms may occur from an intermetatarsal bursitis rather than a neuroma. The neurovascular bundle lies close to the bursa.[47]

Conservative treatment requires increased plantar flexion at the metatarsal heads obtained by use of a metatarsal support, metatarsal bar, or a comma-shaped metatarsal shoe insert.[65] Although symptoms are unilateral in 85% of cases, external appliances should be placed on both shoes so that the patient walks evenly.[1] A broad-toed shoe that allows spreading of the metatarsal heads is helpful. Intermetatarsal bursitis may cause similar symptoms. A local corticosteroid injection into the site of compression may be beneficial. Surgical removal of the neuroma *and nerve* may be required in patients who are resistant to nonoperative therapy.[15,65]

Joplin's Neuroma

Perineural fibrosis of the plantar proper digital nerve may follow a bunionectomy or trauma to the first metatarsophalangeal joint.[2] This results in pain and paresthesia at the plantar aspect of the first metatarsophalangeal joint of the great toe. A Tinel test may be positive beneath the first metatarsophalangeal joint. Relief occurs with foot rest or removal of the shoe. Surgical excision of the nerve may be necessary.

NIGHT CRAMPS

Benign nocturnal cramps in the legs and feet may be a distressing complaint (for detailed explanation see Chapt. 11). Acute symptoms may be prevented by prophylactic use of quinine, or at times, diphenhydramine (Benadryl). A warm bath or foot soaks at bedtime may be helpful. Structural disorders of the feet should be sought and treated appropriately in an effort to prevent recurrences. The Daniell Exercise #1, Table 12–3, may be helpful.[77]

REFERENCES

1. Mann RA: Conservative treatment and office procedures. *In* DuVries' Surgery of the Foot. 4th Ed. Edited by RA Mann. St. Louis, CV Mosby, 1978.

2. Giannestras NJ: Foot Disorders: Medical and Surgical Management, 2nd Ed. Philadelphia, Lea & Febiger, 1973.

3. Miller WE: Nonoperative approach to foot problems. Orthop Rev 7:19–21, 1978.

4. Dagnall JC, Calabro JJ: Chiropody (podiatry) and arthritis. Bull Rheum Dis 23:692–695, 1972.

5. Jahss MH: The abnormal plantigrade foot. Orthop Rev 8:31–34, 1978.

6. Cracchiolo A: The use of shoes to treat foot disorders. Orthop Rev 8:73–83, 1979.

7. Raymakers R: The painful foot. Practitioner 215:61–68, 1975.

8. Mayer PJ: Pes cavus: A diagnostic and therapeutic challenge. Orthop Rev 7:105–116, 1978.

9. Glick JM: Traumatic injuries to the soft tissues of the foot and ankle. *In* DuVries' Surgery of the Foot. 4th Ed. Edited by RA Mann. St. Louis, CV Mosby, 1978.

10. Harrington KD: Degenerative arthritis of the ankle secondary to long-standing lateral ligament instability. J Bone Joint Surg 61:354–361, 1979.

11. Cass JR, Morrey BF: Ankle instability: current concepts, diagnosis, and treatment. Mayo Clin Proc 59:165–170, 1984.

12. Duthie RB, Ferguson AB: Mercer's Orthopedic Surgery, 8th Ed. Baltimore, Williams & Wilkins, 1985.

13. Mann RA, DuVries HL: Acquired nontraumatic deformities of the foot. *In* DuVries' Surgery of the Foot, 4th Ed. Edited by RA Mann. St. Louis, CV Mosby, 1978.

14. Lipscomb PR: Nonsuppurative tenosynovitis and paratendinitis. Am Acad Orthop Surg Instructional Course Lectures, Vol 7. Ann Arbor, 1950.

15. Turek, SL: Orthopaedics; Principles and Their Application. 4th Ed. Philadelphia. JB Lippincott, 1984.

16. Parvin RW, Ford LT: Stenosing tenosynovitis of the common peroneal tendon sheath. J Bone Joint Surg 38A:1352–1357, 1956.

17. Johnston JO: Affections of the foot. *In* DuVries' Surgery of the Foot. 4th Ed. Edited by RA Mann. St. Louis, CV Mosby, 1978.

18. Norris SH, Mankin HJ: Chronic tenosynovitis of the posterior tibial tendon with new bone formation. J Bone Joint Surg 60:523–526, 1978.

19. Sartoris DJ, Resnick DL: Tarsal coalition. Arth Rheum 28:331–338, 1985.

20. Inman VT, Mann RA: Major surgical procedures for disorders of the ankle, tarsus, and midtarsus. *In* DuVries' Surgery of the Foot, 4th Ed. Edited by RA Mann. St. Louis, CV Mosby, 1978.

21. Maclellan GE, Vyvyan B: Management of pain beneath the heel and achilles tendonitis with viscoelastic heel inserts. J Sports Med 15:117–121, 1981.

22. Goldman AB, Katz MC, Freiberger RH: Posttraumatic adhesive capsulitis of the ankle: arthrographic diagnosis. Am J Roentgenol 127:585–588, 1976.

23. Sorrells RB: Heel pain. J Arkansas Med Soc 74:494–497, 1978.

24. Shelley WB, Rawnsley HM: Painful feet due to herniation of fat. JAMA 205:308–309, 1968.

25. Dickinson PH, Coutts MB, Woodward EP, Handler D: Tendo achillis bursitis. J Bone Joint Surg 48:77–81, 1966.

26. Gerster JC, Saudan Y, Fallet GH: Talalgia; a review of 30 severe cases. J Rheumatol 5:210–216, 1978.

27. Fiamengo SA, et al: Posterior heel pain associated with a calcaneal step and achilles tendon calcification. Clin Orth 167:203–211, 1982.

28. Layfer LF: "Last" bursitis—A cause of ankle pain. Arth Rheum 23:261, 1980.

29. Canoso JJ, Wohlgethan JR, Newburg AH, Goldsmith MR: Aspiration of the retrocalcaneal bursa. Ann Rheum Dis 43:308–312, 1984.

30. Heneghan M, Pavlov H: The Haglund painful heel syndrome. Clin Ortho Related Research 187:228–234, 1984.

31. Furey JG: Plantar Fasciitis: The painful heel syndrome. J Bone Joint Surg 57A:672–673, 1975.

32. Michetti ML, Jacobs SA: Calcaneal heel spurs: etiology, treatment, and a new surgical approach. J Foot Surg 22:234–239, 1983.

33. Katoh Y, Chao ETS, Morrey BF, Laughman RK: Objective technique for evaluating painful heel syndrome and its treatment. Foot Ankle 3:227–237, 1983.

34. Spiegl PV, Johnson KA: Heel pain syndrome: which treatments to choose? J Musculoskeletal Med 1:66–72, 1984.

35. Satku K, Pho RWH, Wee A, Path MRC: Painful heel syndrome—an unusual cause. J Bone Joint Surg 66A:607–609, 1984.

36. Siebert JS, Mann RA: Dermatology and disorders of the toenails. *In* DuVries' Surgery of the Foot, 4th Ed. Edited by RA Mann. St. Louis, CV Mosby, 1978.

37. Moskowitz RW: Clinical Rheumatology. 2nd Ed. Philadelphia, Lea & Febiger, 1982.

38. Campbell JW, Inman VT: Treatment of plantar fasciitis and calcaneal spurs with the UC-BL shoe insert. Clin Orthop 103:57–62, 1974.

39. Fry RM: Dance and orthopaedics—each type has its special medical problems. Ortho Rev 12:49–56, 1983.

40. Riggs BL, Hodgson SF, Hoffman DL, et al: Treatment of primary osteoporosis with fluoride and calcium. JAMA 243:446–449, 1980.

41. Lester DK, Buchanan JR: Surgical treatment of plantar fasciitis. Clin Orthop 186:202–205, 1984.

42. Kahn C, Bishop JO, Tullos HS: Plantar fascia release

and heel spur excision via plantar route. Ortho Review 4:69–72, 1985.

43. Baxter DE, Mann RA: Bones of the foot and their afflictions. In DuVries' Surgery of the Foot, 4th Ed. Edited by RA Mann. St. Louis, CV Mosby, 1978.

44. Inmann VT, Mann RA: Principles of examination of the foot and ankle. In DuVries' Surgery of the Foot, 4th Ed. Edited by RA Mann. St. Louis, CV Mosby, 1978.

45. Milgram JE, Jacobson MA: Footgear; therapeutic modifications of sole and heel. Orthop Rev 7:57–62, 1978.

46. Epps CH: Fractures of the forepart and midpart of the adolescent foot. Orthop Rev 7:63–69, 1978.

47. Bossley CJ, Cairney PC: The intermetatarsophalangeal bursa—its significance in Morton's metatarsalgia. J Bone Joint Surg 62:184–187, 1980.

48. Greenfield J, Rea J, Illfeld FW: Morton's interdigital neuroma. Indications for treatment by local injections verus surgery. Clin Orthop 185:142–145, 1984.

49. Gross RH: Foot pain in children. Pediatr Clin N Am 24:813–823, 1977.

50. Chapman MW: Fractures and fracture-dislocations of the ankle and foot. In DuVries' Surgery of the Foot, 4th Ed. Edited by RA Mann. St. Louis, CV Mosby, 1978.

51. Garcia A, Parkes JC: Fractures of the foot. In Foot Disorders: Medical and Surgical Management, 2nd Ed. Edited by NJ Giannestras. Philadelphia, Lea & Febiger, 1973.

52. James SJ, Bates BT, Osternig LR: Injuries to runners. Am J Sports Med 6:40–50, 1978.

53. Baugher WH, Balady GJ, Warren RF, Marshall JL: Injuries of the musculoskeletal system in runners. Contemp Orthop 1:46–54, 1979.

54. Brady DM: Running injuries. Clinical Symposium (CIBA) 32(No. 4)2–36, 1980.

55. Mann RA: Biomechanics of the foot and ankle. Orthop Rev 7:43–48, 1978.

56. Giannestras NJ: Principles of bunion surgery. Orthop Rev 7:83–86, 1978.

57. Jacobson MA: Simple footgear corrections useful in office emergencies. Orthop Rev 8:63–68, 1979.

58. Shields MN,, RPT: Disorders of the foot. Postgraduate Clinical Seminar, 44th Annual Meeting, Am Rheum Assoc. Atlanta, May 28, 1980.

59. Goodwin C, OTC: Personal communication.

60. Kernohan J, Levack B, Wilson JN: Entrapment of the superficial peroneal nerve. J Bone Joint Surg 67B:60–61, 1985.

61. Lowdon IM: Superficial peroneal nerve entrapment, a case report. J Bone Joint Surg 67B:58–59, 1985.

62. Feldman RG, Goldman R, Keyserling WM: Peripheral nerve entrapment syndromes and ergonomic factors. Am J Indus Med 4:661–681, 1983.

63. Keck C: The tarsal tunnel syndrome. J Bone Joint Surg 44:180–182, 1962.

64. Kopell HP, Thompson WAL: Peripheral Entrapment Neuropathies. Huntington NY, RE Krieger, 1976.

65. Curtiss PH: Neurologic diseases of the foot. In Foot Disorders; Medical and Surgical Management, 2nd Ed. Edited by NJ Giannestras. Philadelphia, Lea & Febiger, 1973.

66. Goodgold J, Kopell HP, Spielholz NI: The tarsal-tunnel syndrome. N Engl J Med 273:742–745, 1965.

67. Wilemon WK: Tarsal tunnel syndrome. Orthop Rev 8:111–118, 1979.

68. Mann RA: Diseases of the nerves of the foot. In DuVries' Surgery of the Foot, 4th Ed. Edited by RA Mann. St. Louis, CV Mosby, 1978.

69. Janecki CJ, Dovberg JL: Tarsal-tunnel syndrome caused by neurilemoma of the medial plantar nerve. J Bone Joint Surg 59:127–128, 1977.

70. McGill DA: Tarsal tunnel syndrome. Proc R Soc Med 57:23–24, 1964.

71. Mackinnon SE, Dellon AL, Daneshvar A: Tarsal tunnel syndrome: histopathologic examination of a human posterior tibial nerve. Contemp Ortho 9:43–48, 1984.

72. Gretter TE, Wilde AH: Pathogenesis, diagnosis, and treatment of the tarsal-tunnel syndrome. Cleve Clin Q 37:23–29, 1970.

73. Fu R, DeLisa JA, Kraft GH: Motor nerve latencies through the tarsal tunnel in normal adult subjects. Arch Phys Med Rehabil 61:243–248, 1980.

74. Albrektsson B, Rudholm A, Rudholm U: The tarsal tunnel syndrome in children. J Bone Joint Surg 64:215–217, 1982.

75. Gessini L, Jandolo B, Pietrangeli A: The anterior tarsal syndrome. J Bone Joint Surg 66-A:786–787, 1984.

76. Lassmann G, Lassmann H. Stockinger L: Morton's metatarsalgia. Virchows Arch [Pathol Anat]370:307–321, 1976.

77. Daniell HW: Simple cure for nocturnal leg cramps. N Engl J Med 301:216, 1979.

78. Sheon RP: A joint protection guide for nonarticular rheumatic disorders. Postgrad Med 77 (5):329–338, 1985.

13

Generalized Soft Tissue Rheumatic Disorders

Many systemic illnesses can affect the periarticular soft tissue structures; most of these can be specifically categorized. What is left for inclusion here are what Smythe has termed the "Pain Amplification Syndromes", psychiatric somatization disorders, eosinophilic fasciitis, and polymyalgia rheumatica. The conditions included by Smythe under the title of Pain Amplification Syndromes include fibrositis, steroid withdrawal, sympathetic reflex dystrophy, and malignant hyperthermia.[1]

The term *fibrositis* has had many uses in the past. At present, an alternative term, *fibromyalgia* has been offered by some investigators. For this edition, we have stayed with the term fibrositis, but include the findings and data published under both terms.

The inclusion of eosinophilic fasciitis and polymyalgia rheumatica are included despite their known inflammatory pathogenesis because they are important causes of widespread pain and disability and they are important in the differential diagnosis of this disease group. Furthermore, some of our colleagues want them included!

FIBROSITIS SYNDROME

The fibrositis syndrome is the epitome of the soft tissue rheumatic pain disorders. The term "fibrositis syndrome" refers to a disorder with variable features that includes widespread aching and stiffness accompanied by localized sites of deep tenderness (tender points), sleep disturbance, fatigue, a characteristic personality, and chronicity.[1] "Fibrositis" should not be used merely to describe widespread soft tissue pain symptoms.[2] Essential to the diagnosis are the localized tender points first described over a century

ago.[3] The syndrome often begins in mid-life, although persons of any age may become symptomatic. Fibrositis may follow a precipitating life stress, such as a demotion at work, another illness, or trauma. Sometimes the patient is so overwhelmed by pain, the term "fibrositis storm" has been used.[4] Fibrositis has been divided into *primary* or *secondary* according to whether the symptoms could result from another underlying disease. But the separation may be questionable.[5]

Since Smythe suggested the use of a tender point count to help diagnose fibrositis,[2] a number of controlled studies have shown that the presence of widespread axial pain and aching, stiffness and fatigue, and the presence of tender points will separate out fibrositis from other disorders.[6–9] The tender points are the essential feature of fibrositis. Figure 13–1 and Table 13–1 present some of these accepted tender points.[2] The necessary number of tender points needed for diagnosis range from 4 or more;[7] and in most patients from 7 to 12 tender points can be detected.[2,6,9,10]

Fibrositis is the third most common rheumatic disorder seen among some rheumatology practices;[5,11] as many as 3 million women might be afflicted in the U.S.[11] The condition is a frequent cause for disability payments. Once diagnosed, the rate of hospitalization is reduced significantly.[9a] The diagnosis by itself may reduce anxiety and stress-related symptoms.

Reynolds published a history of fibrositis and muscular rheumatism.[12] He noted the increasing interest in muscular rheumatism in conjunction with the use of massage throughout Europe in the last century. This popular form of therapy led to the wide interest in

267

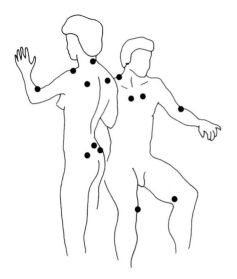

Fig. 13–1. The tender point map represents the 14 points recommended for use by Smythe and Moldofsky as a standard for diagnostic or therapy studies. These have been widely accepted among rheumatologists studying fibrositis.[28] (After Smythe, Moldofsky,[2] with permission.)

the muscles as the primary site of involvement in the genesis of muscular rheumatism. The tender hard places were suspected to cause pain in a "target zone" at some distance from the "trigger point".[13–15] Trigger points and tender points have been discussed more

completely in the Introduction and in Chapter 1.

The term "fibrositis," introduced by Gowers in 1904,[16] was applied to regional painful conditions thought to arise at the points of fascial and tendinous attachment. The tissues were thought to have suffered irritation and inflammation, perhaps from overstretching. Gowers used the term "inflammation" in a broad sense (see Chapt. 14). He applied "fibrositis" as a descriptive term that included "traumatic fibrositis" or "cervical fibrositis." At first the term was used to imply any pain of muscle origin and was to some extent used interchangeably with fasciitis, myofibrositis, myofasciitis, muscular rheumatism, and muscular strain.[17]

Presently, the term fibrositis syndrome is reserved for a specific soft tissue pain syndrome with the following characteristics:

Aching, Stiffness, and Fatigue. Soft tissue aching is widespread in broad regions of the cervical and lumbar spinal segments. The symptoms are aggravated by fatigue, tension, excessive work activity, immobilization, and chilling.[1,2,6–8,10] Heat, massage, programmed activity, and vacations are helpful in symptom relief. Although these symptoms may vary from day to day, they are nevertheless always present, and these patients rarely have "nor-

Table 13–1.   Examination for Tender Points (from Wolfe F, Sheon RP[10])

Point	Location
Trapezius	Midpoint of the upper fold
Second costochondral junctions	Just lateral to junctions on upper surface for maximum effect
Lateral epicondyles	Tennis-elbow sites: 1–2 cm distal to epicondyles, within muscle that tenses when long finger is actively extended
Supraspinatus	At origins, above scapular spine near the medial border
Low cervical	Anterior aspects of interspinous spaces C4 to C6
Low lumbar	Interspinous ligaments L4 to S1
Gluteus medius	Upper outer quadrants of buttocks, in anterior fold of muscle
Medial fat pad	Overlying medial collateral ligament of the knee, proximal to the joint line

mal" days. Trunk pain usually is bilateral and symmetric, although use may cause one side to be more tender than the other. Leg cramps are frequent. Stiffness occurs more diffusely than in specific joint areas. (This differs from the pattern of morning stiffness in rheumatoid arthritis in which stiffness is maximally localized to joints.) Neck pain and stiffness, and muscle contraction headache often occur in the early morning hours. Fatigue occurs much more often as a major complaint in fibrositis than in other rheumatic diseases or control groups. Often the patient wakes up more tired than when she retired.[18] Paresthesia of the lower extremities occurs commonly after prolonged sitting, or after performing any prolonged activity. Paresthesia and the *sensation* of swelling of the hands and arms are common. Rings feel tight in the morning. *Visible swelling does not occur*, at least to the physician observer.

Tender Points. Essential to the diagnosis of fibrositis are the presence of tender points, usually four or more.[1,2,5–8,8a,10,15,19,20] Similar *but painless* areas of firmness have been noted in normal persons,[21,22] but the key finding is *pain reproduction* after tender-point palpation.[20–24] The number of tender points directly correlates with the presence of other features of the syndrome. Thus, with an increasing number of tender points, the patient is likely to have neck pain, skin fold tenderness, and headache.[10,25]

Tender points are reproducible areas of tenderness that occur in precise locations. Melzack noted that 71% of tender points occur at acupuncture points.[26] Muscle areas at locations other than points are not more tender than in normal persons.[1] Common sites for tender points are deep cervical points near the transverse processes of cervical vertebrae 4, 5, 6; within the muscle belly of the right and left trapezius muscles; at the second costochondral junction of either side, approximately 1 cm lateral to the junction or on the superior surface of the rib; at the origin of the supraspinatus muscle near the medial border of the scapula of either side; within the muscle belly of the rhomboids, levator

scapulae, or infraspinatus muscles of the scapulae; 1 or 2 cm distal to the lateral epicondyle of the elbow in the extensor communis tendons; the upper lateral quadrant of the buttocks in the gluteal fascia; the lumbar interspinous ligaments to either side of lumbar vertebrae 4, 5, S1; the medial fat pad proximal to the joint line overlying the collateral ligament of the knee; and bony points, particularly the tip of the acromion or at the greater trochanter.[2] When patients with established rheumatoid arthritis have more than 4 tender points, their pain and fatigue may be due to concomitant fibrositis. Wolfe, et al studied those rheumatoid patients with more than 4 tender points and found that these patients had features compatible with fibrositis; much of their symptomatology of widespread aching and fatigue, and morning stiffness were thought to be the result of the fibrositis rather than inflammation.[9,28]

Sleep Disturbance. If the patient does not volunteer that she suffers sleep disturbance, the patient's spouse often volunteers that the patient "moves all over the bed all night long." The patient may fall asleep promptly but then awakens frequently throughout the night. Characteristically, the patient feels more tired in the morning than when she went to bed. Sleep is not restful. Moldofsky noted that non-rapid eye movement (non-REM) sleep was disturbed and contaminated by alpha rhythms in patients with the fibrositis syndrome.[29] Furthermore, by depriving volunteers of non-REM sleep, the characteristic tender points were produced.[29–30] Patients with fibrositis do not enter deep sleep (stage 4 sleep); they often feel that if they could keep moving and not stop, they would be better off. However, fatigue develops quickly. Others find this pattern less often in patients with fibrositis; also, other abnormal EEG patterns may be noted.[31,32]

Perfectionistic Personality. The patients tend to be compulsive at work, at home, at hobbies, or at social activities. They live with rigid time deadlines. When presented with an appointment, they are characteristically conscientiously prompt. They dislike tranquilizers and are sparse users of drugs or alcohol.[1] Features of compulsive grooming may be evident including precise hair arrangement, plucked eyebrows, and fastidious nail care. They are rarely obese. They tend to be of above-average intelligence. Living the compulsive life often leads to depression, particularly at midlife. Migraine headaches are often noted in the patients' family or in the patients themselves. The application of three standardized psychologic tests to 22 fibrositis patients versus a matched control group revealed no differences overall or to individual responses.[33] However, other studies of fibrositis patients using MMPI testing had variable results.[28,34–36] Patients with fibrositis were not found to be more anxious nor to have enhanced pain perception when compared to a matched control group.[37]

Normal Laboratory Tests. Studies that are characteristically normal include complete blood counts, erythrocyte sedimentation rate, serum proteins, muscle enzyme studies, and antinuclear and rheumatoid factor determinations.[1] Laboratory abnormalities are inconsistent with a diagnosis of primary fibrositis.

Primary Fibrositis

When making a diagnosis of fibrositis, the physician should consider all of the five features outlined. When other disorders coexist, the clinician should determine whether or not that diagnosis can explain the fibrositis features. If not, fibrositis may be diagnosed as an additional condition. However, some will disagree; they would prefer that primary fibrositis be limited to patients with the features detailed above and without osteoarthritis or trauma or other rheumatic disease.[7,38,39] Additional features that may occur include autonomic dysfunction with dermographism,[24] cutis anserina ("goose skin"— contraction of the arrectores pilorum muscles that causes elevation of hair follicles)[17] or cutis marmorata (a transitory purplish mottling of the skin), and excessive sweating.[19] Raynaud's phenomenon and a past history of depression were common in one series of patients.[40]

Skinfold tenderness with hyperesthesia over the upper scapular region may be noted. Following testing for skinfold tenderness performed by rolling the patient's skin in a gentle pinching fashion, a marked hyperemia sometimes occurs.[1]

During the physical examination the patient appears unhappy, but is generally not overtly depressed and usually is forthright without much grossly evident neurotic behavior. Joint examination reveals normal range of active and passive motion. However, general musculoskeletal discomfort is evident. Grip testing is approached hesitantly and is carried out slowly, but usually the patient demonstrates full or low normal levels of strength.[1]

The five criteria previously defined serve to distinguish fibrositis from pain that is a malingering pretense or that is neurotically symbolic.[1] The fibrositis syndrome can be added upon other systemic disease; the compounded symptoms then may lead to more complex, inappropriate, and at times, hazardous medical or surgical treatment than the primary systemic disease would have required. If fibrositis is identified as a concomitant problem, therapy should be directed toward both disorders.[1] For example, the addition of features of the fibrositis syndrome to patients suffering from rheumatoid arthritis or systemic lupus erythmatosus often results in treatment with drugs far stronger than signs of inflammation would warrant. Following treatment of the fibrositis syndrome, the anti-inflammatory drugs or corticosteroids can be significantly reduced or even eliminated.

Secondary Fibrositis. About 6% of patients with symptoms of fibrositis will develop or have another rheumatic disease. In particular, rheumatoid arthritis and systemic lupus erythematosus may underlie the symptoms of fibrositis.[24] Widespread osteoarthritis, Forestier's disease (DISH), ankylosing spondylitis, polymyositis, polymyalgia rheumatica, and vasculitis may be found also. Other diagnoses that can give rise to symptoms of fibrositis include neuropathy, paraneoplastic syndromes, hypothyroidism, hyperparathyroidism, inflammatory bowel disease, and anemias.[18] Drugs that might be incriminated include clofibrate, diuretics, cimetidine, lithium, cytotoxic drugs, alcohol, and amphetamines.[41]

Etiology. Fibrositis syndrome may be the result of an interaction of local factors, reflex phenomena associated with chronic pain of deep origin, disturbed sleep, or factors involved in the "gate theory" of pain persistence.[1]

Local lesions have been suspected, but are found inconsistently. In these patients, the episacroiliac lipoma (described in Chapt. 8) is not likely responsible for the widespread pain in the lumbar region.[1] Histopathologic changes described in uncontrolled studies of tender points include a metachromatic substance in interfibrillar spaces,[42] masses of mucoid amorphous substances between muscle fascicles, platelet clots or clusters, and mast cells discharging granules into intercellular spaces.[43] Type II fiber atrophy, a moth-eaten appearance in Type I fibers, electron microscopic evidence of segmental muscle fiber necrosis[44] with lipid and glycogen deposition in some and subsarcolemmal mitochondrial accumulation in all samples examined, was also described.[44,45,45a] In one report,[46] the lactic dehydrogenase isoenzymes, LD 3-5 fractions were found to be increased in tissue and blood.[46] Venous myoglobin, determined by radioimmunoassay, was found to significantly increase when determined 1 to 3 hours after tender muscle area massage, whereas the determination after massage of nonsymptomatic areas remained normal.[47] This suggests a disorder of the muscle fibers.

The possibility that autoimmune mechanisms might be involved is suggested by recent reports of immunoglobulin deposition in the dermo-epidermal junction of sun exposed forearm skin of patients with primary fibrositis. The patients had reticular skin discoloration (cutis marmaratus).[4,48–52] McBroom et al. also noted immunoglobulin deposition in cutaneous blood vessels as well.[50] Caro reported less intense immunofluorescence when compared to lupus patients; therefore fibrositis patients did not have a positive lupus band test by the usual brilliant fluorescence observed in lupus skin.[48,48a,48b] Whether these deposits are passively deposited on previously injured tissue, or are pathogenetically involved in vascular injury is not known. Serum IGG_4 and IGE levels were reported within normal limits.[4] The muscle fiber changes are interpreted to represent the results of chronic muscle spasm and ischemia.[45]

Reflex phenomena as contributing factors in pathogenesis have been the subject of much speculation since Travell's mapping of the tender point locations. She suggested a reflex pain cycle,[19] further elaborated as a pain-spasm-pain cycle.[17,53] The persistence of the reflex phenomenon might result from anti-pain centers within the central nervous system as advocated by Melzack.[53] However, increased levels of beta endorphin in the plasma of fibrositis patients was reported.[54] But the theory of a pain amplification syndrome would suggest that the patients' beta endorphin levels would be decreased rather than increased.[54] Yunus, Denko, and Masi in a subsequent report did not detect abnormal serum beta endorphin in fibrositis.[55] The gate theory suggests an abnormality in receptor sites, or other areas within the midbrain areas of these patients.[54a] A concept of a circular physiologic mechanism in which emotional stress enhances muscle spasm with local vasoconstriction and with further induced muscle spasm has been the subject of intense speculation.[56,56a,56b,56c] Tender points and trigger points may follow trivial injury.[57] Bursitis of motor-unit action potentials was reported.[58,59] More recent electrodiagnostic studies failed to confirm this finding.[60] The persistence of pain and reflex muscle spasm are associated with inhibition of voluntary movement, increased blood flow, and cutaneous or deep hyperalgesia. These changes may be found in sites far removed from the area of deep pain.[1]

In a controlled study utilizing a standardized task, patients suffering from chronic muscle tension produced 50% more electrical activity in performing the task than did normal controls. The patients' estimations of the degree of muscle tension were lower than measured. This misperception of muscle tension may require a reeducation program.[61]

The sleep disturbance seen in patients with the fibrositis syndrome may not simply be the result of pain. Rather, Moldofsky has provided evidence that deprivation of stage 4 non-REM sleep may induce lesions comparable to tender points.[2,29,30] These investigations suggest that an endogenous arousal system is activated by stressful life situations. In turn, this disturbed sleep, pain, and fatigue become locked into a self-perpetuating cycle.[2,23] Psychologic abnormalities, noted earlier, are unlikely involved except that established pain might be enhanced by mood, stress, fatigue, or depression.[23a] (See Psychogenic Rheumatism.) Pain threshold assessment at nontender point areas and psychologic tests in these patients reveal normal findings, but pain thresholds at tender point locations was significantly reduced.[62]

Although osteoarthritis is found in many patients with the fibrositis syndrome,[24] symptoms do not appear to correlate with degenerative changes of the spinal apophyseal joints, or disc degeneration.[63,64] Although most persons over the age of 40 will have developed osteoarthritis, these radiographic features should be interpreted with caution. This caveat has been discussed in previous chapters.

Laboratory and Radiographic Examination. As mentioned earlier, a requirement for the diagnosis of primary fibrositis is the finding of normal laboratory tests. In addition to the erythrocyte sedimentation rate, complete blood count, urinalysis, and muscle enzymes, we commonly utilize a chemical battery or profile that includes tests of thyroid function. Metabolic disorders such as hypo- or hypercalcemia, diabetes mellitus, thyroid dysfunction, and hyperlipidemias are ruled out at small cost. Dysproteinemia and hematologic malignancies can similarly be excluded. Radiographic examination of patients with fi-

brositis sometimes reveals calcification of the lower costal cartilages; the association to fibrositis is unclear.[65] Straightening of the cervical spine may also be noted. Bone scans are normal when examined with 99m Tc pertechnetate followed by 99m Tc methylene diphosphonate.[66]

Differential Diagnosis. The fibrositis syndrome is not synonymous with psychogenic rheumatism. It differs significantly from the latter by the presence, the location, and the constancy of tender points. The fibrositic patient often relates symptoms to changes in her *external* environment including weather, heat, cold, humidity, rest, or exercise. These external factors influence the patient's symptoms for better or for worse. Conversely, the patient with psychogenic rheumatism is at the mercy of changes in her *internal* environment; symptoms vary with mood, psyche, pleasure, excitement, mental distraction, worry, or fatigue. A problem exists when a patient with the fibrositis syndrome also has a marked neurosis. The patient with psychogenic rheumatism frequently exhibits the "touch me not" reaction when a physical examination is performed.[67] Such patients react excessively to the examiner's touch anywhere on the body (see Psychogenic Rheumatism).

Secondary fibrositis has been discussed. Other conditions that can be confused with fibrositis include polymyalgia rheumatica (see discussion following), rheumatoid arthritis in the myalgic prodromal stage, the hypermobility syndrome, Forestier's disease (diffuse idiopathic skeletal hyperostosis, DISH), idiopathic edema, and parkinsonism.[24,68–74]

Symptoms of fatigue, myalgia, and malaise may develop before the onset of joint symptoms in patients with rheumatoid arthritis[70] or other connective tissue diseases.[24] The test for rheumatoid factor may be positive despite the absence of evident articular inflammation. Careful inquiry for morning stiffness in true joint locations, particularly in the fingers and toes, careful palpation of digits for joint synovitis, and examination for finger flexor tendinitis should be carried out. Although response to aspirin therapy is nonspecific, patients with fibrositis secondary to rheumatoid arthritis generally show a better response than do patients with primary fibrositis.

Other occult early connective tissue disease must also be excluded.[21] One of the common causes for similar symptoms is a hypothyroid myopathy (Hoffman's syndrome).[57] These patients have painful muscle spasm and the characteristic slow relaxation phase of myxedema reflexes in addition to features of fibrositis; myoedema presumably underlies these features. Occasionally the use of laxatives may result in a similar constellation of findings, as they may induce hypokalemia and give rise to a state of muscle irritability.[68] Various myopathies might be misdiagnosed as fibrositis. In McArdle's syndrome, exertional muscle pain and stiffness, cramps, and limb involvement should not be confusing.[75] A screening test can be performed. A sphygmomanometer cuff placed around the upper arm is inflated above systolic pressure; the patient exercises the forearm muscles by gripping forcefully for 20 to 30 times in 1 minute. In patients with defective glycolysis of McArdle's disease, a painful contracture develops, and persists until the cuff is deflated.[75]

Patients with fibrositis require a careful examination with several observations in order to exclude serious underlying disease, even though symptoms may have persisted for several months or even years. See Table 13–2, Danger list for generalized soft tissue rheumatic pain.

Management. Identification of tender points that reproduce the patient's pain is a great moral victory for the patient. Family members, tired of hearing the patient complain without seeing evidence of disease, have usually inferred a psychogenic pain state. The clinician may now direct the patient away from a purely psychologic cause for the symptomatology.[1]

The patient comes to the physician feeling threatened by her illness. Treatment should begin with reassurance, explanation, and relief from mechanical stress to the neck and low-back areas.[1] A fibrositis pamphlet, available from the local chapter of the Arthritis Foundation, is helpful in patient education and understanding of disease considerations in treatment goals. Initial therapy should include proper sleep position with support under the arch of the neck, use of a firm mattress, and development of strong abdominal muscles to provide back support.

Pain relief enables the patient to enter a general mobilization-exercise program. Identifying tender points and injecting them with a corticosteroid-anesthetic mixture is helpful for some patients and can often be advised on the first visit.[20,24] Each tender point can be injected with $\frac{1}{2}$ to 1 ml of procaine/methylprednisolone (not to exceed 60 to 80 mg steroid total dosage.) A one-inch #23 needle is usually adequate for use except for the gluteus area in which a 3.5 inch #20 spinal needle can be used. No controlled observations are available comparing the results of a corticosteroid-anesthetic injection to results obtained when a local anesthetic is used alone. A total maximum of 40 mg of methylprednisolone or equivalent can be administered into multiple sites at any one time. The steroid may be suspended in 1 to 10 ml of a local anesthetic, depending on the amount of corticosteroid used. Alternatively the tender points may be injected with procaine alone, massaged with ice, or if few in number, sprayed with fluorimethane while the involved muscle is stretched.[76,77] Narcotics do not play a role in the treatment of the fibrositis syndrome, and indeed they do not work. Similarly, oral corticosteroids are not helpful.[79] Cyclobenzaprine (Flexeril) 5 to 40 mg/day has been helpful during flareups.[80,80a] Other drugs that are useful include mepro-

Table 13–2. Danger List, Generalized Soft Tissue Rheumatic Pain

1. Fever, sweats, weight loss.
2. Lymphadenopathy, organomegaly.
3. Raynaud's phenomenon.
4. Neuropathy.
5. Joint swelling or tenderness.
6. Limitation of joint or spine motion.
7. Bruits or diminished pulse.
8. Any unexplained laboratory abnormality.

bamate, carisoprodol, and diazepam to depress the brainstem activating systems and provide a sedative effect. Furthermore, they may act centrally as skeletal muscle relaxants.[81] Nocturnal sedation with amitriptyline, 25 to 100 mg at bedtime, is helpful for sleep disturbance.[81a] On occasion amitriptyline may result in a stimulating rather than a sedative effect and patients should be warned that if this occurs, amitriptyline should be discontinued and another tricyclic tried (see Chapt. 14). Joint protection advice for the neck, back, and shoulder may be of value (see Chapts. 2, 4, 8, and 16).

Attitudinal changes should be approached with the patient.[78] The clinician should urge the patient to recognize perfectionistic features and impatience with activities of daily living, since these patients tend to complete a task no matter what the physical cost. These patients should be taught to pace physical activity, housekeeping, or hobbies. They should pursue a physical fitness activity such as cardiovascular fitness training,[78a] swimming, roller skating, tennis, and racquetball depending on overall assessment. These activities tend to involve considerable muscular stretching as well as toning up. Tension should be dealt with by rest, programmed exercise, and emotional escape. Biofeedback relaxation and learning to appreciate tension perception are often helpful.[61]

Physical therapy with mobilizing exercises should be part of the regimen of every patient with the fibrositis syndrome. Patients often find a hot bath or ice pack rewarding. Such measures should be utilized immediately before performing a stretching-mobilizing exercise program. Additional exercises for posture correction, and exercises to correct any functional deficit should be individually tailored to the patient's needs.[23] We recommend that a 10- to 15-minute exercise regimen be performed in the morning before dressing and be repeated in the evening following undressing.[1,82] If muscle irritability prevents the patient from performing exercises, then a physical therapist may administer deep massages and rhythmic stabilization exercise.[77]

When joint laxity co-exists, therapeutic exercise is very important in order to prevent severe disability.[77a] If the fibrositis syndrome overlies another associated disease, the fibrositis must be managed concomitantly with the basic disease.[24]

Outcome and Additional Suggestions. The patient should know at the onset that a multidisciplinary approach as outlined will take several months before significant benefit is realized. Loss of all symptoms is unusual,[1] and the longer the patient has suffered before entering treatment, the less favorable the outcome.[24] It is wise for the clinician to inform the patient that during the first month the pain may actually seem worse. This can result from vigorous stretching, or simply from changing the patient's routine.

If the exercises are done with a gradual prolonged initiation of the stretching portion of each exercise, less irritation will occur.

Interruption of employment can be a disaster. The patient should be kept both psychologically and physically active, keeping in mind the value of a job as a positive distraction. If fired or forced to resign because of failure to perform as a result of pain and exhaustion, these patients seldom return to full productive capacity.[1] After an interval of 4 to 6 weeks, night pain or persistent regional pain reproduced by tender-point palpation may indicate the need for another corticosteroid tender-point injection. Some clinicians prefer multiple repeated injections with only a local anesthetic.

The expertise of the Bureau of Vocational Rehabilitation may be utilized for the purpose of evaluating the effect of chronic pain on the job performance and the psychosocial makeup of the patient. We have had good results when the patient is brought in contact with a knowledgeable vocational counselor. Work should not require prolonged sitting or standing. Rather, these patients should be provided jobs that require variation in body positions. They seem to function better as secretaries, store managers, hostesses, or teachers, and less well as bookkeepers, accountants, and physicians!

In our experience many of these patients do obtain gratifying relief of symptoms. We have followed hundreds of these patients for many years; we remain amazed at their diligence in performing the exercise program twice daily, and often they no longer require drug therapy. A subgroup requires amitriptyline or cyclobenzaprine (Flexeril) during stressful situations. Total cures are rare. This is in sharp contradistinction to the results of rheumatoid arthritis and other connective tissue disease in which a significant minority have remissions.[1] The young woman who develops the fibrositis syndrome shortly after the establishment of a family has a less satisfactory outlook for remission than a similar patient with lupus or rheumatoid arthritis.[1] Current research into endorphins, antipain regions in the central nervous system, and gate controls may lead to more satisfactory solutions.

PSYCHOGENIC RHEUMATISM

The complaint "I hurt all over" or "The pain is so bad, you just don't know how bad it is!" will often put the clinician on the defensive; or, provoke a massive diagnostic workup. What is called "psychogenic rheumatism" includes many manifestations of mental illness and exaggerated psychophysiologic responses to internal stress. The somatoform disorders include the following:[11]

1. Somatization disorder (including classic hysteria).
2. Hypochondriasis
3. Conversion disorder (hysterical neurosis)
4. Psychogenic pain disorder (includes psychogenic rheumatism)

Wallace also described a number of epidemics of pain attacks that he believes were forms of mass hysteria. These included epidemic fibromyalgia in British and American armed forces during World War II, and epidemic neuromyasthenia during polio epidemics.[11]

Psychogenic rheumatism often is regional or generalized pain so severe that the body cannot be touched, the "touch-me-not" syndrome.[67] The scalp, face, trunk, and limbs may share the pain-to-touch equally. Tender points are not present. The patient usually can relate the onset to an emotionally charged situation. Whereas fibrositis has exacerbations brought on by the external milieu, psychogenic rheumatism relates to internal stress. The patient has an ache in the body when there is an ache in the mind. Other times, the patient feels just fine. Often the patient will say "Before this, I couldn't have felt better." That, too, differs from fibrositis, in that fibrositis symptoms rarely return completely to normal.

Other features of psychogenic rheumatism include:[83]

1. Previous diagnosis of "arthritis"
2. Predominantly female
3. Have been seen by multiple physicians
4. Report "swelling" but no objective signs
5. Have great concern for family history of "arthritis"
6. Depressed, apprehensive, anxious
7. May have other rheumatic disease
8. Have normal laboratory tests
9. Pain in regions (e.g., whole left side of body)
10. Pain terms are bizarre (e.g., searing, pulsating, burning)
11. Location of pain changes, or becomes the touch-me-not response
12. May vigorously deny emotional factors
13. Refractory to medical and physical therapy
14. Often tearful, the symptoms are "so bad"

Conversion reactions are more impressive in focusing on a specific disability. In our experience, they usually involve the upper or lower limb, and can be confused with a reflex sympathetic dystrophy. Bone scans are helpful in differential diagnosis (see Reflex Sympathetic Dystrophy). To further complicate the problem, reflex dystrophy and conversion may improve with use of a transcutaneous electric nerve stimulator! When confronted with an obvious conversion problem, the patient can be informed of the diagnosis, and given an explanation to the effect that stress created so much "charging up" of the nervous system that the condition was the result. If that stress can be handled in other ways, such as with a relaxation program, the symptoms may gradually disappear.

Somatic delusions in schizophrenia are easily recognized if other delusions or hallucinations are brought out during the history.

Treatment begins with an examination to exclude other diagnoses. Then provide some gentle exercise or warm baths, or both. Be empathetic. When the crisis is over, and the patient more amenable, begin to counsel the patient about stress and symptoms. Obtain psychiatric consultation if needed.

POLYMYALGIA RHEUMATICA

Widespread stiffness and aching of the shoulder girdle and/or the pelvic girdle are the usual complaints. The condition is rarely seen in persons younger than age 55. The onset is usually abrupt, and shoulder motion may rapidly become limited. The key distinction from fibrositis is the limitation of motion and a rapid erythrocyte sedimentation rate.[84] Bone scans may demonstrate uptake by the involved joints.[85–89] The distinction from giant cell arteritis is difficult, and we recommend temporal artery biopsy to exclude this diagnosis. Three to 4 cm or longer segments of the vessel are obtained, and the entire segment specially examined for arteritis. The biopsy may be done as an outpatient procedure. Some rheumatologists routinely recommend bilateral biopsy if frozen section studies of the initially biopsied vessel are normal. We find 20% of patients with polymyalgia have an abnormal biopsy: 10% have frank giant cell arteritis, and 10% have less defined features of arteritis such as fibrosis and disruption of the internal elastic membrane. A therapeutic trial with 10 to 20 mg of prednisone daily provides dramatic symptomatic benefit but may not be enough to prevent vascular occlusion if vasculitis is present. Blindness is a feared complication. The pa-

tient usually will note significant symptomatic benefit after a few days of steroid therapy.

Other connective tissue disorders that have polymyalgia symptoms include rheumatoid arthritis and Sjogren's syndrome.[90] Such patients usually do not respond as strikingly to the steroid trial. Also to be ruled out are paraneoplastic musculoskeletal syndromes, hypertrophic osteoarthropathy, Paget's disease, ankylosing spondylitis, calcium apatite deposition disease, and pseudogout.

EOSINOPHILIC FASCIITIS

Usually pain, swelling, and tenderness followed by severe induration of the skin and subcutaneous tissue occur. The skin at first is erythematous and warm; later it becomes hyperpigmented and nodular. The extremities are the usual site for involvement. Circulating eosinophilia is regularly present. Biopsy reveals inflammation and fibrosis, frequently with eosinophils in the deep fascia. Immunoglobulin and complement is deposited in the subcutaneous fascia. Contractures and sclerodermatous skin changes or morphea may occur.[91] Pulmonary fibrosis, autoimmune anemia, thrombocytopenia, Raynaud's phenomenon, Sjogren's syndrome, carpal tunnel syndrome, and myelofibrosis may occur.[92,93] A wedge biopsy including skin and muscle should be examined. Treatment with low dose corticosteroids has been helpful in some cases.[91,93,94] Toxic oil syndrome, due to ingestion of adulterated oil, can similarly result in scleroderma, eosinophilia, neuropathy, myalgia, rash, and pulmonary edema.[95]

REFERENCES

1. Smythe HA: Nonarticular Rheumatism and Psychogenic Musculoskeletal Syndromes. *In* Arthritis and Allied Conditions, 10th Ed. Edited by DJ McCarty. Philadelphia, Lea & Febiger, 1985.
2. Smythe HA, Moldofsky H: Two contributions to understanding of the 'fibrositis' syndrome. Bull Rheum Dis 28:928–931, 1977.
3. Simons DG: Muscle pain syndromes—part II. Am J Phys Med 55:15–42, 1976.
4. Caro XJ, Quismorio FP: Immunological studies of skin and circulating autoantibodies in primary fi-

brositis syndrome. 1985: Paper presented to Nonart Rheum Study Group, Los Angeles, June 5, 1985.

5. Wolfe F, Cathey MA, Kleinheksel SM, Amos SP, et al: Psychological status in primary fibrositis and fibrositis associated with rheumatoid arthritis. J Neurol Sci 58:73–78, 1983.

6. Campbell SM, Clark S, Tindall EA, Forehand ME, Bennett RM: Clinical characteristics of fibrositis. Arth Rheum 26:817–824, 1983.

7. Yunus M, Masi AT, et al: Primary fibromyalgia: Clinical study of 50 patients with matched normal controls. Arth Rheum 11:151–170, 1981.

7a. Calabro JJ, Eyvazzadeh C, Weber C: Primary fibromyalgia in children. (Abstract #D58) Arth Rheum 29 (No 4)(Supp), 1986.

8. Yunus MB, Masi AT: Juvenile primary fibromyalgia syndrome: a clinical study of 33 patients and matched normal controls. Arth Rheum 28:138–145, 1985.

8a. Simms R, Mason J, Felson D, Goldenberg D: Tenderness in 75 anatomic sites: Distinguishing fibromyalgia from controls. (Abstract #D33) Arth Rheum 29 (No. 4) (Supp), 1986.

9. Wolfe F, Cathey MA: The epidemiology of tender points: A prospective study of 1520 patients. J Rheum 12:1164–1168, 1985.

9a. Cathey MA, Wolfe F, Kleinheksel SM, Hawley DJ: The socio-economic impact of fibrositis (Abstract #B34) Arth Rheum 2 (No 4)(Supp), 1986.

10. Wolfe F, Sheon RP: When aching is generalized, consider fibrositis. Diagnosis July:44–61, 1984.

11. Wallace DJ: Fibromyalgia: Unusual historical aspects and new pathogenic insights. Mt Sinai J Med 51:124–131, 1984.

12. Reynolds MD: The development of the concept of fibrositis. J Hist Med & Allied Sci 38:5–35, 1983.

13. Travell J, Rinzler S, Herman M: Pain and disability of the shoulder and arm. JAMA 120:417–422, 1942.

14. Edeiken J, Wolferth CC: Persistent pain in the shoulder region following myocardial infarction. Am J Med Sci 191:201–210, 1936.

15. Simons DG: Muscle pain syndromes—Part I. Am J Phys Med 54:289–311, 1975.

16. Gowers WR: Lumbago: Its lessons and analogues. Br Med J 1:117–121, 1904.

17. Bonica JJ: Management of myofascial pain syndromes in general practice. JAMA 164:732–738, 1957.

18. Beetham WP Jr: Diagnosis and management of fibrositis syndrome and psychogenic rheumatism. Med Clin N Am 63:433–439, 1979.

19. Travell J, Rinzler SH: The myofascial genesis of pain. Postgrad Med 11:425–434, 1952.

20. Travell J: Myofascial trigger points: clinical view. In Advances in Pain Research and Therapy. Vol. I. Edited by JJ Bonica, D Albe-Fessard. New York, Raven Press, 1976.

21. Slocum CH: Fibrositis. Clinics 2:169–178, 1943.

22. Copeman WSC: Aetiology of the fibrositic nodule: a clinical contribution. Br Med J 2:263–264, 1943.

23. Smythe HA: 'Fibrositis' as a disorder of pain modulation. Clin Rheum Dis 5:823–832, 1979.

23a. Yunus MB, Masi AT: Association of primary fibromyalgia syndrome (PFS) with stress-related syndromes. (Abstract #D34) Arth Rheum 29 (No 4)(Suppl), 1986.

24. Kraft GH, Johnson EW, LaBan MM: The fibrositis syndrome. Arch Phys Med Rehabil 49:155–162, 1968.

25. Wolfe F: Tender points, trigger points, and the fibrositis syndrome. Clin Rheum Pract Jan/Feb: 36–38, 1984.

26. Melzack R, Stillwell DM, Fox EJ: Trigger points and acupuncture points for pain: Correlations and implications. Pain 3:3–23, 1977.

27. Reynolds MD: Myofascial trigger point syndromes in the practice of rheumatology. Arch Phys Med Rehabil 62:111–114, 1981.

28. Wolfe F: Non-articular symptoms in fibrositis. Rheumatoid arthritis, osteoarthritis, and arthalgia syndrome. (Abstract #E45) Arth Rheum 25 (No. 4) [Supp], 1982.

29. Moldofsky H, Scarisbrick P, England R, et al.: Musculoskeletal symptoms and Non-REM sleep disturbances in patients with "fibrositis syndrome" and healthy subjects. Psychosomat Med 37:341–351, 1975.

30. Moldofsky H, Scarisbrick P: Induction of neurasthenic musculoskeletal pain syndrome by selective sleep stage deprivation. Psychosomat Med 38:35–44, 1976.

31. Golden H, Weber SM, Bergen D: Sleep studies in patients with fibrositis syndrome. (Abstract #142) Arth Rheum 26 (No. 4) [Supp], 1983.

32. McBroom P, Ware JC, Russell IJ: Sleep disturbances in primary and secondary fibromyalgia syndrome. Paper presented to the Nonarticular Rheumatism Study Group, American Rheumatism Association, Minneapolis, 1984.

33. Clark S, Campbell SM, Forehand ME, Tindall EA, Bennett RM: Clinical characteristics of fibrositis. Arth Rheum 28:132–137, 1985.

34. Payne TC, Leavitt F, Garron DC, et al: Fibrositis and psychologic disturbance. Arth Rheum 25:213–217, 1982.

35. Ahles TA, Yunus MB, Riley SD, Bradley JM, Masi AT: Psychological factors associated with primary fibromyalgia syndromes. Arth Rheum 27:1101–1106, 1984.

36. Reynolds MD: The definition of fibrositis. Arth Rheum 25:1506–1507, 1982.

37. Clark SR, Forehand ME: Pain perception and anxiety with fibrositis. (Abstract #16) Arth Rheum 26 (No. 4) [Supp], 1983.

38. Yunus MB: Primary fibromyalgia syndrome: current concepts. Comprehensive Therapy 10:21–28, 1984.

39. Yunus MB: Fibromyalgia syndrome: a need for uniform classification. J Rheum 10:841–844, 1983.

40. Dinerman H, Goldenberg DL, Felson DT: A prospective evaluation of 118 patients with the fibromyalgia syndrome: Prevalence of Raynaud's phenomenon, sicca symptoms, ANA, low complement, and Ig deposition at the dermal-epidermal junction. J Rheum 13:368–373, 1985.

41. Lane RJM, Mastaglia FL: Drug-induced myopathies in man. Lancet 2:562–566, 1978.

42. Brendstrup P, Jespersen K, Asboe-Hansen G: Morphological and chemical connective tissue changes in fibrositic muscles. Ann Rheum Dis 16:438–440, 1957.

43. Awad EA: Interstitial myofibrositis: Hypotheses of

the mechanism. Arch Phys Med Rehabil 54:449–453, 1973.

44. Henriksson KG, Bengtsson A, Larsson J, et al: Muscle biopsy findings of possible diagnostic importance in primary fibromyalgia (fibrositis, myofascial syndrome). Lancet 2:1395, 1982.

45. Kalyan-Raman UP, Kalyan-Raman K, Yunus MB, Masi AT: Muscle pathology in primary fibromyalgia syndrome: A light microscopic histochemical and ultrastructural study. J Rheum 11:808–813, 1984.

45a. Bartels EM, Danneskiold B: Histologic abnormalities in muscle from patients with certain types of fibrositis. Lancet 1:755–757, 1986.

46. Ibrahim GA, Awad EA, Kottke FJ: Interstitial myofibrositis: serum and muscle enzymes and lactate dehydrogenase isoenzymes. Arch Phys Med Rehab 55:23–28, 1974.

47. Danneskiold-Samsoe B, Christiansen E, Lund B, Andersen RB: Regional Muscle Tension and Pain (Fibrositis). Scand J Rehab Med 15:17–20, 1982.

48. Caro XJ: Immunofluorescent detection of IgG at the dermal-epidermal junction in patients with apparent primary fibrositis syndrome. Arth Rheum 27:1174–1179, 1984.

48a. Caro XJ, Schroeter AL: Cutaneous vascular immunofluoresence in primary fibrositis syndrome. (Abstract #D31) Arth Rheum (No 4) (Supp), 1986.

48b. Caro XJ, Quismorio FP: IgG subclass distribution of deposits at the dermal-epidermal junction (DEJ) of skin in primary fibrositis syndrome (PFS), (Abstract #D32) Arth Rheum 29 (No 4) (Supp), 1986.

49. Caro XJ, Quismorio FP, Jr: Immunological studies of skin and circulating autoantibodies in primary fibrositis syndrome. (Abstract #E61) Arth Rheum 25 (No. 4) [Supp], 1985.

50. McBroom P, Kolb WP, Kolb LM: Cutaneous vascular immunofluorescence in patients with fibromyalgia syndrome: correlation with circulating immune complexes. Paper presented to the Nonarticular Rheumatism Study Group, American Rheumatism Association, Minneapolis, 1984.

51. Dinerman H, Felson DT, Goldenberg DL, Solomon J: Lupus band test and antinuclear antibodies in fibromyalgia (Abstract #A58) Arth Rheum 28 (No. 4) [Supp], 1985.

52. Dinerman H, Felson D, Goldenberg D: A randomized clinical trial of naproxen and amitriptyline in primary fibromyalgia. (Abstract #159) Arth Rheum 28 (No. 4) [Supp], 1985.

53. Melzack R: Myofascial trigger points: relation to acupuncture and mechanisms of pain. Arch Phys Med Rehabil 62 114–117, 1981.

54. Hall S, Littlejohn GO, Jethwa J, Copolov D: Plasma beta-endorphin (BEP) levels in fibrositis. (Abstract #A6) Arth Rheum 26 (No. 4) [Supp], 1983.

54a. Wilke WS, Mackenzie AH: Proposed pathogenesis of fibrositis. Cleve Clin Q 52:147–154, 1985.

55. Yunus MB, Denko CW, Masi AT: Serum B-Endorphin in primary fibromyalgia syndrome. 1985. Paper presented to Nonarticular rheumatism study group. Los Angeles, June 5, 1985.

56. Bonica JJ: Neurophysiologic and pathologic aspects of acute and chronic pain. Arch Surg 112:750–761, 1977.

56a. Littlejohn GO, Weinstein C, Helme RD: Increased

neurogenic inflammation in fibrositis syndrome (FS). (Abstract #D30) Arth Rheum 29 (No 4)(Supp), 1986.

56b. Lewis T, Kellgren JH: Observations relating to referred pain, visceromotor reflexes and other associated phenomena. Clin Sci 4:47–71, 1939.

56c. Kelly M: The Nature of Fibrositis: I. The myalgic lesion and its secondary effects: a reflex theory. Ann Rheum Dis 5:1–7, 1945.

57. Fowler WM, Taylor RG: Differential diagnosis of muscle diseases. In Musculoskeletal Disorders. Edited by RD D'Ambrosia. Philadelphia, JB Lippincott, 1977.

58. Simons DG: Electrogenic nature of palpable bands and "jump sign" associated with myofascial trigger points. In Advances in Pain Research and Therapy, Vol. I. Edited by JJ Bonica, D Albe-Fessard. New York, Raven Press, 1976.

59. Cobb CR, deVries, HA, Urban RT, et al: Electrical activity in muscle pain. Am J Phys Med 54:80–87, 1975.

60. McBroom P, Russell IJ, Kepler JL: Electromyography in primary and secondary fibromyalgia syndrome. Paper presented to the Nonarticular rheumatism study group, American Rheumatism Association, Minneapolis, 1984.

61. Fowler RS Jr, Kraft GH: Tension perception in patients having pain associated with chronic muscle tension. Arch Phys Med Rehabil 55:28–30, 1974.

62. Tindall E, Campbell SM, Clark S, Moore M, Bennett RM: Pain threshold and psychological disorders in fibrositis: a blinded control study. (Abstract #C92) Arth Rheum 25 (No. 4) [Supp], 1982.

63. Lawrence JS, Bremner JM, Bier F: Osteoarthrosis: prevalence in the population and relationship between symptoms and x-ray changes. Ann Rheum Dis 25:1–24, 1966.

64. Lawrence JS: Disc degeneration: its frequency and relationship to symptoms. Ann Rheum Dis 28:121–138, 1969.

65. Lovshin L: Personal communication.

66. Yunus M, Kalyanaraman UP, et al: Microscopic and radioactive bone scan studies in primary fibromyalgia. (Abstract #E47) Arth Rheum 25 (No. 4) [Supp], 1982.

67. Hench PS, Boland EW: The management of chronic arthritis and other rheumatic diseases among soldiers of the United States Army. Ann Rheum Dis 5:106–114, 1946.

68. Kahn MF: Joint pain complaints linked to three commonly used medications. Orthop Rev 4:73, 1975.

69. Healey LA: Polymyalgia rheumatica and giant cell arteritis. In Arthritis and Allied Conditions, 10th Ed. Edited by DJ McCarthy. Philadelphia, Lea & Febiger, 1985.

70. Williams RC: Clinical picture of rheumatoid arthritis. In Arthritis and Allied Conditions. 10th Ed. Edited by DJ McCarty. Philadelphia, Lea & Febiger, 1985.

71. Carter C, Wilkinson J: Persistent joint laxity and congenital dislocation of the hip. J Bone Joint Surg 46:40–45, 1964.

72. Kirk JA, Ansell BM, Bywaters EGL: The hypermobility syndrome; musculoskeletal complaints as-

sociated with generalized joint hypermobility. Ann Rheum Dis 26:419–425, 1967.

73. Pinals RS, Dalakos TG, Streeten DHP: Idiopathic edema as a cause of nonarticular rheumatism. Arth Rheum 22:396–399, 1979.

74. St John Dixon A: Soft tissue rheumatism: concept and classification. Clin Rheum Dis 5:739–742, 1979.

75. Layzer RB: McArdle's disease in the 1980's. N Engl J Med 312:370–371, 1985.

76. Travell JG, Simons DG: Myofascial Pain and Dysfunction. The Trigger Point Manual, Baltimore, Williams & Wilkins, 1983.

77. Rubin D: Myofascial trigger point syndromes: an approach to management. Arch Phys Med Rehabil 62:107–110, 1981.

77a. Goldman JA: Hypermobility—the missing link to fibrositis. (Abstract #E64) Arth Rheum 28 (No. 4) [Supp], 1985.

78. Hester G, Grant AE, Russell IJ: Psychological evaluation and behavioral treatment of patients with fibrositis. (Abstract #E62) Arth Rheum 25 (No. 4) [Supp], 1982.

78a. McCain GA, Bell D, Mai F, Zilly C: The effects of a double blind supervised exercise program in the fibrositis/fibromyalgia syndrome (FS), (Abstract #D29) Arth Rheum 29 (No 4) (Supp), 1986.

79. Clark S, Tindall E, Bennett R: A double blind crossover study of prednisone in the treatment of fibrositis. (Abstract #D1) Arth Rheum 27 (No. 4) [Supp], 1984.

80. Campbell SM, Gatter RA, Clark S, Bennett RM: A double blind study of cyclobenzaprine versus placebo in patients with fibrositis. (Abstract #D3) Arth Rheum 28 (No. 4) [Supp], 1985.

80a. Brown BR Jr, Womble J: Cyclobenzaprine in intractable pain syndromes with muscle spasm. JAMA 240:1151–1152, 1978.

81. Domino EF: Centrally acting skeletal-muscle relaxants. Arch Phys Med Rehabil 55:369–373, 1974.

81a. Carette S, McCain GA, Bell DA, Fam AG: Evaluation of amitriptyline in primary fibrositis. Arth Rheum 29:655–659, 1986.

82. Lewit K: The needle effect in the relief of myofascial pain. Pain 6:83–90, 1979.

83. Kaplan H: Fibrositis and psychogenic rheumatism. Arthron 3:3–7, 1984.

84. Hunder GG, Hazleman BL: Giant Cell Arteritis and polymyalgia rheumatica. In Textbook of Rheumatology. 2nd Ed. Edited by William N Kelley et al. Philadelphia. WB Saunders, 1985.

85. O'Duffy JD, Warner HW, Hunder GG: Joint imaging in polymyalgia rheumatica. Mayo Clin Proc 51:519–524, 1976.

86. O'Duffy JD: Increasing evidence suggests PMR is not a muscle disease. Wellcome trends in rheumatology 1:1–2, 1979.

87. O'Duffy JD, Hunder GG, Wahner HW: A followup of polymyalgia rheumatica: Evidence of chronic axial synovitis. J Rheumat 7:685–693, 1980.

88. Miller LD, Stevens MD: Skeletal manifestations of polymyalgia rheumatica. JAMA 240:27–29, 1978.

89. Chou CT, Schumacher HR: Clinical and pathologic studies of synovitis in polymyalgia rheumatica. Arth Rheum 27:1107–1117, 1984.

90. Bennett RM: Fibrositis: Does it exist and can it be treated? J Musculo Med June:57–72, 1984.

91. Shulman LE: Diffuse fasciitis with hypergammaglobulinemia and eosinophilia: A new syndrome? J Rheum Supp: 82, 1974.

92. Medsger TA Jr: Systemic Sclerosis (Scleroderma), Eosinophilic Fasciitis, and Calcinosis. In Arthritis and Allied Conditions, 10th Ed. DJ McCarty, Ed. Philadelphia, Lea & Febiger, 1985.

93. Jacobs MB: Eosinophilic fasciitis, reactive hepatitis, and splenomegaly. Arch Intern Med 145:162–163, 1985.

94. Hoffman R, Young N, Ershler WB, Major E, Gewirtz A: Diffuse Fasciitis and Aplastic Anemia: a report of our cases revealing an unusual association between rheumatologic and hematologic disorders. Medicine 61:373–381, 1982.

95. Marinez Tello FJ, et al: Pathology of a new syndrome caused by ingestion of adulterated oil in Spain. Virchows Arch (Pathol Anat) 397:261–285, 1982.

14

Chronic Persistent Pain

Pain is a suffering of the body and mind[1] that can only be known to an individual in his consciousness.[2] Like hunger, pain is an awareness-of-a-need state. It is a drain upon the physical, the emotional, and the economic resources of the patient.[3]

When a person is injured, pain is not always perceived.[4] Consider a football player whose rib is fractured during a tackle; during subsequent active play, the football player may feel no pain. The pain is experienced after play when his attention returns to himself. Thus, pain perception and pain thresholds appear alterable.[5,6] The phenomena of persistent pain in phantom limbs, or magnification of pain by emotion have stimulated researchers to look beyond a simple conduction system within the central nervous system. Experiments to quantify pain thresholds are actively being pursued.[7–9] Anti-pain impulses from the brain areas that descend to the spinal cord have recently been discovered. These and other factors that influence pain are described in this chapter.

The patient with pain as a chief complaint may have a systemic or local illness, a psychiatric illness, or pain that is characteristic for a medical condition but persists after the usual time and treatment. Trigger points usually are absent or are not constant in location or presence. The patients described in this chapter have pain of long duration (more than 6 months) and are unresponsive to any single treatment modality.[10] Persons with chronic persistent pain may have a *primary* psychologic factor or disorder, or may be deemed psychologically normal, but still suffering from pain without foundation. These latter persons are of interest in that they are frequently encountered in medical practice. They do not have features that satisfy a di-

agnosis of fibrositis, or other classifical rheumatic disease; often they began with a backache or headache that slowly progressed over months or years. As will be pointed out, personality changes may be the result of the pain, rather than the cause of the pain.[11]

PSYCHOGENIC PAIN DISORDER

Recently, a classification for chronic pain has been proposed. The American Psychiatric Association has developed the Diagnostic and Statistical Manual of Mental Disorders, 3rd Edition (DSM III). This innovative classification is based upon:

A psychologic and historic component

The medical diagnosis

Numerical scales to quantitate the severity of the psychosocial stress (from 1 to 7) and the highest level of adaptive functioning during the past year (from 1 to 7).

Included are a group of diagnoses, the somatoform disorders where the patient with pain has a significant psychologic component.[12] The psychologic diagnoses may be among the affective disorders, drug dependency, or personality disorders. The method for diagnosis is to list all five axes.

Somatoform Disorders. Criteria for diagnosis include pain that is chronic and severe; the location of the pain fails to correlate with known anatomic distributions; the severity is out of proportion to what one would anticipate; and psychologic factors are implicated as the primary etiology.[12]

Hypochondriasis. The individual has an obsessive rumination over symptoms combined with an inordinate fear of a serious, debilitating illness despite lack of confirmatory findings and medical reassurances.[12]

Conversion Disorder. The patient presents

with an alteration of his physical condition suggestive of an organic disorder. The etiology lies in a definable psychologic factor.

Other features that will suggest psychologic abnormality include excessive "pain talk"; increased anxiety; inappropriate medication; decreased activity or movement; increased bed rest; and unemployment.[10]

Briquet's Syndrome. Patients must have the following to satisfy this diagnosis: A dramatic, vague, complicated medical history with symptoms of physical sickness beginning before age 25. Of the following six groups of symptoms, women must report at least five, and men, four:

1. Sick most of his or her life
2. Loss of sensation, aphonia, walking, pseudoneurologic conversion symptom (e.g., paralysis, blindness) or amnesia (or loss of consciousness)
3. Abdominal pain, vomiting spells
4. More severe than in other women: dysmenorrhea, menstrual irregularity
5. Sexual indifference, lack of sexual pleasure, or pain during intercourse
6. Back pain, joint pain, limb pain, headaches (more than most people)[13]

Pain Prone Disorder. The patient, usually the strongest personality within the family or work group, develops a complaint that never improves. They no longer can function. Features include:

1. A somatic complaint: Pain of obscure origin, hypochondriacal preoccupation; a desire for surgery
2. Patient is a solid citizen: denies conflicts; idealizes self and family relations; was a workaholic
3. Depression: loss of initiative; fatigue; loss of the joy of life
4. History of depression or alcoholism in self or family; abuse by spouse; a crippled relative; or a relative with chronic pain

The condition results from a conflict in which the rigidly maintained ego desires to be independent and to care for others while the emotional needs seek to be dependent and passive.[14]

Alexithymia. Within the group of patients who have a long standing personality disorder and with a generalized or localized pain complaint, are some who cannot express their psychologic conflicts. They have difficulty expressing mood verbally. Alexithymia refers to patients with a limited ability to describe emotions verbally; a paucity of inner fantasy life; their speech and thought are tied to external events; they describe physical symptoms, not emotions.[15]

Other types of purely psychological pain include hysteria, phobic pain (pain that prevents the hand from doing harm), assertive pain (e.g., a compulsive rebel who uses pain to assert control over others),[16] or delusional pain (a psychosis with a well circumscribed delusional system and with pain as the central complaint).[17] The importance of these syndromes lies in early recognition of the need for psychologic care if the physical problems are to be managed. If the workup is nonrevealing, then psychologic evaluation is needed. Often the patient will then, for the first time, tell you that psychologic counseling had occurred in the past; or is on-going! Usually a call to the psychiatrist will confirm the basis of the problem. When the patient first denies any past psychologic care, the reason later given is that "I didn't trust (or like) the psychiatrist and I wanted another opinion." Meantime, another $10,000 workup went down the tube! Fortunately, these patients are not the majority of persons with chronic pain.

PSYCHOLOGIC FACTORS IN PATIENTS WITH CHRONIC PERSISTENT PAIN

Pain may cause temporary changes in personality.[18] Psychologic evaluation of persons who suffer from chronic pain reveals several common deviations including neuroticism and depression. These personality patterns do not, however, relate to future disability or disease outcome.[19-22] In fact, these deviations tend to normalize following relief of the pain.[18] Anxiety, hostility, denial, fear, guilt, hysteria, and depression are associated with changes in pain perception.[16]

In one study, six different personality patterns were defined, yet none of these related to chronicity or to "illness behavior patterns."[21] In another study, examining patients who were undergoing surgery for treatment of painful disorders, affirmative answers to two questions were useful as predictors of a poor outcome: (1) "Has your appetite decreased recently?", and (2) "Has your sexual interest lessened?"[41] In other reports of patients treated nonsurgically, certain other characteristic features were also found that were predictive of an unsuccessful outcome. These included guilt, particularly if related to a supernatural reason given for the illness; projection of guilt onto others, particularly the therapist,[24,25] and pretreatment medication dependency, accident proneness, and expressed dissatisfaction with previous therapy.[26] During care in a comprehensive pain center, these patients opposed psychologic approaches, used circumscribed delusions, and resisted many attempts at treatment. The pain center utilized formal and informal psychologic approaches in an effort to alleviate a "negative—resigned" attitude in such patients.[24]

GATE CONTROL THEORY UPDATED

Melzack and Wall in 1965 suggested that *modulation* of nerve synapses within the dorsal horn of the spinal cord occurs with a feedback control system from other parts of the nervous system. They suggested that each synapse or "gate" may be closed or open to the pain impulses. Thus pain perception is subdued or enhanced by "gates" all along the nerve pathway.[27]

Nerve impulses produced by noxious injury excite "central transmission cells," which receive both excitatory and inhibitory messages from other parts of the nervous system.[28] Substance P, an 11-amino-acid peptide, resides in neurons in the superficial layers of the dorsal horn of the spinal cord.

Following stimulation of peripheral nerves, substance P is released into the spinal fluid. Depletion of substance P produces analgesia to noxious chemical and thermal stimuli.[29] Other mediators include bradykinin, prostaglandins, and hydrogen ions. They arise from tissue injury. Descending anti-pain impulses come from the brainstem and higher centers, such as the analgesic center in the mesencephalon.[5,9,30-35] The analgesic center and its descending anti-pain controls to the spinal cord "gates" are stimulated by non-noxious impulses such as a gentle breeze, love stroking, soft speech, or other soothing sensations. Pain perception results from an interplay of all these influences and is perceived only if the "gates" allow the message to reach the brain.[36] The gate theory has provoked much criticism, debate, and research in the past decade.[37] The criticism was that the system was too simple. Mechanical, thermal, and other sensory systems were probably also involved.

The search for neurotransmitter substances involved in anti-pain transmission led researchers to the discovery of *endogenous* morphine-like peptides, the endorphins,[38-46] which arise within the central nervous system.[41-44] The morphine-like action of these substances is blocked or suppressed by morphine antagonists (e.g., naloxone).[34] Endorphins provide not only a naturally-occurring analgesia but are also involved in regulation of mood and affect. Thus the perception of pain and its modification by emotion have been related to a complex and fascinating neurochemistry.[45] Attempts to prove this remain elusive. Measurement of cerebrospinal fluid beta endorphin yielded an inverse relationship to pain (as expected) but no correlation with mood factors as should also occur.[45] In pain of psychologic origin, cerebrospinal fluid endorphin levels were elevated.[46]

Pain is associated with abnormal firing patterns or after-discharges both in spinal cord cells and in cells of the brainstem reticular formation. Transmitter cells then set up a "pattern-generating mechanism" *for contin-*

ued bursts of firing[9] or reverberating circuits in the internuncial pool.[48] These cells and synapses can be modulated by changes in emotion and behavior (e.g., "rest can relieve pain"). Furthermore, emotional factors may provoke liberation of substances that enhance sympathetic nervous system reflexes.[3] Pain can be modulated further by brainstem inhibitory anti-pain areas. Imbalance in the feedback regulation of the central nervous system results in changes in the sensitivity of pain receptors.

Pain occurs when the number of nerve impulses per unit of time carried from peripheral nerves to the brain areas exceeds a critical level, or when there is a *decreased* input of anti-pain impulses from the analgesic centers located in the mesencephalon. The mesencephalon requires *stimulation* by non-noxious stimuli in order to respond with analgesia.

Because of the intimate relation of stress to illness and the suggestion that stress is linked to ACTH, corticosteroids, and endorphins, we may someday recognize associations of a patient's basic temperament to a specific disease.[44] Quantitative and qualitative determinations of these anti-pain substances perhaps may lead to a better understanding of the relation of tension and anxiety to stress reactions.

DIFFERENTIAL DIAGNOSIS

Virtually any organic disease can cause perplexing pain. Both physical and psychiatric diagnoses must be considered. Often, a relatively common disorder presents in an uncommon fashion. The conditions can only be diagnosed by a comprehensive history and physical examination followed by judicious laboratory and roentgenographic examination. Some categories of diseases to be considered include the connective tissue diseases, neoplastic diseases. occult infections, metabolic disorders, and hematologic diseases. Psychologic causes include affective psychoses, personality disorders, somatoform disorders, organic brain disorders, drug de-

pendency, and neuroses. Often, the patient fits none of these categories and chronic benign pain is an appropriate diagnosis.

THE EXAMINATION

Pain that has persisted longer than 6 months will be approached differently than acute pain. For example, acute infectious processes or fracture are unlikely but not impossible as a cause. The following evaluation must be tailored to each patient.[49]

1. A pain history: Review problem in regard to location, duration, severity; relation to rest or motion; quality; what helps, what makes it worse; what treatment has been tried, with what result.

2. Drug history: occupational history; social factors; psychologic history. Has the patient had psychologic tests or evaluation in the past? Are there any "brick walls": stressful ongoing factors such as a daughter having been raped, an inlaw with organic brain syndrome. Does the patient feel he is exceptionally "charged up" emotionally by any outside factor or event? See Neustadt's series of questions, page 11.

3. General medical history for allergy, other health problems.

4. Physical examination: In addition to a general examination, the patient should be observed arising from a chair, bending over, walking. Note range of joint and spinal motion. The neurologic exam should be thorough. Also, the examination includes palpation for trigger points (Figs. 14–1 and 14–2, and Plates XIV and XV), and sensitivity to palpation noted in nontrigger point areas (such as mid triceps, face, scalp).

5. Psychologic consultation and evaluation should be done when the medical examination has eliminated major disease.

6. Special studies: Certainly a chemical battery that includes a blood sugar, alkaline phosphatase, transaminases, albumen, globulin, and serum iron; CBC; urinalysis; and Westergren erythrocyte

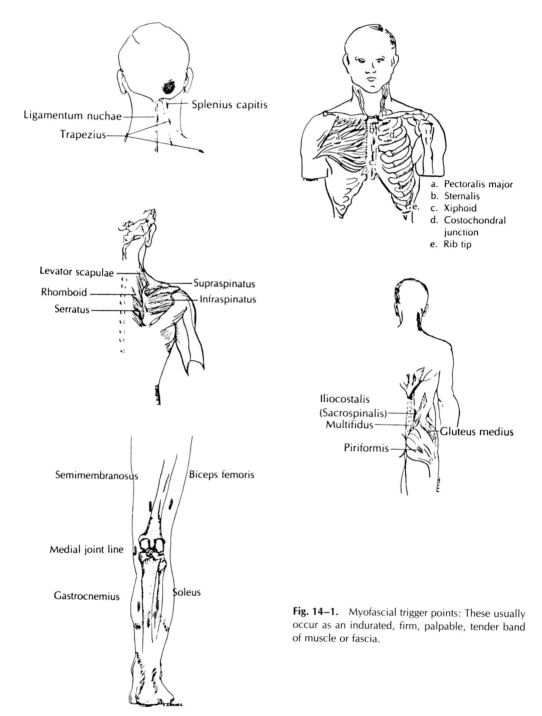

a. Pectoralis major
b. Sternalis
c. Xiphoid
d. Costochondral
   junction
e. Rib tip

Fig. 14–1. Myofascial trigger points: These usually occur as an indurated, firm, palpable, tender band of muscle or fascia.

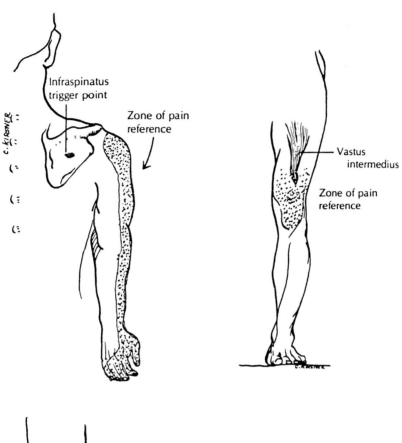

Infraspinatus
trigger point

Zone of pain
reference

Vastus
intermedius

Zone of pain
reference

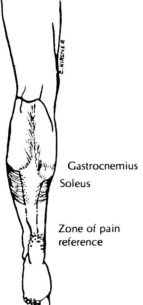

Gastrocnemius
Soleus

Zone of pain
reference

Fig. 14–2. Zones of reference: Upon palpating the trigger point, pain is produced at some distant point. This zone of reference is quite characteristic for each trigger point.

sedimentation rate are appropriate. If indicated, roentgenographic examinations, CT scans, bone scan, electrodiagnostic studies, and specialty consultation may be carried out.

Pain quantification can only be subjectively measured presently. The method most easily used is a visual analogue scale[50] that consists of a horizontal line with each end defined in terms of pain relief ("worst possible pain" at one end, "no pain" at the other end). The patient then draws a hatch line across the horizontal line approximating the severity of pain at that point in time. This technique is in wide use in evaluating drugs under study. The technique is undergoing evaluation for sensitivity and bias.[51] We have found the visual analogue scale to be a fair assessment of the functional severity of pain. When the pain is the "worst possible" in a patient who moves quite well, then psychologic factors are highly likely, in our experience.

MANAGEMENT

Before you begin treatment, decide whether you are treating a predominant physical or psychologic problem. Are drugs or litigation likely to be an issue? Can you reasonably expect to work with the patient for months or possibly, for years? If you do not believe the patient, or feel that you cannot work with the patient, do not accept management; refer the patient to someone more likely to help.[52] Pain games result in the physician calling the patient a "crock", while the patient calls the physician a "quack!" The "Quack-Crock" syndrome arises from an improper approach both by the patient and the physician.[53] You must get the patient off the symptom and on to the medical determination for disability, disease, or etiology. Posner suggests the following to facilitate communication:[53]

—Tell the patient that he should feel free to express needs, ask questions, and express anger.
—Tell the patient that you believe the pain is real.

—Honesty, the ability to teach, and the willingness to listen are essential to the physician-patient relationship.
Provide education techniques
—Write out names, dosage, and intervals of usage of medications for future reference
—Provide backup care—if the medication doesn't work, then call the office.
—Assist the patient to change pain behavior.

At the first visit, we will often employ the six basic points of treatment described in the Introduction of this book. After a careful examination, we have reasonably excluded an organic persisting lesion. (Point One)

We will have run through the patient's "average day" of activities, and interpersonal relationships, looking for aggravating factors. (Point Two)

We will have told the patient that we believe they hurt, and that the pain has persisted for more than an expected duration because. . . . For patients with longstanding psychologic impairment, or with features of a somatoform disorder, we would enlist the aid of a psychiatrist.[53a] (Point Three)

We will provide self-help exercises. Often, getting the patient into a water exercise program using the "Y" programs, the Arthritis Foundation programs, or other health club programs is helpful. (Point Four)

Pain relief is provided with either non-narcotic analgesics, tricyclic antidepressants, nonsteroidal anti-inflammatory drugs, or intralesional soft tissue injections. Local heat, ice, counterirritants may also help. (Point Five)

An expected outcome without perfection is provided. The duration of this program may last for 3 or 4 months. If not helpful, we tell the patient on the first visit that if they try this conscientiously, and it fails, then we will move up to utilizing a psychologist for assisting in relaxation techniques (we have our occupational therapist teach relaxation), biofeedback training, or referral to a pain clinic.

Thus we move from total self help to a support team. (Point Six)

ANTI-PAIN MODALITIES

It has been stated that if *acute* painful disorders were managed more astutely, there would be less *chronic* pain.[54] Pain centers must often deal with the results of less than adequate prior management in these patients. An institution or pain center that provides only one modality of care for these patients is doomed to failure; this inadequate care may likely exhaust the patient's emotional and financial resources.

Oral Drug Therapy

We have emphasized throughout this book that oral medication often plays a minor role in the management of many musculoskeletal soft tissue pain syndromes. When inappropriately used, drug dependence may be as great a problem as the underlying pain disorder. In addition to analgesics and nonsteroidal anti-inflammatory agents, we generally use two additional classes of oral medication. First are the skeletal muscle relaxants such as meprobamate, carisoprodol, and diazepam. These agents are thought to depress the brainstem activating system, to provide a sedative effect, and to have central-acting skeletal muscle relaxant properties.[55] Often they are used only when initiating an exercise program.

The second class of drugs, the tricyclic antidepressants such as amitriptyline, imipramine, desipramine, doxepin, and protriptyline are beneficial for selective patients, particularly those with chronic pain or the fibrositis syndrome. These agents may provide increased relief from pain and reduced need for analgesics.[56–62] It is difficult to separate the pain-sparing effects from the antidepression effect.[63] The tricyclic drugs are generally well tolerated. However, drug interactions have been reported. These include an increased anti-depressant effect with thyroxin, decreased anti-depressant effect as well as marked sedation with alcohol, additive anti-cholinergic effect with anti-Parkinsonism drugs, increased anti-coagulant effect with dicumarol, increased hypotensive effect with guanethidine, and decreased anti-depressant effect with propranolol or methyldopa.[64] Contraindications include glaucoma, urinary retention, and previous hypersensitivity to the drug. They should not be given concomitantly with a monoamine oxidase inhibitor. Central nervous system stimulation with nervousness, insomnia, and heart palpitations occur but are infrequent. Appetite stimulation is a definite problem. These drugs are generally given in small doses before retiring. The initial starting dose should be low, followed by gradual increases until restful sleep is noted. The dose may then be reduced to the lowest effective maintenance dosage; every-other-day dosage may maintain the beneficial effect. The effect on pain management does not fall off with continued use, even after 2 years.[62] We have used amitriptyline for over 20 years in patients with persistent pain (most often, tension vascular headache) and have monitored blood chemistries yearly without a single untoward event thus far!

Placebo therapy also cannot be ignored. If a noneffective harmless medication is given by a physician with an aura of empathy, strength, and assuredness, the patient will more likely evidence a placebo response. Add the same degree of physician "professionalism" to a worthwhile drug and the effect may be dramatic.[65] Caffeine enhances analgesic effects;[66] many patients use too much caffeine, however, and overuse should be avoided.

Rub-ons generally contain salicylates or other counterirritants. They are of short term benefit; the major side effect is local irritation or contact allergy. Arnica, used as a liniment suffers from bad odor as does DMSO.[67] Dimethylsulfoxide (DMSO) has enjoyed a wide press but is of little real therapeutic value.[68] Double blind studies are made difficult by the bad odor (garlic-like) of this agent. Available as a solvent, the analgesic effect has had wide claim but little substance. Percy and Carson employed a 5% placebo compound versus a 70% active compound to test the effect in patients with tennis elbow and shoulder pain. No difference in effect was noted.[69]

EXERCISE THERAPY

Runner's high, and even addiction, attest to the effect of exercise on mood. Part of the pain patient's depression is from the inability to perform tasks, the loss of strength and endurance, and the loss of muscle tone. If pain prevents a resistive exercise, we will often begin with a pool exercise, or a supervised weight-assistive program. Such conditioning might possibly activate the "anti-pain" system.[70] Other pleasant and undemanding sports include fishing, boating, bicycling, (or tricycling) swimming, walking, camping, or pool exercises particularly for persons with lower limb arthritis.

Transcutaneous Electrical Nerve Stimulators (TENS)

Studies have attempted to quantify the role of TENS units in pain therapy. Although they do suggest that use of a TENS unit modifies pain, well demonstrated placebo effects complicate interpretation of the data. Studies are further complicated by the large number and types of TENS units available and the types of pain problems being evaluated.[71-77] Whether the effect is real or placebo, TENS use may at times be beneficial in the treatment of persistent pain if the patient supplements this modality with a total therapeutic program. Placebo response may represent a specific therapeutic modality in that stimulation of endogenous endorphins results.[78,79] The effect does not often last longer than 2 months.[80] TENS units dating from 1854 have been of interest to one of us (RPS)[81] (see Chapter 16 for further discussion and Fig. 16–1).

Implantable (dorsal spinal column) stimulators have been the subject of interest, debate, concern, and guarded enthusiasm and should be considered only in select patients.[72,82]

Acupuncture

Acupuncture and electro-acupuncture received initial enthusiasm in the lay press a few years ago. As previously noted, acupuncture sites often overlap myofascial trigger points. Some 365 acupuncture points have been reported.[83] Pain thresholds may be raised by acupuncture.[5,84] In some studies, short-term pain relief was associated with acupuncture treatment; similar relief occurred in patients treated with placebo acupuncture.[83,85,86] The initial enthusiasm for acupuncture in myofascial and soft tissue pain syndromes has waned.

Biofeedback Training

The application of biofeedback training to relieve muscle tension has been the subject of considerable interest over the last two decades.[87,88] A visual feedback method to facilitate muscle relaxation was first reported a decade ago.[89] Biofeedback training is essentially a reinforcement of muscle reeducation. It attempts to modify autonomic functions, pain, and motor disturbances by acquired volitional control.[87] The technique employs sequential voluntary muscle contraction and relaxation. Electromyography (EMG) provides audible or visible feedback to the patient.[90] Biofeedback training is generally used only as an adjunct to another treatment in order to enhance that therapy.[91] A controlled study of EMG monitored biofeedback for relaxation training recognized that the taking of frequent rest breaks by the anxiety-tension-prone individual may be of equal importance to that of the biofeedback training.[92] In one study of patients with regional musculoskeletal pain, biofeedback resulted in significant muscle relaxation. Subjective pain improved in both the control and treatment sequences.[93] Biofeedback training for reinforcement of muscle reeducation is also helpful in cases of hysterical paralysis, in modifying autonomic nervous system function and pain, and in developing control of motor disturbances.[87] Using biofeedback training for raising skin temperature in patients with Raynaud's phenomenon has been noted (see Chapt. 6).

Biofeedback cannot be used as a single modality to treat patients with complex psychophysiologic abnormalities that often exist in these patients.[94]

Another simple relaxation technique uses a meditation procedure that can be practiced independent of a therapist.[95] The patient is taught how to relax body segments by deep concentration. This technique facilitates rehabilitation, particularly in patients with features of hopelessness and depression.

Transcutaneous nerve stimulators, acupuncture, biofeedback training, and psychotropic drugs are still undergoing clinical evaluation and are to be considered only as adjuncts to a comprehensive treatment plan.[96]

Further Measures

The decade following the publication of the "gate control" theory has been fruitful. The therapeutic measures described in preceding chapters will help the vast majority of patients. For the present, the physician can often *prevent* a chronic pain state by following the six points of management presented in the Introduction. When pain has become chronic (defined as longer than 6 months in duration),[16] the clinician should seek factors that compensate the patient for having pain. Occasionally a state of conflict and anxiety may produce a self-destructive injury-producing act ("the accident process").[97] Such patients may respond best to a group psychotherapy program including role changes in home and work, acquiring new social or personal skills, and other measures to improve the patient's "self image."[98] Biofeedback relaxation or transcutaneous nerve stimulation may improve pain:antipain imbalance. Such measures can succeed only if the physician and patient cooperate in a comprehensive therapeutic endeavor.

Chronic pain may require efforts to correct abnormal learned behavior. Operant conditioning, or behavior modification, as recommended by Fordyce[99] has been helpful in reducing the patient's awareness of pain and in allowing the patient to return to a more natural social existence. Operant conditioning refers to the recognition and removal of anything that enforces or encourages pain. Provision of rewards for proper attitude and behavior may prod a poorly motivated patient.[100]

Pain clinics have been established for many years. John Bonica is perhaps the first to have utilized a multidiscipline approach to pain. His pioneering efforts centered on application of his knowledge as an anesthesiologist but rapidly grew to incorporate the disciplines of psychology, pharmacology, orthopedic surgery, and education specialists. He has, more than anyone, fathered the multiple treatment approach to pain.[3] Pain clinics can be inpatient or outpatient facilities but usually require 3 to 4 weeks of daily attendance. Mood usually improves more than pain; the patient often says "Now I can handle the pain." Employment status, medication use, and other parameters of wellness show improvement.[61,101,102] Few controlled studies are available. Sturgis et al. assessed outcome of patients treated at a pain center compared with patients who had been eligible for such treatment but who had declined the treatment; the followup was obtained by telephone interview an average of 30 months later. No statistical differences were noted in current pain levels, employment status, use of medication or surgery since referral.[103] Sometimes the patient spontaneously improves after several years even without further medical care. When asked what had helped, the patient often does not know; the pain just gradually subsided.

Use of a behavioral diary can be helpful. In it, the patient records daily behavior and subjective experiences. This makes the patient more active in monitoring and assuming responsibility. The physician then becomes an advisor.[52]

Most patients with chronic pain can achieve relief and become effective members of their community and family. To achieve this, the patient, clinician, psychiatric therapist, vocational counselor, insurance personnel, and other "third-party" persons must work together by communicating, trying, and trusting one another.

REFERENCES

1. Webster: The New American Webster Handy College Dictionary. New York, New American Library, Inc., 1972.
2. Merskey H: Psychiatric aspects of the control of pain. *In* Advances in Pain Research and Therapy, Vol I. Edited by JJ Bonica, D Albe-Fessard. New York, Raven Press, 1976.
3. Bonica JJ: Neurophysiologic and pathologic aspects of acute and chronic pain. Arch Surg *112*:750–761, 1977.
4. Wall PD: On the relation of injury to pain: The John J Bonica lecture. Pain 6:253–264, 1979.
5. Mayer DJ, Price DD: Central nervous system mechanisms of analgesia. Pain 2:379–404, 1976.
6. Malow RM, Olson RE: Changes in pain perception after treatment for chronic pain. Pain *11*:65–72, 1981.
7. Lynn B, Perl ER: A comparison of four tests for assessing the pain sensitivity of different subjects and test areas. Pain 3:353–365, 1977.
8. Sternbach RA: Evaluation of pain relief. Surg Neurol 4:199–201, 1975.
9. Melzack R, Loeser JD: Phantom body pain in paraplegics: Evidence for a central "pattern generating mechanism" for pain. Pain 4:195–210, 1978.
10. Addison RG: Chronic pain syndrome. Am J Med 77(3A):54–58, 1984.
11. Hendler N, Fink H, Long D: Myofascial syndrome: response to trigger-point injections. Psychosomatics 24:993–999, 1983.
12. Reich J, Tupin JP, Abramowitz SI: Psychiatric diagnosis of chronic pain patients. Am J Psych *140*:1495–1498, 1983.
13. DeFigueiredo JM, Baiardi JJ, Long DM: Briquet syndrome in a man with chronic intractable pain. Johns Hopkins Med J *147*:102–106, 1980.
14. Blumer D, Heilbronn M: Chronic pain as a variant of depressive disease, the pain-prone disorder. J Nerv & Ment Dis *170*:381–431, 1982.
15. Lesser IM: Current concepts in psychiatry, alexithymia. N Engl J Med *312*:690–692, 1985.
16. Millman BS: Managing intractable pain: Resources and recourses. Drug Ther 8:65–80, 1978.
17. Swanson DW, Swenson WM, Maruta T, McPhee MC: Program for managing chronic pain. Mayo Clin Proc *51*:401–408, 1976.
18. Bond MR: Pain and personality in cancer patients. *In* Advances in Pain Research and Therapy. Vol. I. Edited by JJ Bonica, D Albe-Fessard. New York, Raven Press, 1976.
19. Crown S: Psychological aspects of low back pain. Rheumatol Rehabil *17*:114–122, 1978.
20. Waring EM, Weisz GM, Bailey SI: Predictive factors in the treatment of low back pain by surgical intervention. *In* Advances in Pain Research and Therapy, Vol I. Edited by JJ Bonica, DG Albe-Fessard. New York, Raven Press, 1976.
21. Pilowsky I, Spence ND: Is illness behavior related to chronicity in patients with intractable pain? Pain 2:167–173, 1976.
22. Pheasant HC. The problem back. Curr Pract Orthop Surg 7:89–115, 1977.
23. Forrest AJ, Wolkind SN: Masked depression in men with low back pain. Rheumatol Rehabil *13*:148–153, 1974.
24. Khatami M, Rush AJ: A pilot study of the treatment of outpatients with chronic pain: symptom control, stimulus control and social system intervention. Pain 5:163–172, 1978.
25. Diamond MD, Weiss AJ, Grynbaum B: The unmotivated patient. Arch Phys Med Rehabil *49*:281–284, 1968.
26. Swanson DW, Swenson WM, Maruta T, Floreen AC: The dissatisfied patient with chronic pain. Pain 4:367–378, 1978.
27. Melzack R, Wall PD: Pain mechanisms: A new theory. Science *150*:971–979, 1965.
28. Smukler NM: Pain perception. Bull Rheum Dis *35*(1):1–8, 1985.
29. Levine J: Pain and Analgesia: the outlook for more rational treatment. Ann Intern Med *100*:269–276, 1984.
30. Reynolds DV: Surgery in the rat during electrical analgesia induced by focal brain stimulation. Science *164*:444–445, 1969.
31. Dennis SG, Melzack R: Pain-signalling systems in the dorsal and ventral spinal cord. Pain 4:97–132, 1977.
32. Bloom F, Segal D, Ling N, Guillemin R: Endorphins: Profound behavioral effects in rats suggest new etiological factors in mental illness. Science *194*:630, 1976.
33. Liebeskind JC: Pain modulation by central nervous system stimulation. *In* Advances in Pain Research and Therapy, Vol. I. Edited by JJ Bonica, D Albe-Fessard. New York, Raven Press, 1976.
34. Adams JE: Naloxone reversal of analgesia produced by brain stimulation in the human. Pain 2:161–166, 1976.
35. Procacci P: A survey of modern concept of pain. *In* Handbook of Clinical Neurology, Vol. 1. Edited by PJ Vinken, GW Bruyn. Amsterdam, North-Holland, 1969.
36. Wall PD: Modulation of pain by nonpainful events. *In* Advances in Pain Research and Therapy, Vol. I. Edited by JJ Bonica, D Albe-Fessard. New York, Raven Press, 1976.
37. Nathan PW: The gate-control theory of pain. Brain 99:123–158, 1976.
38. Pert CB, Pasternak G, Snyder SH: Opiate agonists and antagonists discriminated by receptor binding in brain. Science *182*:1359–1361, 1973.
39. Simon EJ, Hiller JM, Edelman I: Stereo-specific binding of the potent narcotic analgesic (^{3}H) etorphine to rat-brain homogenate. Proc Natl Acad Sci USA 70:1947–1949, 1973.
40. Terenius L: Characteristics of the receptor for narcotic analgesics and a synaptic plasma membrane fraction from rat brain. Acta Pharmacol Toxicol 33:377–384, 1973.
41. Guillemin R: Beta-lipotropin and endorphins: Implications of current knowledge. Hosp Pract *13*:53–60, 1978.

42. Guillemin R: Endorphins, brain peptides that act like opiates. N Engl J Med 296:226–228, 1977.
43. Basbaum AI, Fields HL: Endogenous pain control mechanisms: Review and hypothesis. Ann. Neurol 4:451–462, 1978.
44. Rosch PJ: Stress and illness. JAMA 242:427–428, 1979.
45. Bunney WE, Pert CB, Klee W, et al: Basic and clinical studies of endorphins. Ann Intern Med 91:239–250, 1979.
46. Cleeland CS, Shacham S, Dahl JL, Orrison W: CSF endorphin and the severity of pain. Neurology 34:378–380, 1984.
47. Terenius L: Endorphins and modulation of pain. Adv Neurol 33:59–64, 1982.
48. Luce JM, Thompson TL, Getto CJ, Byyny RL: New concepts of chronic pain and their implications. Hosp Pract 14:113–123, 1979.
49. Rowlingson JC, Stehling L: Anesthesia Update #10, the evaluation and treatment of the patient with chronic pain. Orthopaedic Review 11:79–85, 1982.
50. Huskisson EC: Measurement of Pain. Lancet 2:1127–1131, 1974.
51. Carlsson AM: Assessment of Chronic Pain. I. Aspects of the Reliability and Validity of the Visual Analogue Scale. Pain 16:87–101, 1983.
52. Weddington WW Jr: Longitudinal management of chronic pain. Comp Therapy 9:14–20, 1983.
53. Posner RB: Physician-patient communication. Am J Med 78:59–64, 1984.
53a. Smith GR Jr, Monson RA, Ray DC: Psychiatric consultation in somatization disorders. New Engl J Med 314:1407–1413, 1986.
54. Cailliet R: Chronic pain: is it necessary? Arch Phys Med Rehabil 60:4–7, 1979.
55. Domino EF: Centrally acting skeletal-muscle relaxants. Arch Phys Med Rehabil 55:369–373, 1974.
56. Halpern LM: Analgesic drugs in the management of pain. Arch Surg 112:861–869, 1977.
57. Duthie AM: The use of phenothiazines and tricyclic antidepressants in the treatment of intractable pain. S Afr Med J 51:246–247, 1977.
58. Beaumont G: The use of psychotropic drugs in other painful conditions. J Int Med Res 4:56–57, 1976.
59. Richardson JW, Richelson E: Antidepressants: a clinical update for medical practitioners. Mayo Clin Proc 59:330–337, 1984.
60. Spiegel K, Kalb R, Pasternak GW: Analgesic activity of tricyclic antidepressants. Ann Neuro 13:462–465, 1983.
61. Aronoff, GM: Pain units provide an effective alternative technique in the management of chronic pain. Orthop Review 11:95–100, 1982.
62. Blumer D, Heilbronn M: Second-year follow-up study on systematic treatment of chronic pain with antidepressants. Henry Ford Hosp Med J 29:67–68, 1981.
63. Ward NG, Bloom VL, Friedel RO: The effectiveness of tricyclic antidepressants in the treatment of coexisting pain and depression. Pain 7:331–341, 1979.
64. Rosenbaum AH, Maruta T, Richelson E: Drugs that alter mood, tricyclic agents and monoamine oxidase inhibitors. Mayo Clin Proc 54:335–344, 1979.
65. Fields HL, Levine JD: Biology of Placebo Analgesia. Am J Med 70:745–746, 1981.
66. Laska EM, et al: Caffeine as an analgesic adjuvant. JAMA 251:1711, 1984.
67. Penrod DS, Bacharach B, Templeton JY: Dimethyl sulfoxide for incisional pain after thoracotomy. Ann NY Acad Sci 141:493–495, 1967.
68. Committee on Drugs and Committee on Sports Medicine, Am Acad Ped: Dimethyl Sulfoxide (DMSO). Pediatrics 71:76–77, 1983.
69. Percy EC, Carson JD: The use of DMSO in tennis elbow and rotator cuff tendonitis: a double-blind study. Med Sci Sports Exer 13:215–219, 1981.
70. Mellion MB: Exercise therapy for anxiety and depression. Postgrad Med 77:91–98, 1985.
71. McKelvy PL: Clinical report on the use of specific TENS units. Phys Therapy 58:1474–1477, 1978.
72. Eriksson MBE, Sjolund BH, Nielzen S: Long term results of peripheral conditioning stimulation as an analgesic measure in chronic pain. Pain 6:335–347, 1979.
73. Thorsteinsson G, Stonnington HH, Stillwell GK, Elveback LR: The placebo effect of transcutaneous electrical stimulation. Pain 5:31–41, 1978.
74. Sternbach RA, Ignelzi RJ, Deems LM, Timmermans G: Transcutaneous electrical analgesia: a follow-up analysis. Pain 2:35–41, 1976.
75. Timmermans G, Sternbach RA: Human chronic pain and personality: A canonical correlation analysis. In Advances in Pain Research and Therapy, Vol. I. Edited by JJ Bonica, D Albe-Fessard. New York, Raven Press, 1976.
76. Schuster GD, Infante MC: The efficacy of TENS; noninvasive postoperative analgesia. Orthop Rev 8:143–149, 1979.
77. Serrato JC: Pain control by transcutaneous nerve stimulation. South Med J 72:67–71, 1979.
78. Levine JD, Gordon NC, Fields HL: The mechanism of placebo analgesia. Lancet 2:654–657, 1978.
79. Benson H, Epstein MD: The placebo effect: A neglected asset in the care of patients. JAMA 232:1225–1227, 1975.
80. Richardson RR, et al: Transcutaneous electrical neurostimulation in functional pain. Spine 6:185–188, 1981.
81. Sheon RP: Transcutaneous Nerve Stimulation: A not so new panacea. Postgrad Med 75 (No. 5): 71, 1984.
82. Long DM: Electrical stimulation for the control of pain. Arch Surg 112:884–888, 1977.
83. Murphy TM, Bonica JJ: Acupuncture analgesia and anesthesia. Arch Surg 112:896–902, 1977.
84. Ulett GA: Acupuncture treatments for pain relief. JAMA 245:768–769, 1981.
85. Kepes ER, Chen M, Schapira M: A critical evaluation of acupuncture in the treatment of chronic pain. In Advances in Pain Research and Therapy, Vol I. Edited by JJ Bonica, D Albe-Fessard. New York, Raven Press, 1976.
86. Waylonis GW: Long-term follow-up on patients with fibrositis treated with acupuncture. Ohio State Med J 73:299–302, 1977.

87. Rusk HA: Rehabilitation Medicine, 4th Ed. St. Louis, CV Mosby, 1977.
88. Peck CL, Kraft GH: Electromyographic biofeedback for pain related to muscle tension. Arch Surg 112:889–895, 1977.
89. Jacobs A, Felton GS: Visual feedback of myoelectric output to facilitate muscle relaxation in normal persons and patients with neck injuries. Arch Phys Med Rehabil 50:34–39, 1969.
90. Kottke FJ: Therapeutic exercise. In Handbook of Physical Medicine and Rehabilitation, 2nd Ed. Edited by FH Krusen. Philadelphia, WB Saunders, 1971.
91. Shapiro D, Schwartz GE: Biofeedback and visceral learning: clinical applications. Semin Psychol 4:171–183, 1972.
92. DeVries HA, Burke RK, Hopper RT, Sloan JH: Efficacy of EMG biofeedback in relaxation training. Am J Phys 56:75–81, 1977.
93. Large RG, Lamb AM: Electromyographic (EMG) feedback in chronic musculoskeletal pain: a controlled trial. Pain 17:167–177, 1983.
94. Turner JA, Chapman CR: Psychological interventions for chronic pain: a critical review. I. Relaxation training and biofeedback. Pain 12:1–21, 1982.
95. Grzesiak RC: Relaxation techniques in treatment of chronic pain. Arch Phys Med Rehabil 58:270–272, 1977.
96. deJong RH: Central pain mechanisms. JAMA 239:2784, 1978.
97. Hirschfeld AH, Behan RC: The accident process: etiological considerations of industrial injuries. JAMA 186:193–199, 1963.
98. Steinhart MJ: Conversion hysteria. Am Fam Pract 21:125–129, 1980.
99. Fordyce WE: An operant conditioning method for managing chronic pain. Postgrad Med 53:123–128, 1973.
100. Licht S: History. In Therapeutic Exercise. 3rd Ed. Edited by JV Basmajian. Baltimore, Williams & Wilkins, 1978.
101. Cinciripini PM, Floreen A: An evaluation of a behavioral program for chronic pain. J Behav Med 5:375–389, 1982.
102. Bohan A, Wright D, Pewell T, et al: Treatment of chronic pain in the arthritic with rehabilitation and behavioral medicine techniques. (Abstract #E61) Arth Rheum 25 (No. 4) [Supp], 1982.
103. Sturgis ET, Schaefer CA, Sikora TL: Pain center follow-up study of treated and untreated patients. Arch Phys Med 65:301–303, 1984.

15

Intralesional Soft Tissue Injection Technique

Over two decades of experience in the use of local anesthetics or corticosteroid suspensions for soft tissue injection have established both its safety and its effectiveness in therapy.[1] Although it has been stated by some that no statistically valid data are available to support the use of local injection of corticosteroids in the treatment of musculoskeletal disorders,[2] observations by other clinicians support the safety and prolonged benefit of this therapy.[2-4] Furthermore, in this era of concern for cost containment, soft tissue injection is recognized for its value in reducing the need for more complex prolonged medical measures and for surgical intervention.[5-7] Use of intralesional corticosteroids for tendinitis and myofascial disorders involving the shoulder, elbow, hip, knee, and foot has been widely reported. The importance of careful localization of the site of involvement before injection has been pointed out. Carpal tunnel syndrome has been reported amenable to local corticosteroid injections. At least 60%[8,9] of patients treated conservatively can avoid surgical intervention. Tendinitis is particularly helped by intralesional steroid injection. For example, over 70% of patients with stenosing tenosynovitis, "trigger finger," can be successfully treated with this modality without resorting to surgical intervention.[6,7,10] Use of local corticosteroid and lidocaine was more effective and for a longer duration than use of lidocaine alone in the treatment of anserine bursitis.[11] Local injection for myofascial pain is more controversial. Janet Travell popularized the use of procaine and still strongly recommends it for trigger point injection.[12] Trigger points and acupuncture points are at similar locations.[13] Perhaps for that reason,

needle puncture alone may suffice for symptomatic relief.[14,15] But dry needling requires multiple sessions (average is 8 treatments).[15] In a study comparing repeated injections of saline solution with mepivacaine for myofascial pain more pain relief occurred after the first injection in the saline solution group. The subsequent injections resulted in similar pain relief with either saline or mepivacaine lasting 1.5 to 4.5 hours.[16] In another double blind cross-over trial, bupivacaine and etidocaine were superior to saline solution and dry needling.[17] Studies documenting the safety and efficacy of local soft-tissue injections with a crystalline corticosteroid and local anesthetic agent have been reviewed in each chapter. In our experience, a single trigger point injection using a local corticosteroid and a short acting local anesthetic mixture, along with joint protection advice, and the other points in management as detailed in this book, will usually eliminate the trigger point and pain indefinitely (fibrositis excepted). At least 80% of patients respond to this regimen in our experience. Local post-injection pain is alleviated with the application of ice. Obviously the hazards and frequency of injection as detailed in this chapter are important. Patients with fibrositis may require 1 to 6 injections per year.

Epidural steroid injections for the treatment of lumbar disc disease and lumbar spinal stenosis is under investigation. In one study of spinal stenosis patients, pain relief occurred in 11 of 25 patients. The relief persisted for 4 to 16 months.[18] In a controlled study of patients with chronic back pain and sciatica, epidural steroids were compared with procaine alone; no difference was noted.[19] But simple deep paravertebral muscle and presacral/sacroiliac injections using a #22 needle 2.0–3.5 inches long will also provide relief at much less expense. Hollander reported on the safety of local soft tissue and joint injection therapy in over 100,000 injections in 4000 patients.[3] The incidence of infection was less than 1 per 16,000 injections. Others report 3000 or more injections per year (Mayo Clinic) with no untoward reactions,[2,4] In the past 20 years we too have performed thousands of *soft tissue* injections with few complications.

The technique of soft tissue injection has been presented in each chapter. We recommend combining a corticosteroid with a local anesthetic. Some package inserts accompanying the corticosteroid agents suggest that other agents should not be mixed with them; in our experience no untoward reactions have occurred when local anesthetics are mixed in the same syringe with the corticosteroid suspension. The addition of the local anesthetic has the advantage of providing immediate symptomatic relief and also dilutes the steroid preparation, allowing a more diffuse distribution of the drug with less hazard of local tissue atrophy. The total amount of local anesthetic administered to the patient should be kept to less than 6 to 8 ml if possible. Use of local anesthetics without corticosteroids has been advocated by some; this requires more frequent injections[20–22] and is less often effective in subacute or chronic disorders. Recently introduced longer-acting local anesthetic agents, such as bupivacaine and etidocaine, may prove more effective and improve injection technique.[23] Longer acting agents, bupivacaine in particular are cardiotoxic.[24] Sudden death has occurred during their administration. Used for stellate ganglion block, we have seen one cardiac arrest occur. Magnetic resonance imaging revealed myotoxicity of bupivacaine with the abnormality persisting for up to 10 days.[25]

The addition of a corticosteroid suspension is recommended for the following reasons: (1) benefit is often longer lasting and in most cases one injection suffices, (2) the safety of infrequent injections has been established by time, (3) more frequent injections with a local anesthetic alone increase the risk of inadvertent intravenous instillation of the anesthetic, (4) reactions to local anesthetics are proportional to the number of sites injected as well as the volume and total dosage utilized at any one time, and (5) the addition of the corticosteroid reduces the necessity to locate and inject every trigger point; rather, only the most prominent trigger point need be injected; the less significant lesions usually also improve.

A local anesthetic-corticosteroid injection facilitates an exercise and physical therapy regimen. It is one of the few regional analgesic-anti-inflammatory techniques that is suitable for everyday practice and requires little special training.[1,20] In the treatment of entrapment neuropathies, tendinitis, tenosynovitis, or bursitis, the local anesthetic-corticosteroid injection results in such predictable benefit that diagnosis is assisted by the resulting benefit.

INDICATIONS

Use of soft tissue injection is indicated in traumatic, inflammatory, or degenerative processes of the musculoskeletal system, especially when associated with local tenderness or trigger points;[4,20] to assist in confirming the diagnosis of bursitis, tendinitis, and entrapment neuropathies; and in certain periarticular soft tissue conditions that can lead to limitation of motion. In these situations, injection is helpful in providing a more rapid resumption of active range of motion, thus preventing more serious sequelae.[2]

CONTRAINDICATIONS

Hypersensitivity to any anesthetic preparation is rare but can occur.[1,26] Dermal allergy is less common with lidocaine and its derivatives.[26] Soft tissue injection is obviously contraindicated in the vicinity of infections. A relative contraindication is an extremely apprehensive or neurotic patient.[20] Injections into tendon areas are contraindicated in any-one who tends to overuse these structures, which may result in tendon rupture.[27]

HAZARDS

A corticosteroid agent for soft tissue injection should be used with some caution in patients who have had previous peptic ulcers or diabetes, or who are using anticoagulants. The diabetic who is taking insulin may be advised to use a sliding scale of increased insulin dosage for 1 or 2 days following the injection based upon the result of fractional urine sugar determinations. Aggravation of the diabetic state is rarely a problem. Application of local compression following soft tissue injection avoids significant hematomas in most patients receiving anticoagulants. An *active* peptic ulcer is a relative contraindication to a local corticosteroid injection. Local injections with corticosteroids should also be used with caution, if at all, in patients with recent thromboembolic disease, pneumonia, or active systemic infection.[20] Introducing infection has become remarkably rare since the introduction of disposable needles and syringes.[3]

The complications of systemic corticosteroids are widely recognized. The interval between injections as recommended in this chapter should prevent systemic complications known to result from prolonged corticosteroid use. Furthermore, the problem of corticosteroid pseudorheumatism will be avoided.[25]

Certain hazards are related to the specific site of injection. A pneumothorax may result when soft tissue injections are made into the chest or trapezius regions.[29] Intravascular injection or hematoma formation is a risk following injection of the popliteal, antecubital, or groin regions. Reflex sympathetic dystrophy and nerve injury with paralysis may follow inadvertent injection of a neurovascular bundle, but are rare complications.

Although tendon rupture following local steroid injection may occur, this complication is infrequent if injections are made around, rather than directly into the tendon, and if overexertion is avoided for a week or longer. Most research supports the finding that harmful effects of corticosteroids on tendons generally result from use of massive corticosteroid doses.[30] In one study, rabbits' Achilles tendons were partially transected and then injected with 0.3 mg/kg triamcinolone acetonide at 2, 8, 14, and 20 days, and compared to a control group that were injected with equal volumes of normal saline solution. The saline treated animals had a greater final tendon weight, 66% more adhesions, and superior mechanical properties of failure load, strain and energy to failure as compared to the steroid injected animals. Thus, repeated administration of local steroids should be performed with caution, and in the lowest possible dose for palliation of tendon injuries.[31] In other studies comparing soluble versus relatively insoluble steroid preparations injected into musculotendinous junctions of rabbits, then examined up to 30 days later, findings revealed the insoluble corticosteroids were associated with more local inflammation and calcium deposits than that seen with the soluble steroids; however, when these agents were mixed with lidocaine, no calcium deposits had developed.[32] When physiologic doses of steroids are injected directly into rabbit tendons, the injury returned toward normal after 2 weeks. Therefore, athletes who receive intralesional steroid injections are urged to rest the involved limb for at least 2 weeks.[30] Bowstring deformity of a digit following corticosteroid injections for flexor tenosynovitis has been described but is rare.[33] Corticosteroid injections into the region of the Achilles tendon should never be performed, since tendon rupture at this site is a disastrous complication. Patellar tendon rupture following a corticosteroid injection is a distinct hazard in athletes.[34] Experimental studies of corticosteroid injections into rabbit tendons using usual therapeutic doses revealed disorganization of collagen and a 35% loss of tendon strength; this healed within 14 days.[30]

The use of these agents as described here

may be associated with specific pharmacologic or hypersensitivity reactions:

Local Anesthetics. (Table 15–1.) Accidental intravenous introduction of the local anesthetic agent may result in central nervous system or cardiovascular reactions. These effects may depend on the blood levels of the agents, which in turn depend upon the site of the injections, the number of sites injected, and the dose. A linear relationship exists between reactions and the total dose of the local anesthetic.[26]

Central nervous system effects include lightheadedness, dizziness, visual or auditory (tinnitus) complaints, slurred speech, muscle twitching, or muscle tremors, particularly about the face.[26] Cardiovascular effects include prolongation of the conduction time with resultant bradycardia, and stimulation of vascular smooth muscle contractions. Another rare hazard of local anesthetics is anaphylaxis.[26] More severe reactions following intravenous injection include clonic and tonic convulsions, shallow respirations, diminished blood pressure and pulse rate, and finally, cardiorespiratory collapse. These reactions may begin 5 to 15 minutes or even several hours following the injections.[20] Serious hypersensitivity or toxic reactions are more likely to occur when large amounts of local anesthetic are used for soft tissue injection therapy.

The clinician should have an airway, oxygen, intravenous diazepam, short-acting parenteral barbiturates, phenylephrine, epinephrine, and rapid-acting intravenous corticosteroids available for emergency use.[20,26]

More common than the serious reactions described is the more immediate vasovagal reaction seen in patients with vasomotor instability. The vasovagal reaction occurs within seconds following the injection. The patient becomes pale, sweaty, and lightheaded, and may faint. The pulse rate is slow but blood pressure remains normal. A crushable ampule of ammonia is helpful for use in such patients.

Table 15–1. Local Anesthetics in Current Use[26]

Anesthetic agents	Concentrations available	Duration of action (Min)
Procaine (Novocaine)	1–2 mg/ml	50
Lidocaine (Xylocaine) (Dilocaine) (L-Caine) (Nervocaine) (Nulicaine) (Ultracaine)	10–15–20 mg/ml	100
Chloroprocaine (Nesacaine)	10–20 mg/ml	60
Mepivacaine (Carbocaine)	10–20 mg/ml	100
Prilocaine (Citanest)	10–20–30 mg/ml	60
Bupivacaine (Marcaine)	2.5–5 mg/ml	175
Etidocaine (Duranest)	2.5–5–10 mg/ml	200

Table 15–2. Corticosteroids in Current Use

Corticosteroids	Concentrations available	Dose range
Prednisolone tebutate (Hydeltra TBA)	20 mg/ml	5–15 mg
Betamethasone acetate and disodium phosphate (Celestone Soluspan)	6 mg/ml	1.5–3 mg
Methylprednisolone acetate (Depomedrol)	20–40–80 mg/ml	10–20 mg
Triamcinolone acetonide or diacetate (Kenalog, Aristocort)	10–25–40 mg/ml	5–15 mg
Triamcinolone hexacetonide (Aristospan)	5–20 mg/ml	5–20 mg
Dexamethasone acetate suspension (Decadron-LA)	8 mg/ml	0.8–3.2 mg

Focal muscle injury, which is proportional to the potency and duration of action of the local anesthetic agent, may occur and is usually reversible.[26] Localized nerve damage has not been seen following use of a local anesthetic agent unless the injection is inadvertently made into a nerve.

Corticosteroids. Systemic toxicity from local injections of corticosteroids is infrequent if the interval between subsequent injections is longer than 6 weeks and the number of injections is less than 8 per year.[35] Adrenal suppression may occur but is usually transient.[36] Local complications include infections, which will be rare if the clinician uses disposable equipment and careful aseptic techniques.[35] Although infection is a rare complication, the patient should report any post-injection development of pain, redness, or swelling.[20] Local cutaneous atrophy or depigmentation may occur;[20,37] the atrophy usually resolves but may require weeks or months to regress. A postinjection "flare" or local crystal reaction occurs in 1 to 2% of patients receiving steroid injections, and is ameliorated with ice packs.[38] When triamcinolone preparations are used for injection in women, menstrual irregularity, breast tenderness, and skin flushing can occur.

Corticosteroids used for local injections

Table 15–3. Soft Tissue Injection—Helpful Points on Technique[40]

1. Mark site of injection with circular end of ball point pen.
2. Prepare a sterile field; use gloves or sterile technique.
3. Use the shortest needle that will reach the lesion.
4. For injecting tender points, use the needle as a probe.
5. For injecting tendon sheaths, insert the needle parallel to the tendon.
6. At site of nerve entrapment, wait a moment after needle is inserted; be certain the needle has not penetrated a nerve or vessel.
7. Use 1 or 2% local anesthetic *without epinephrine.*

should be the repository preparations in suspension.[20] We generally use the dose ranges given in Table 15–2 for any given injection site depending on the size of the area and the total number of sites to be injected.[1] Although we prefer to use procaine or lidocaine in a 1% solution and the methylprednisolone acetate or triamcinolone acetonide, the preparations, cost, availability, and personal experience will assist each clinician in choosing the most suitable agents. The addition of ep-

Table 15–4. Soft Tissue Injection Technique[40]

Injection site	Needle size, no.	Needle length, inches	Local anesthetic, ml	Crystalline steroid, mg	Comments
Temporomandibular joint	25	¾	0.5	10–20	Have mouth open
Cervical TP	23	1	0.5–1.0	5–20	Use needle as a probe
Trapezius or scapular TP	20–23	1	0.5–1.0	10–20	
Shoulder tendons	22	½–2	1.0–2.0	20	Watch for twitch response
Epicondyle elbow	23	1	1.0	20	Inject tender spot and tendon
Carpal tunnel	23	1	1.0	20–40	Inject radial side of palm. Longus
Hand tendons	25–27	½	0.25	5–10	Distal to tendon nodule
Chest or thorax TP	25	1	1.0	20	Inject intercostal nerve, also
Erector spinae TP	20	2	1.0–2.0	20	Determine if needle site
Gluteus TP	20	2–3½	1.0	20	reproduces sciatica, if present
Trochanteric bursitis	20	1½–3½ (spinal)	1.0–3.0	40	Use needle as probe for TP
Fascia lata fascitis	20	2	0.5–1.0	5–10	May have 6–12 sites along fascia
Knee and foreleg	20	1–2	1.0	20	Avoid peroneal nerve
Tarsal tunnel	23	1	1.0	20–40	Avoid nerve and vessels
Plantar fascia	23	1	0.5	10–20	Locate at least 3 TPs
Intermetatarsal bursitis	25	¾	0.5	5–10	Just proximal to web of toes

Note: TP = trigger point.

inephrine to the local anesthetic is not recommended.

TECHNIQUE

Prior to injection the point of maximum-
tenderness should be located by palpation.
Then the clinician can use the open end of
the needle container cover to indent and
mark the trigger point location.[39] Strict skin
sterilization is essential. If iodine is used, a
history of iodine sensitivity should be sought
prior to skin preparation. We do not routinely
use sterile gloves, although the clinician may
feel more comfortable doing so. The use of a
sterile finger cot may be helpful. Raising a
skin wheal before deep injection is not as essential since the introduction of disposable
needles that are sharp and without barbs. A
vapocoolant spray such as ethylchloride may
provide surface anesthesia if desired.

A No. 20 spinal needle 4 inches long may
be necessary for injecting the piriformis muscle, the trochanteric bursa, or the low back
region. On the other hand, a No. 25, No. 26,
or No. 27 dermal needle $\frac{1}{2}$ inch long is most
appropriate for a "trigger finger" tendon injection. Between these extremes is carpal
tunnel injection with a No. 22 or No. 23
needle, 1 inch long. In myofascial pain disorders, the needle point may be used as a
probe to reproduce the patient's pain.

Although we much prefer use of a corticosteroid-anesthetic mixture, some clinicians
may wish to use a local anesthetic agent alone.
A total of 1 to 20 ml of a local anesthetic
repeated daily or as required for relief has
been recommended.[20] Reportedly, 5% of persons are refractory in response to procaine
and similar local anesthetic compounds.[20] Use
of jet injectors or similar devices has been
limited by the necessity for daily care and
cleaning of the delivery instrument.[20]

Pitfalls to Injection Therapy. These injections are not solvents for hypertrophic or degenerated tissue![20] The injection must be part
of a comprehensive program for soft tissue
rheumatic pain as described throughout each
section of this book. Among the pitfalls lead-

ing to failure are the following:[20] (1) a wrong
diagnosis or incorrect localization of the soft
tissue rheumatic pain site, (2) advanced or
irreversible changes, (3) uncorrected contrib-
utory factors such as poor body mechanics,
or systemic factors that are unrecognized or
untreated, (4) multiple lesions that are unrecognized, (5) refractoriness to "caine" drugs
if used alone, (6) treatment of subjective complaints without findings, and (7) persons who
are hypersensitive or who have low pain
thresholds.

If infection is suspected, local injection
therapy should not be used until infection has
been excluded. A previous mild crystal reaction or a vasovagal reaction is not an absolute contraindication to future reinjection.

Frequency of Injections. How often and
how many times a soft tissue lesion should be
injected requires common sense. Disorders
known to be occasionally stubborn in their
response, such as a carpal tunnel syndrome
or a thickened olecranon bursitis, may best
be treated by surgery rather than by many
repeated local injections.

Repeated need for injection of the same site
should raise the possibility of continued strain
or aggravation. Review of work, hobby, sport,
or homemaking activity should be undertaken. In general, more than 3 corticosteroid-
anesthetic injections over a short period of
time into the same site should be avoided.

REFERENCES

1. Moskowitz RW: Clinical Rheumatology. 2nd Ed.
   Philadelphia, Lea & Febiger, 1982.
2. Fitzgerald RH: Intrasynovial injection of steroids;
   uses and abuses. Mayo Clin Proc 51:655–659, 1959.
3. Hollander JL, Jessar RA, Brown EM: Intra-synovial
   corticosteroid therapy: A decade of use. Bull Rheum
   Dis 11:239–240, 1961.
4. Finder JG, Post M: Local injection therapy for rheumatic diseases. JAMA 172:2021–2030, 1960.
5. Alexander SJ: Cost containment in carpal tunnel syndrome. Arthritis Rheum 22:1415–1416, 1979.
6. Phalen GS: Soft tissue affections of the hand and
   wrist. Hosp Med 7:47–59, 1971.
7. Clark DD, Ricker JH, MacCollum MS: The efficacy
   of local steroid injection in the treatment of stenosing
   tenovaginitis. Plast Reconstr Surg 51:179–180, 1973.
8. Wolin I: The management of tenosynovitis. Surg
   Clin N Am 37:53–62, 1957.

9. Moore L, Bernat J, Taylor T: Carpal tunnel syndrome: A conservative management program. (Abstract #143) Arth Rheum 26 (No. 4) [Supp], 1983.

10. Janecki CJ: Extra-articular steroid injection for hand and wrist disorders. Postgrad Med 68:173–181, 1980.

11. Larrson L, Baum J: The syndrome of anserina bursitis: An overlooked diagnosis. Arth Rheum 28:1062–1065, 1985.

12. Simons DG, Travell JG: Myofascial origins of low back pain—1. Principles of diagnosis and treatment. Postgrad Med 73:66–108, 1983.

13. Melzack R, Stillwell DM, Fox EJ: Trigger points and acupuncture points for pain: Correlations and implications. Pain 3:3–23, 1977.

14. Lewit K: The needle effect in the relief of myofascial pain. Pain 6:83–90, 1979.

15. Gunn CC, Milbrandt WE, Little AS, Mason KE: Dry needling of muscle motor points for chronic lowback pain. Spine 5:279–291, 1980.

16. Frost FA, Jessen B, Siggard-Anderson J: A Control, Double-Blind comparison of mepivacaine injection versus saline injection for myofascial pain. Lancet 1:499–501, 1980.

17. Hameroff SR, Crago BR, Blitt CD, Womble J, Kanel J: Comparison of Bupivacaine, Etidocaine, and Saline for Trigger-Point Therapy. Anesthesia Analgesia 60:752–755, 1981.

18. Hozman R, Eisenberg G, McLaughlin D, Arnold W: Epidural steroid injection (ESI) in the treatment of lumbar spinal stenosis (SS). (Abstract #93) Arth Rheum 27 (No. 4) [Supp], 1984.

19. Cuckler JM, Bernini PA, Wiesel SW, Booth RE, Rothman RH, Pickens GT: The use of epidural steroids in the treatment of lumbar radicular pain. J Bone Joint Surg 67A:63–66, 1985.

20. Steinbrocker O, Neustadt DH: Aspiration and Injection Therapy in Muscoloskeletal Disorders. New York, Harper and Row, 1972.

21. Swezey RL, Weiner SR: Rehabilitation Medicine and Arthritis. In Arthritis and Related Conditions, 10th Ed. Edited by DJ McCarty. Philadelphia, Lea & Febiger, 1985.

22. Brown BR: Myofascial and musculoskeletal pain. Inst Anesthiol Clin 21:139–151, 1983.

23. Brown BB: Diagnosis and therapy of common myofascial syndromes. JAMA 239:648, 1978.

24. Health: Adverse reactions with Bupivacaine. Health Human Services Bull, pg 23, 1983.

25. Newman RJ, Radda GK: The myotoxicity of bupivacaine, a ^{31}P N.M.R. investigation. Br J Pharmac 79:395–399, 1983.

26. Covino BG, Vassallo HG: Local Anesthetics: Mechanisms of Action and Clinical Use. New York, Grune and Stratton, 1976.

27. Sweetnam R: Corticosteroid arthropathy and tendon rupture. J Bone Joint Surg ₹1:397–398, 1969.

28. Rotstein J, Good RA: Steroid pseudorheumatism. Arch Intern Med 99:545–555, 1957.

29. Shafer N: Pneumothorax following "trigger point" injection. JAMA 213:1193, 1970.

30. Kennedy JC, Willis RB: The effects of local steroid injections on tendons: A biomechanical and microscopic correlative study. Am J Sports Med 4:11–21, 1976.

31. Kapetanos G: The effect of the local corticosteroids on the healing and biomechanical properties of the partially injured tendon. Clin Ortho Research 163:170–179, 1982.

32. Trapp RG, Hill JJ, Su C, Mody N: Effects of injectable corticosteroids on extra-articular soft tissues of the extremities (Abstract #D56) Arth Rheum 28 (No. 4) [Supp], 1985.

33. Gottlieb NL, Riskin WG: Complications of local corticosteroid injections. JAMA 243:1547–1548, 1980.

34. Ismail AM, Balakrishnan R, Rajakumar MK. Rupture of patellar ligament after steroid infiltration. J Bone Joint Surg 51B:503–505, 1969.

35. Hollander JL: Arthrocentesis technique and intrasynovial therapy. In Arthritis and Allied Conditions. 10th Ed. Edited by DJ McCarty. Philadelphia, Lea & Febiger, 1985.

36. Reeback JS, Chakraborty J, English J, et al: Plasma steroid levels after intra-articular injection of prednisolone acetate in patients with rheumatoid arthritis. Ann Rheum Dis 39:22–24, 1980.

37. Cassidy JT, Bole GG: Cutaneous atrophy secondary to intra-articular corticosteroid administration. Ann Intern Med 65:1008–1018, 1966.

38. McCarty DJ, Hogan JM: Inflammatory reaction after intrasynovial injection of microcrystalline adrenocorticosteroid esters. Arth Rheum 7:359–367, 1964.

39. Finkel RI: Personal communication.

40. Sheon RP: Chapter 8. Non-Articular Rheumatism and Nerve Entrapment Syndromes in Rheumatic Therapeutics, edited by S.H. Roth. New York, McGraw-Hill Book Co., 1985.

16

Physical and Occupational Therapy

Physical therapy including physical modalities, and passive and active exercise has been emphasized in every chapter. Disuse leads to cellular and tissue deterioration; in one writer's opinion, lifetime physical exercise holds more promise for sustained health than does any drug in current or prospective use.[1]

Exercise might also act to stimulate the immune system! There is some evidence that exercise increases granulocytosis, lymphocytosis, interleukin-1 and in turn, this increases host defense mechanisms.[2]

Occupational therapy refers to joint work rather than on-the-job work. We will review the principles for joint protection, and the common sense advice that has been gleaned from real life experience of living with arthritis and chronic soft tissue rheumatic disorders.

This chapter presents the rationale for exercise of various types, and the modalities that might help ease pain and provoke more rapid use of an exercise program. Much of this therapy is empiric; we have presented in other chapters the data we could find to support or weaken the argument for the use of these methods of adjunctive care.

Patients with soft tissue rheumatic pain syndromes often become sedentary as a result of their chronic symptoms. Frequently they have poor muscle tone, or they have used muscles inappropriately. However, soft tissue rheumatic pain can also occur in active people and athletes. The goal of an exercise program is to correct local or general body pathophysiology that has resulted in loss of normal function.[3,4] The specific exercise program must be individualized, based on a prior appropriate evaluation of the musculoskeletal system in each patient.[5]

There is much to learn in the science of conditioning exercise. Whether exercises are performed for correction of a postural disorder or for development of endurance, a fundamental knowledge of the basic aspects of rehabilitation are necessary. For example, stretching exercises cannot be performed effectively without first providing for relaxation of the involved muscles. Sometimes assisted stretching exercise must be augmented by using brief contractions of agonist muscles in order to induce relaxation of antagonists.[4] More simply, we tell patients that they must obtain increased muscle length before they can accomplish muscle strength.

Ligamentous and capsular structures tend to shorten when normal tension or stretching forces are interrupted.[4] The strength and length of flexor muscles should be in balance with opposing extensor muscles. An exercise program must also provide proper posture and proper rest positions in order to prevent muscle fatigue.

Flexibility is the ability to yield to passive stretch and then to relax; flexibility helps to facilitate action with minimal resistance to the tissues. Flexibility in boys increases from ages 6 to 10 and then declines at age 16. In girls flexibility peaks at age 12. In studies of 16-year-old athletes, swimmers and baseball players had greater flexibility, whereas wrestlers were least flexible.[6] After age 25 there is a general and steady loss of flexibility. Stretching exercises designed to produce a greater range of motion have resulted in significant improvement in flexibility; the improvement continues for many weeks after the cessation of exercises. Lack of flexibility may lead to muscle "brittleness" and soft tissue rheumatic complaints.

GOALS OF THERAPEUTIC EXERCISE

The obvious overall goal is to obtain maximum independent function and efficiency within the limits imposed by the musculoskeletal condition.[1] The specific objectives may be listed as follows:[5]

1. Develop a sense of good body alignment.
2. Relax unneeded musculature to permit smooth coordinated efficient motion.
3. Increase muscular strength as needed to attain and maintain good alignment and function.
4. Achieve flexibility within a normal range.
5. Maintain and increase joint range of motion.

EVALUATION FOR AN EXERCISE PLAN

Therapists should determine the potential response capabilities of the patient's musculoskeletal system. This potential is based on an assessment of strength, range of movement, functional ability, and any abnormal skeletal motion.[3] Range of motion determination has already been described. Numerous methods and standards for range of motion determination have been critically analyzed, and the interested reader should refer to the chapter "Clinical Assessment of Joint Motion" by Margaret L. Moore in Basmajian's excellent test, Therapeutic Exercise.[7]

THE TYPE OF EXERCISE

Most likely the clinician will refer the patient to a qualified physical therapist. The clinician should provide the therapist with the diagnosis, which body regions are of concern, and what goals the clinician and patient have established. The physical therapist should evaluate the patient and then develop an exercise plan which should be communicated to the clinician. Most of the exercises we are concerned with in soft tissue rheumatic pain conditions involve mobilizing and stretching exercises.

Exercises are categorized as passive, active, active assisted, and resistive. These terms refer to the amount of effort the patient undertakes in performing a therapeutic exercise. If the therapist alone performs a movement of the patient's musculoskeletal system, the activity is "passive." If the patient performs the activity with some help by the therapist the exercise is "active assisted." If the patient performs without assistance, the exercise is "active." And if the exercise is performed against weight, it is defined as "resistive."[4]

Strengthening as opposed to mobilizing exercise has been the subject of much research in recent years. This modality may be added to the exercise program once the muscles have responded favorably to the mobilizing exercise plan. Strengthening exercises may be categorized as static or isometric, dynamic or isotonic, or isokinetic. These refer to the performance of a resistive exercise without joint motion (static-isometric); exercise with joint motion and against resistance (dynamic or isotonic); or exercise against a machine that provides a defined time and rate of movement of the joint (isokinetic).[8] A technique recommended for myofascial pain syndromes is postisometric relaxation. Lewit and Simons studied this in 244 patients and noted immediate pain relief in 94%.[9] The technique begins by placing the muscle in a stretched position followed by an isometric contraction; then relaxation and again, a gentle stretch.

Recommendations regarding the pace of exercise vary. In the DeLorme system,[10,11] a gradually increasing amount of resistance is applied to achieve strength; in the modified DeLorme (Oxford) technique,[12] a maximum resistance weight is determined for a given exercise, and then after performing with maximum weight, the load is gradually reduced. The number and duration of repetitions of resistance exercise are further components of the specifically prescribed program. The isokinetic exercise machine (e.g., the Nautilus equipment) is helpful because it provides a quantitative evaluation of the patient's progress.[8]

Throughout this text, certain brief exercises utilizing activities of 5 to 10 seconds' duration with momentary rest between efforts have been described. We wish to stress that muscle training is an extremely complex process; there is no one right way. Different techniques have been effectively utilized to achieve the same goal for a given condition. It is wise to urge the patient to allow the therapist to develop an exercise plan unique for that patient. This can seldom be provided on a single visit. Some clinicians prefer to take the time to teach the patient the exercise program themselves, rather than depend upon a physical therapist. If this is done, we recommend the patient return and demonstrate the exercises after several weeks of unsupervised therapy at home. A planned graduated exercise program must be based on periodic reevaluation.[3]

Therapeutic exercise can be overdone. Pain may result from improper performance, improper diagnosis, or too vigorous a program. We ask the patient to accept discomfort that lasts no longer than 20 minutes following the exercise performance. Others will allow up to 3 hours of discomfort.[3] Short periods of exercise repeated during the day are preferred to a prolonged single daily session.[4] We recommend that the exercise program take no more than 20 to 30 minutes per session. Most of our patients require less than 10 minutes of exercise twice daily. An overly prolonged muscle contraction is self-defeating since ischemia induced by the contraction reduces the muscle's own blood supply.[13] When strength is desired, the exercise should eventually be carried to the point of muscle fatigue.[8] Strengthening exercises are not nearly as painful as are mobilizing exercises of tissues that suffer from adhesions, such as in adhesive capsulitis or frozen shoulder.

EXERCISES FOR CONDITIONING AND FITNESS

The physical fitness goals of aging Americans have led to a whole new industry that centers around aerobic exercises. The goal is to improve health, control weight, and improve mood.[14] Certainly, the effects of aerobic exercise on reduction of coronary thrombosis are well established. Running or jogging 2 or 3 days a week for a total weekly mileage of 15 or 20 miles is acceptable if lower limb alignment is satisfactory. Swimming is nearly as good. For those with less stable lower limbs, bicycling, swimming, or cross-country skiing may be advisable. For persons with lower limb arthritis, water aerobics, or the Arthritis Foundation water exercise program provided by the "Y" 's (YMCA/YWCA) may be acceptable. Encourage the patient to begin gradually. Just walking 30 minutes in divided sessions is a beginning. Then adding 3 to 10 pound hand weights can help condition for further effort.

Aerobic exercise uses large muscles and achieves a heart rate about 80% of the maximum for the person's age. It improves tendon elasticity, muscle efficiency, and vital capacity. In addition, studies of dance aerobics demonstrated that participants had an increase in high density lipoprotein, and a decrease in percent of body fat and low density lipoprotein. A well-designed program will provide a warm-up and cool-down of sufficient duration.[15] In addition, asthmatics, hypertensives and those with stress are helped by aerobic exercise.

Exercises for the traveler during prolonged sitting may help relax muscles, prevent stiffness, tension, and headache:[16]

1. Cross left leg over right. Make circle with your left foot, first one direction, then reverse. Reverse legs—cross right leg over left and perform rotation with right foot.

2. Lift right knee off seat as far to the chest as possible; hold. Repeat with left knee. Repeat. Stretch right leg out in front, stretch and repeat with left leg.

3. Sit with toes on the floor, heels slightly raised. Keep back straight, stomach muscles tight. Slowly lower heel to floor, first the left then the right. Then raise each heel. Repeat.

4. Sit straight, shoulders back. Rotate head on a full circle. Reverse. Move head side to side; touch chin on chest; hold. Stretch

head back as far as possible; hold; then flex chin; repeat.

5. Stretch arms in front at shoulder level. Flex wrists up and down. Bend elbows, touch shoulders with fingers, bring elbows straight up, then down. Repeat.

6. Bend elbows, point palms outward. Stretch fingers open, then close. Repeat. Make hands into fists. Hold. Repeat. Press palms together in front of you, hold. Repeat. Hook fingers and pull arms as hard as you can. Repeat.

7. Reach for ceiling with right hand, hold. Repeat with left hand.

8. Sit up straight. Draw in stomach. Clasp arms in front of you, bend forward and stretch clasped arms toward floor. Repeat.

9. Make a circle with your right shoulder—up, down, around. Repeat with left shoulder.

10. Clasp arms at elbows. Turn to left side 3 times. Turn to right side 3 times. Repeat.

If you are annoying your neighbor passenger, buy him a drink!

Of course there are contraindications to exercise. Some that should be under consideration include a history of unstable angina, arrhythmias, excessive medication effect, heart failure, severe aortic stenosis, other severe cardiovascular diseases, thrombophlebitis, recent infection, and use of high dose of phenothiazine agents.[17] A careful history and consideration for any health problem should precede an exercise prescription.

ADJUNCTS TO AN EXERCISE PROGRAM

In order to provide increased blood flow, reduce muscle irritability, and raise the pain threshold, either moist heat or ice may be applied before performing the exercise.[4] Diathermy is a rather expensive form of heat. Ultrasound, also a heat modality, may facilitate extensibility of soft tissues.[18] Biofeedback training and transcutaneous nerve stimulation may increase general relaxation before performing an exercise.

A controlled study of biofeedback in patients with regional pain of 6 months' duration

revealed significant improvement in pain and in electromyographic activity of the involved muscles.[19] However, the control group noted pain relief without improved electromyographic activity. In a similar group of patients, auriculotherapy (electrical stimulation of the outer ear) failed to provide significant pain relief.[20]

Ice massage, friction massage, or vapo-

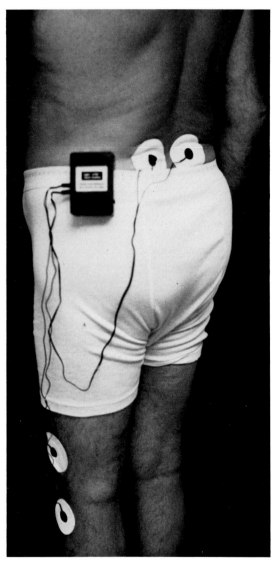

Fig. 16–1. One of several types of transcutaneous electric nerve stimulators with electrodes in place for sciatica.

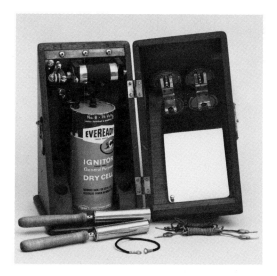

Fig. 16–2. Battery run transcutaneous nerve stimulator manufactured between 1900 and 1910.

coolant spray can be simple but effective measures for pain control that permit an exercise plan to proceed. These techniques have been described in previous chapters. They require the assistance of another person or therapist. Two rather recent high tech techniques for pain control include the TENS unit and the cold laser.

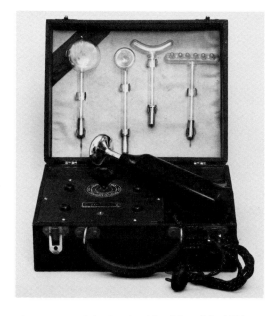

Fig. 16–3. "Violet Ray Machine," Swedish, 1931.

TENS (Transcutaneous nerve stimulation) can induce a change in neuronal activity. The use of electricity for medical purposes was recently reviewed.[21] Electric eels were used by the ancients; hand cranked (produced in 1856) and battery operated TENS models sold through mail order catalogs (1900–1910) were in wide use for the treatment of numerous illnesses. (Figs. 16–1 to 16–4). Present day models provide low current frequency with a longer pulse width. Proper placement of the electrodes and proper amplitude is essential and may require a trained therapist to test the device applied to several locations.[22,23] In one study intraarticular temperature rose significantly following application of TENS to rabbit joints.[24] This would suggest a physiologic tissue effect of the TENS unit. However O'Brien et al. could find no evidence that TENS altered experimental pain threshold or plasma Beta endorphin levels.[25] Studies to date have suggested a strong placebo effect; but in many cases the TENS unit was the best of many analgesic measures.[26,27] In a controlled study of patients with fibrositis and tendinitis, TENS use has been helpful.[28] Similarly, a controlled study suggested that a TENS unit may provide pain relief for patients with osteoarthritis of the knees, although a significant number of patients also had relief of at least 3 weeks' duration with a placebo unit.[27]

Patients with persistent pain and spasm may respond to transcutaneous nerve stimulation; however, many investigators remain skeptical. One author states that use of percutaneous currents has been resurrected by the desire for alternatives to traditional physical therapy and to provide a market for the electronics industry.[24] Another author states that transcutaneous stimulation is a safe placebo.[30] If so, it is expensive. Yet transcutaneous nerve stimulation, if successful, does allow the patient to participate in treatment (Fig. 16–1). Instructions regarding the proper variation of the electric current and frequencies, and the regions of application such as to painful areas, dermatomes, or distal sites must be provided.[29,31]

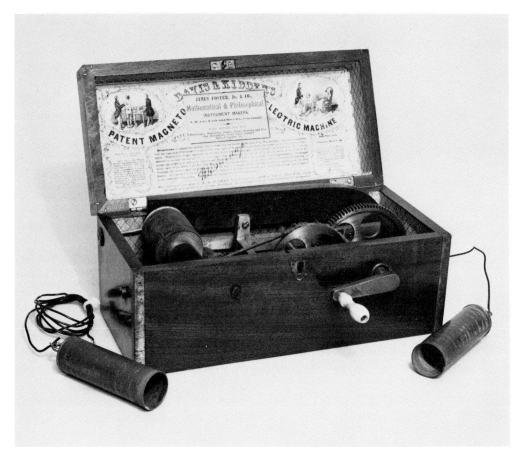

Fig. 16–4. Hand cranked electric nerve stimulator, 1856.

Laser (Light Amplification by Stimulated Emission of Radiation) therapy is not an approved form of treatment in humans at this time. Anecdotal reports of benefit followed application for tendinitis, osteoarthritis, backache, and other soft tissue disorders. The use in humans occurred as a result of the use of an infrared diode laser to treat race horses. The literature accompanying this unit, the Pegasus II laser, states that it has a wavelength of 904 nanometers, and can penetrate 35 mm depth. It is claimed that it does not increase tissue temperature to serious levels. Thus the term "cold laser". The claim for therapeutic benefit rests on a presumption that it increases blood flow, modifies intracapillary pressure, and stimulates immune processes. Also, it is alleged that this energy results in increased mitotic activity and tissue regeneration.[32] A double blind study with placebo control using a helium neon laser in the treatment of osteoarthritis suggested benefit. In addition, treatment of trigeminal neuralgia, post-herpetic neuralgia, and sciatica resulted in pain relief without drug therapy in 19 of 26 patients. Sham treatment resulted in no pain relief.[33,34] Use of Gallium aluminum sulfate laser treatments compared to sham control treatments applied to osteoarthritic hand joints also demonstrated significant pain relief with laser treatment.[35]

PASSIVE EXERCISES

Laying on of hands is an act of religious and loving connotation. Caressing, stroking, or rubbing can stimulate endorphin production and perhaps induce analgesia. The use of massage, friction massage, manipulation, and traction therapy are extensions of this idea. A technique for friction massage helpful in tendinitis is shown in Figure 16–5. Swezey provides an extensive review of these techniques.[36] As was pointed out in Chapter 8, spinal manipulation should be restricted to the trunk; manipulation of the cervical spine is hazardous. Manipulation of the low back works best in acute back pain, no leg pain, and no neurologic deficits.[37] Patients who have recurrences tend to have longer duration of pain and underlying psychologic abnormality.[38] Acupuncture, acupressure, rolfing, moxa, and cupping have been used in various societies up to the present time. Most studies suggest that their major benefit lies in a powerful placebo effect.

Sports medicine and conditioning accidents are treated with a time honored RICE regimen:[39] Rest, Ice, Immobilization, Compression, and Elevation. These passive measures are used to reduce the inflammation of injury, and allow resumption of training once healing has progressed.

Probably the most important adjunct to physical therapy is the relationship developed between the therapist and the patient.

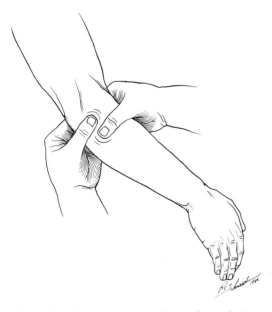

Fig. 16–5. Friction massage technique for tendinitis.

A therapy program achieves success only after a proper evaluation, the establishment of reasonable goals, individualization of the exercise prescription, proper pacing of the exercise program, and last and most importantly, motivation of the patient to the performance of a diligent exercise plan. If a patient is looking for a "magic bullet," less effective results are to be anticipated. We can help best those patients most willing to help themselves.

OCCUPATIONAL THERAPY

The occupational therapist assists by teaching patients how to perform tasks with less joint work and stress. The therapist uses a discipline known as joint protection. Joint protection measures may provide an immediate reduction in pain, inflammation, and stress to the joints, and are easily demonstrated for use in the clinic or office. Although they are widely accepted as important to the care of patients with deforming arthritis,[40–43] the techniques have not been widely adapted to patients with non-articular rheumatic problems.

The aims of joint protection are[43] *disability prevention* and the *enhancement of performance*. These aims require that joint protection reduce local joint stress and preserve joint integrity. The use of pain as a signal for the patient to moderate activity is important. Therapy must provide for the use of proper body mechanics, posture, and positioning. Work simplification, reduction of musculoskeletal effort, and avoidance of staying in one position are also important. Lastly, these programs teach the use of stronger and larger joints where possible.[40] Patient compliance in using these principles and techniques is essential.

Implicit in these measures is the ability to recognize and avoid those aggravating habits and activities that can initiate or perpetuate symptoms.[44] Whether the regional disorder is a bursitis, tendinitis, fasciitis, myofascial pain, structural disorder, or a nerve entrapment problem, they share similar aggravating factors that are common to each body region.

Table 16–1. A Joint Protection Guide for Non-Articular Rheumatism (from Sheon[44])

Harmful	Helpful
Head and Neck	
■ Sitting or standing for more than 30 minutes can induce more neck strain than lifting heavy objects.	■ Alternate tasks in which the body does not move (e.g., knitting) with tasks that allow the body greater movement (e.g., sweeping).
■ Lying on a sofa with the head propped forward, falling asleep in a chair and allowing the head to drop forward, or lying on more than one thin pillow stretches the muscles at the back of the neck. Hours later, these muscles may go into spasm, resulting in headache, stiff neck, or limited neck movement.	■ Align the entire trunk, chest, and head on a slanted wedge or a very large pillow to watch television or read in a reclining position. Anyone with hiatus hernia, sinus trouble, or heart disease who has been told to sleep in a propped-up position should elevate the entire mattress or the head of the bed rather than simply putting two or three pillows under the head.
■ Sleeping on the stomach can strain the neck.	■ Sleep on the side or the back, keeping the arms below the level of the chest.
■ Clenching the jaw can cause muscle spasm in the neck.	■ Use a bite spacer, relaxation techniques, or muscle relaxants.
■ Storing items in the kitchen at a level that is too high or too low can strain the neck.	■ Store items that are used daily no higher than shoulder height or lower than knee level. If storage is a problem, use a step stool to avoid tilting the head excessively.
■ Working too close to work materials can strain the neck.	■ Maintain the proper hand-to-eye distance of 16 in. (about 40 cm)). Position work materials in such a way that the neck remains straight. Place a computer screen at eye level.
■ Incorrectly using the telephone can cause neck pain.	■ If both hands must be free during phone conversations, use a speaker phone or a shoulder holder briefly.
Shoulder	
■ Repetitively moving the shoulder to and fro while holding the elbow out to the side pinches tendons inside the shoulder.	■ Frequently interrupt such tasks as washing windows, vacuuming, and working on an assembly line. Keep the elbow close to the body during to-and-fro movement. When raking or sweeping, hold the rake or broom out in front of the body. Doing so changes the angle of shoulder motion.
■ Sleeping with the arms overhead can pinch muscles and nerves in the shoulder region.	■ Sleep with arms below the level of the chest.
■ Similarly, working with the arms overhead for prolonged periods can be injurious.	■ Take frequent breaks when working with the arms overhead.
■ Using the shoulder as a weight-bearing joint (e.g., when leaning on crutches or canes or pushing off from chairs) can lead to shoulder injury.	■ See that crutches fit 2 in. (about 5 cm) below axillae; carry weight on ribs. A forearm cane may be preferred. When arising from a chair, push off with thigh muscles, not the hands.

Table 16–1. *Continued*

Harmful	Helpful
■ Reaching sideways and backward into the back seat of a vehicle to bring a briefcase, grocery bag, or other object forward is a common cause of pain in the shoulder-blade region.	■ Face the object and draw it forward.
■ Repetitively reaching behind for a kitchen utensil and bringing it forward has a similar effect.	■ Turn the body, not just the shoulder, and grasp the utensil.
■ Placing the hands on top of the steering wheel for long periods can be irritating to nerves and muscles in the shoulder region.	■ Keep the hands below the 3- and 9-o'clock positions on the wheel. If possible, use a steering wheel that tilts.

Elbow

Harmful	Helpful
■ Using the elbow to push the body up when arising from bed or to prop it up when sitting	■ Use the abdominal muscles to help roll the body out of bed; when sitting, keep the elbows in space.
■ Repeatedly using tools that must be twisted and forced (e.g., screwdriver, pipe wrench) may injure tendons near the elbow. Improperly gripping golf clubs, rackets, or other pieces of sports equipment may be injurious to the elbow.	■ Grip tools less tightly; use foam-plastic pipe insulation (sold at hardware stores) on tool handles; take frequent short breaks. Learn the proper techniques for gripping various pieces of sports equipment.
■ Unconsciously clenching the hands while sleeping or driving may produce elbow pain.	■ Wear gloves (seams to the outside) to bed. Use a padded steering wheel. Learn to use relaxation techniques.

Wrist and hand

Harmful	Helpful
■ Repetitively moving the fingers excessively, such as occurs in typing, peeling vegetables, knitting, needlepointing, playing cards, and some types of assembly-line work, is the most common cause of carpal tunnel syndrome (numbness, tingling combined with a sensation of swelling, and weak finger grip), tendinitis, trigger finger, and trigger thumb.	■ Restrict repetitive tasks to 20-minute periods separated by a short break. Keep the hands flat and open rather than making tight fists. Pad the handles on utensils and tools and the steering wheel with pipe insulation. Use stronger, larger joints for assistance. Use the palms and forearms to carry heavy objects. Push, slide, or roll objects instead of lifting them. Use both hands as much as possible when lifting heavy objects.
■ Writing, stapling, or using scissors for long periods can cause hand injuries.	■ Use pencil holders and pad the stapler; take frequent breaks.
■ Pushing off from chairs, clenching the hands, writing for prolonged periods, or doing work that requires repetitive wrist or hand motion can result in carpal tunnel syndrome.	■ Keep the hands off chairs when arising; be aware of hand clenching and wear gloves to bed if necessary; interrupt lengthy writing sessions. Consult an occupational therapist about work-induced problems.

Chest wall and upper trunk

Harmful	Helpful
■ Carrying heavy objects (e.g., logs, grocery bags) across the chest can strain muscles in the chest wall and cause sudden, severe chest pain.	■ Turn and face the object, then lift it, and use the body, not just the arms, to carry it.

Table 16–1. *Continued*

Harmful	Helpful
■ Smoking-induced coughing aggravates chest wall pain.	■ Stop smoking!
■ Sleeping with the arms overhead can pinch nerves, which in turn can cause chest wall muscles to tighten up.	■ Sleep with arms below the level of the chest.
■ Arching the spine backward during exercise or while working with the arms overhead (e.g., painting a ceiling) can lead to bursitis of the spine.	■ Cautiously try extension exercises; discontinue if painful. Do not arch backward while working with the arms overhead.

Low back

Harmful	Helpful
■ Having weak abdominal muscles puts a strain on the low back.	■ If possible, perform exercises that strengthen the abdominal muscles and then *use* these muscles. Always keep them contracted.
■ Shoveling snow, weeding the garden, or lifting heavy objects can cause an acute attack of back pain, often referred to as "a catch in the back."	■ Lie on the back and elevate the legs with a sofa cushion placed under the ankles, not the knees; place moist heat packs under the back, then do numerous knee-to-chest lifts.
■ Bending over with the knees locked can injure the back.	■ Always bend at the knees, not at the waist.
■ Twisting at the waist while holding large or heavy objects can cause back strain, as can constantly carrying an object, such as a young child, to one side of the body.	■ Turn or rotate the entire body by moving the feet. Draw the object to the chest, lift it with the arms held stiff, and use the thigh muscles for strength. Hold the object centered in front of you.
■ Standing for prolonged periods, especially on a concrete surface, rapidly tires the back muscles.	■ Place one foot atop a 2 × 4 × 8-in. (about 5 × 10 × 20-cm) wood block for a while and then alternate, thus transferring body weight from one foot to the other. Wear rubber-soled shoes when working or walking on concrete.
■ Having one leg that is more than 0.5 in. (1.3 cm) shorter than the other should not be overlooked as a cause of back pain.	■ Have shoes for the foot of the shorter leg built up.
■ Sitting for too long can strain the back.	■ Sit on a bar stool; doing so is uncomfortable and promotes frequent changes of position. Break up desk work and card games by standing up and moving around every 30 minutes. Use cruise control, if available, when driving long distances.
■ Doing strenuous physical work or engaging in a sports activity on an occasional or weekend basis can lead to back pain.	■ Do trunk-stretching warm-up exercises before engaging in any strenuous activity.
■ Sleeping on the stomach or flat on the back can cause backache.	■ Sleep on one side or on the back with the knees and feet elevated with a cushion or pillow.

Table 16–1. *Continued*

Harmful	Helpful
Coccyx and buttock region	
■ Sitting or falling hard often results in pressure injury to the coccyx, or tailbone.	■ Protect the point of tenderness at the tip of the coccyx by using a foam-rubber or sponge-like cushion that is at least 3 in. (about 8 cm) thick and the size of a seat cushion. Cut a 3-in. circle out of the center of the cushion with a bread knife. For at least a month following injury, place the cushion under the tailbone whenever seated or doing exercises on the floor.
■ Bending over with the knees locked is a very common cause of pain in the buttock region. Persons who can touch the floor with their palms are likely to bend improperly.	■ Always bend at the knees, not at the waist.
■ Applying pressure to the sciatic nerve, such as occurs with a ruptured disk, direct injury, constriction of the spinal canal (spinal stenosis), or muscle spasm adjacent to the nerve, can result in sciatica. Sciatica is a symptom complex of pain, numbness, and tingling radiating from a buttock to below the knee. Another cause of leg pain is bursitis at the side of the hip. Here again, bending over with the knees locked is a common causative factor.	■ Take proper care of the back by strengthening and using the abdominal muscles to support the back, attaining and maintaining ideal weight, avoiding prolonged periods of sitting or standing, wearing rubber-soled shoes when working or walking on concrete, assuming proper rest and sleep positions, and performing trunk-stretching exercises before engaging in strenuous activities.
■ Carrying a large wallet in a back pocket can cause sciatica. Similarly, wearing a tight belt, leaning over a drafting table, or improperly positioning a seat belt can put pressure on a nerve, causing numbness, tingling, and a burning sensation in the lateral hip and thigh region.	■ Check for pressure placed on the pelvic bones by a wallet, belt, or workbench and, if present, remedy the situation. Learn to wear seat belts correctly.
Knee	
■ Pushing off from chairs with the hands wastes the quadriceps muscle.	■ Keep the hands in the lap when arising from a sitting position.
■ Repetitively twisting the knee while dancing or exercising can damage it.	■ Modify or avoid knee-twisting dance steps and exercises.
■ For some persons, bicycling can strain the knee.	■ Pace bicycling if it causes knee pain.
■ Engaging in sports activities on an occasional or weekend basis without proper conditioning or warm-up is potentially harmful to the knee.	■ Engage in sports activities regularly to stay in condition. Do warm-up exercises.
■ Climbing stairs repeatedly is irritating to the knee.	■ Limit stair climbing. If lack of a toilet on the first floor necessitates stair climbing, one solution is to place a portable commode somewhere on the first floor.
■ Sitting for prolonged periods allows the muscles behind the knee to tighten up.	■ Limit sitting to 30 minutes, then move around.

Table 16–1. *Continued*

Harmful	Helpful
■ Having certain foot disorders can result in poor alignment of the leg bones, which in turn affects the knee.	■ Consult a physician.
■ Wearing shoes having worn-down heels can aggravate knee problems.	■ Buy shoes with proper heels and check them for signs of excessive wear.
■ Working on the hands and knees on a hard surface can result in bursitis in the front of the knee. Also known as water on the knee and housemaid's knee, this swelling is visible in front of the kneecap.	■ Instead of working on the hands and knees, use a mechanic's or milker's stool; either one sits low to the ground. Sit with the legs apart and reach forward to perform, with little effort, such tasks as gardening and washing floors.

Leg

■ Some forms of leg cramps appear to be inherited. Persons who have nocturnal leg cramps tend to have similarly afflicted family members, as do those with daytime leg cramps. The precipitating mechanism is not clearly understood.	■ Stretch the calf muscles by performing the following maneuver. Stand 3 ft (about 1 m) from a wall and lean forward, placing the hands on the wall. Keep the bare feet flat on the floor; do *not* allow the heels to rise. With the outstretched arms touching the wall, walk the palms upward on the wall as if climbing the rungs of a ladder. Reach as high as possible, until the heel cords are stretched to the maximum. Maintain this position for 30 seconds, then walk the palms down the wall. Perform this maneuver three times each before supper, after supper, and bedtime, and at bedtime for one week. Doing so often prevents nocturnal leg cramps. To alleviate a cramp in progress, apply ice or a hot shower spray to the most tender muscle.

Ankle and foot

■ Being loose-jointed may provoke repeated ankle injury, with the ligaments at the outside of the ankle giving way and tearing.	■ Wear low-heeled shoes that tie up close to the ankle; high-necked shoes that tie above the ankle may give less support to the ankle. Good walking shoes have rubber soles and stiff heel counters.
■ Having flat arches, a condition common in loose-jointed persons, may cause joint and muscle fatigue. Working on a hard surface, standing in one position for prolonged periods, or being overweight compounds the problem.	■ Use arch supports if deemed necessary by a physician. Many loose-jointed, flat-footed persons have no ankle problems and thus do not need arch-preserving shoes.
■ Wearing shoes with crepe soles, many of which are too flexible to support the metatarsal area, can be injurious.	■ Invest in a pair of running shoes. One of the best-designed types of shoes available, they are cushioned, have a moderate arch, and shift body weight back toward the ankle and away from the metatarsal arch, or ball of the foot.

Table 16–1. *Continued*

Harmful	Helpful
■ Wearing slippers or moccasins or going barefoot aggravates metatarsal and toe pain.	■ Try running shoes for everyday use. Always wear shoes that shift body weight behind the metatarsal arch and that tie or buckle to keep the feet from slipping forward.
■ Walking and/or standing on concrete (which we all are doing increasingly) promotes joint and muscle fatigue. This is true even when the concrete is covered with carpeting.	■ Select shoes with rubber soles, which act as shock absorbers.
■ Squeezing the forefoot, which tends to widen with age, into too narrow a shoe may cause nerves to be pinched between the bones of the toes. Having bunions can also be problematic. Neuralgia, with a burning sensation and aching pain in the forefoot radiating to the toes (usually the third and fourth), is symptomatic of improper shoe fit.	■ Ensure that shoes fit properly. Sometimes, use of an external metatarsal bar helps to spread the toe bones. Wear shoes with enlarged toe boxes to accommodate troublesome bunions. Fortunately, today's specialty shoe stores usually stock shoes having extra depth and enlarged toe boxes.
■ Having burning pain in the feet at night suggests a pinched nerve at the ankle or neuritis caused by diabetes or a nutritional deficiency.	■ Consult a physician.

Recognition and avoidance of the aggravating or perpetuating habit or factor can be a simple therapeutic effort and might eliminate progression of the regional disorder to a more severe and widespread condition of "chronic benign pain".[45] Joint protection along with the removal of aggravating and perpetuating habits may be cost effective. Some examples of joint protection advice for the various body regions are provided in the Table 16–1.[44]

Two other formal programs that incorporate these principles are the back school and work hardening. This educational program for low back pain, when combined with a physical therapy program was superior to placebo treatment.[46] Work hardening is an occupational therapy program for industrial rehabilitation that was discussed previously. The program can result in improved strength, flexibility, endurance, and decreased functional limitations and disability.[47]

REFERENCES

1. Bortz WM: Disuse and aging. JAMA 248:1203–1208, 1982.
2. Simon HB: The immunology of exercise. A brief review. JAMA 252:2735–2738, 1984.
3. Rusk HA: Rehabilitation Medicine. 4th Ed. St Louis, CV Mosby, 1977.
4. Swezey RL, Weiner SR: Rehabilitation medicine and arthritis. In Arthritis and Allied Conditions. 10th Ed. Edited by DJ McCarty. Philadelphia, Lea & Febiger, 1985.
5. Daniels L. Worthingham C.: Therapeutic Exercise for Body Alignment and Function. 2nd Ed. Philadelphia, WB Saunders, 1977.
6. Allman FL: Exercise in sports medicine. In Therapeutic Exercise. 3rd Ed. Edited by JV Basmajian. Baltimore, Williams & Wilkins, 1978.
7. Moore ML: Clinical assessment of joint motion. In Therapeutic Exercise. 3rd Ed. Edited by JV Basmajian. Baltimore, Williams & Wilkins, 1978.
8. DeLateur BJ: Exercise for strength and endurance. In Therapeutic Exercise. 3rd Ed. Edited by JV Basmajian. Baltimore, Williams & Wilkins, 1978.
9. Lewit K, Simons DG: Myofascial pain: relief by postisometric relaxation. Arch Phys Med Rehabil 65:452–456, 1984.
10. DeLorme TL: Restoration of muscle power by heavy-resistance exercises. J Bone Joint Surg 27:645–667, 1945.
11. DeLorme TL, Watkins AL: Techniques of progressive resistance exercise. Arch Phys Med 29:263–273, 1948.
12. Zinovieff AN: Heavy-resistance exercises; the "Oxford techniques." Br J Phys Med 14:129–132, 1951.
13. Liberson WT: Brief isometric exercises. In Therapeutic Exercise. 3rd Ed. Edited by JV Basmajian. Baltimore, Williams & Wilkins, 1978.
14. Leach RE: Rx exercise: Effects and side effects. Hosp Pract 16:(Jan):72a–72w, 1981.

15. Rosenbaum J: What do you know about aerobics? Medical Times (Jan):105–107, 1985.
16. Travel notes: Exercise break. Northwest Orient 15:58, 1984.
17. Kirkendall DT: Exercise prescription for the healthy adult. Primary Care 11:23–31, 1984.
18. Gersten JW: Effect of ultrasound on tendon extensibility. Am J Phys Med 34:362–369, 1955.
19. Large RG, Lamb AM: Electromyographic (EMG) feedback in chronic musculoskeletal pain: a controlled trial. Pain 17:167–177, 1983.
20. Melzak R, Katz J: Auriculotherapy fails to relieve chronic pain. JAMA 251:1041–1043, 1984.
21. Sheon RP: Transcutaneous Nerve Stimulation: A not so new panacea. Postgrad Med 75 (No. 5): 71, 1984.
22. Bengston R, Warfield CA: Physical therapy for pain relief. Hosp Prac (Aug):84e–84s, 1984.
23. Policoff LD: Effective use of physical modalities. Orth Cl No Am 13:579–586, 1982.
24. Weinberger A, Dalith M, Toren A, Volovsky P, Pinkhas J: Intraarticular temperature and pressure changes following transcutaneous electrical stimulation of the rabbit joint. (Abstract #C11) Arth Rheum 27 (No. 4) [Supp], 1984.
25. O'Brien WJ, Rutan FM, Sanborn C, Omer GE: Effect of transcutaneous electrical nerve stimulation on human blood beta endorphin levels. Phys Therapy 64:1367–1374, 1984.
26. Thorsteinsson G, Stonnington HH, Stillwell GK, et al: Transcutaneous electrical stimulation: a double-blind trial of its efficacy for pain. Arch Phys Med Rehabil 58:8–13, 1977.
27. Lewis D, Lewis B, Sturrock RD: Transcutaneous electrical nerve stimulation in osteoarthrosis: a therapeutic alternative? Ann Rheum Dis 43:47–49, 1984.
28. Fitzcharles M, Banks E, St Pierre J, Dent R, Osterland CK: A double-blind comparison of transcutaneous electrical nerve stimulation (TENS) and placebo in soft tissue rheumatism. Ann Rheum Dis 43:110, 1984.
29. Rusk HA: Rehabilitation Medicine, 4th Ed. St. Louis, CB Mosby, 1977.
30. Swezey RL, Weiner SR: Rehabilitation medicine and arthritis. In Arthritis and Allied Conditions. 10th Ed. Edited by DJ McCarty. Philadelphia, Lea & Febiger, 1985.
31. McKelvy PL: Clinical report on the use of specific TENS units. Phys Therapy 58:1474–1477, 1978.
32. Gugger T: The Laser defined. Pegasus II, advertisement.
33. Willner RE, Castel C: Laser beam for arthritic pain. Geriatric consultant (Jan/Feb):21, 1985.
34. Walker J: Relief from chronic pain by low power laser irradiation. Neurosci Letter 43:339–344, 1983.
35. Abeles M, Marlowe S, Ingenito F: Treatment of osteoarthritis of the hand with low power infrared laser. (Abstract #E39) Arth Rheum 28: (No. 4) [Supp], 1985.
36. Swezey RL: The modern thrust of manipulation and traction therapy. Seminars Rheum Dis 12:321–331, 1983.
37. Haldeman S: Spinal manipulative therapy. Clin Orth 179:62–70, 1983.
38. Hoehler FK, Tobis JS: Psychological factors in the treatment of back pain by spinal manipulation. Br J Rheum 22:206–212, 1983.
39. Birrer RB: Sports medicine rheumatology. Clin Rheum in Pract 2:196–208, 1984.
40. Melvin JL: Rheumatic disease: occupational therapy and rehabilitation. FA Davis, Philadelphia, 1982, 351–377.
41. Rossky E: Joint conservation and protection. Rehabilitation management of rheumatic conditions. Edited by G. Ehrlich. Baltimore, Williams & Wilkins, 1980, 234–242.
42. Lorig K, Fries JF: The arthritis helpbook. Reading, Addison-Wesley, 1980, 67–112.
43. de Blecourt JJ, Wood PHN, Badley EM: Aims of rehabilitation for rheumatic patients. Clin Rheum Dis 7:291–304, 1981.
44. Sheon, RP: A joint protection guide for nonarticular rheumatism. Postgrad Med 77 (No. 5):331–337, 1985.
45. Cailliet R: Chronic Pain: Is it necessary? Arch Phys Med Rehabil 60:4–7, 1979.
46. Berquist-Ullman M, Larsson UL: Acute low back pain in industry. A controlled prospective study with special reference to therapy and confounding factors. Acta Ortho Scand 170:1–117, 1977.
47. Matheson LN, Ogden LD, Violette K, Schultz K: Work hardening: occupational therapy in industrial rehabilitation. Am J Occup Therapy 39:314–321, 1985.

Appendix

The following tables are a quick reference for those illustrations that pertain to injections and to exercises.

Illustrations for Intralesional Injections

Figure 2–4.   Temporomandibular joint injection 30
Figure 2–10.   Injection for trapezius trigger point 37
Figure 2–11.   Injection for splenius capitis and upper cervical muscles 38
Figure 2–14.   Injection of intraspinatus bursitis 43
Figure 4–12.   Injection for impingement syndrome (beneath acromioclavicular joint
                into supraspinatus tendon) 78
Figure 4–13.   Injection for biceps tendinitis 79
Figure 4–20.   Four point injection for frozen shoulder 89
Figure 4–22.   Injection for scapular myofascial trigger points 91
Figure 5–2.   Injection for tennis elbow 103
Figure 6–6.   Injection for DeQuervain's tenosynovitis 124
Figure 6–7.   Injection for trigger thumb 125
Figure 6–8.   Injection site for trigger finger 126
Figure 6–12.   Injection for carpal-tunnel syndrome 130
Figure 7–4.   Injection for chest wall myofascial pain and costosternal junctions. . . 149
Figure 8–17.   Injection for low back trigger points 193
Figure 9–6.   Injection for trochanteric bursitis. 213
Figure 10–7.   Injection site for infrapatellar tendon and fat pad 229
Figure 10–8.   Injection for anserine bursa and medial collateral ligament of knee . . 231
Figure 12–5.   Injection for plantar fasciitis and the painful heel 252
Figure 12–12. Injection for tarsal tunnel syndrome 262

Illustrations for Exercises

Figure 2–3.   Isometric jaw exercises 29
Figure 2–6.   Active-resistance shoulder shrugging 32
*Figure 2–7.   Neck-erector strengthening 33
Figure 2–9.   Method for stretching sternomastoid muscle 36
Figure 2–12.   Flexion cervical traction technique 41
Figure 3–7.   Chest wall stretching 55
Figure 4–14.   Pendulum exercise for shoulder cuff stretch 82
Figure 4–15.   Wand exercise for shoulder capsule 82
Figure 4–16.   Wand exercise for biceps stretch 83

---

*Posture improvement exercise

Figure 4–17. Wall ladder exercise for shoulder capsule 86
Figure 4–18. Wand exercises for frozen shoulder 87
Figure 4–19. Strengthening exercise for infraspinatus and teres minor muscles . . . 88
Figure 4–21. Scapular muscle stretching 90
Figure 4–23. Subscapularis strengthening 92
Figure 4–24. Shoulder capsule stretch 93
Figure 4–25. Passive shoulder capsule stretch 93
Figure 4–26. Passive shoulder stretch in a doorway 94
Figure 5–3.   Extensor forearm stretch (for tennis elbow) 105
Figure 5–4.   Strengthening exercise for forearm muscles (for tennis elbow) 105
Figure 5–5.   Flex or forearm stretch (for golfer's elbow) 106
Figure 5–6.   Biceps stretching exercise 106
Figure 5–7.   Resistance exercise for triceps 106
Figure 6–4.   Resistance extension exercises for the hand 123
Figure 6–13. Exercise for carpal-tunnel syndrome 131
Figure 6–17. Stretching exercise for first carpal metacarpal joint and adjacent
              tendons 135
*Figure 7–10. Extension exercise for the thoracolumbar spine 156
*Figure 8–9.   Abdominal strengthening exercise 188
*Figure 8–10. Pelvic tilt exercise. 188
Figure 8–11. Knee chest flexion exercise 189
Figure 8–12. Knee chest exercise performed from sitting position 189
Figure 8–13. Hamstring stretch exercise 189
Figure 8–14. Trunk stretching exercise. An excellent warm up exercise 190
Figure 8–15. The trapeze gravity exercise 191
Figure 8–16. A passive back extension exercise 193
Figure 9–3.   Hip flexor muscle stretch exercise 211
Figure 9–4.   Iliotibial band stretch exercise 212
Figure 9–8.   Pendulum hip capsule stretch exercise 215
Figure 10–5. Resistance quadriceps exercise 227
Figure 10–6. Quadriceps stretch exercise 227
Figure 10–10. Hamstring and posterior leg muscle stretch 232
Figure 11–1. Exercise for leg cramp 240
Figure 12–10. Mobilizing forefoot and ankle exercise 257

_____

*Posture improvement exercise

Index

Page numbers followed by "f" indicate figures; page numbers followed by "t" indicate tables.

Abdomen
 and chest pain, 143
 musculature effect on back support, 162-163
 strengthening exercises in low back pain, 187, 188f
Abdominal cutaneous nerve entrapment, 200
Accident process, 10-11
Achilles tendon, 247-248
 bursitis, 248
 calcific tendinitis, 248
 corticosteroid injection in, 295
 pump bumps, 249
 rheumatoid nodules at, 249
 rupture, 248
 tight, 247-248
Acrocyanosis, in hand, 134
Acromioclavicular joint pain, 93
Active resistive motion, 64
Acupuncture
 in chronic persistent pain, 288
 in low back pain, 195
Adolescents
 patellofemoral pain syndrome in, 229
 psychogenic leg pain in, 239
Adson test, in thoracic outlet syndrome, 50, 51f
Aerobic exercise, 303
Aging, muscle effects, 18-19
Alexithymia, 281
Amitriptyline
 in chronic pain, 287
 in fibrositis, 274
 in low back pain, 191
 in myofascial pain, 10
 in reflex sympathetic dystrophy, 58
Amytal, in reflex sympathetic dystrophy, 58
Anesthesia, frozen shoulder manipulation under, 87-88
Anesthetics
 agents in current use, 296t
 hazards, 296-297
 injection with steroids, 294. *See also*
        Corticosteroids, injection
 injection without steroid, 294
Ankle, 243-265. *See also* Foot
 adhesive capsulitis, 248-249
 danger signs, 244t
 decision chart for, 263t
 examination, 244-246, 246f
 exercises for, 258t
 joint protection, 245t, 312-313t
 sprain, 246-247
 tendinitis, 247

Anserine bursitis, 230
Anterior interosseous nerve syndrome, 131
Antidepressants, tricyclic. *See* Amitriptyline
Antinuclear antibodies, in Raynaud's disease, 132
Apley grinding maneuver, 222
Arthritis, rheumatoid. *See* Rheumatoid arthritis
Arthrography
 in frozen shoulder, 85
 in knee bursitis, 230
 in low back pain, 184
 of shoulder, 75
Arthroscope, 222
Arthroscopy
 of knee, 222, 224
  complications, 222
  meniscus tear, 224
 in rotator cuff disorders, 71
Autonomic nervous system, in erythermalgia, 134

Back
 abdominal and chest musculature in support of, 162-
        163
 danger signs, 161t
 exercises, 156f
 joint protection, 310t
Back pain
 herniated intervertebral disc causing, 156
 in hypermobility syndrome, 118, 163
 lower, 159-200. *See also* Sciatica
  aggravating factors in, 166-167t, 185-186
  anthropomorphic factors in, 161
  clinical presentation, 164
  in coccygodynia, 199-200
  danger signs in, 161t
  decision chart for, 175t
  differential diagnosis, 185
  history-taking in, 173-174, 174f
  hypermobility syndrome and, 163
  incidence, 159
  in ischial bursitis, 200
  lordotic lumbosacral angle and, 163
  management, 185-194, 197
   comprehensive program, 196-197
   corset, 186-187
   exercises, 187-189, 188-191f, 192t, 193f
   fluorimethane spray, 190
   ice massage, 190
   oral medication, 190-191
   pelvic traction, 186
   resting position, 180f, 186

Back pain, management *(Continued)*
    sitting and sleeping positions, 186
    trigger point injection, 191, 193-194
  manipulation of spine in, 195-196
  mechanical, 164-165
    acute attack, 165
    clinical features, 164-165
  muscle spasm causing, 163-164
  myofascial, 163, 169-171, 170f
    examination in, 176, 178f
    in sacrococcygeal joint, 199
    trigger points in, 170-171, 170f
      injection into, 191, 193-194, 193f
  occupational factors in, 160-161
  osteitis condensans ilii causing, 197-198
  osteitis pubis causing, 198-199
  outcome, 194-197
  pathologic changes in, 162
  pathophysiology, 162-164
  pelvic syndromes, 197-200
  physical examination in, 174, 176-183
    disability determination, 182-183
    gait determination, 180
    in malingering, 180, 182
    Naffziger's test, 180
    nerve root evaluation, 180, 181t
    percussion over vertebrae, 176, 179f
    spine movements, 176, 177f
    straight-leg-raising test, 176, 178, 179f, 180
    trigger point palpation, 176, 178f
  pre-employment status of patients with, 161
  pseudosciatica, 165
  psychological factors in, 160, 171-173
  radiographic and laboratory evaluation, 183-185
  referred, 185
  sciatica, 165, 168-169. *See also* Sciatica
  social and environmental factors related to, 159-160
  surgery in, 196
  work hardening in, 195
  zygapophyseal joint abnormalities in, 162
  in Scheuermann's disease, 150
Back school, 186, 313
Baker's cyst, 231, 232f, 233
  aspiration, 231
  examination, 231, 232f
  management, 233
  rupture, 231, 233
Bed rest, in low back pain, 186
Behavior modification, in chronic persistent pain, 289
Biceps tendon
  impingement syndrome, 66-68, 70, 70f
  rupture, 71
  tendinitis, 66, 68, 70-71, 72f, 73f
    corticosteroid-anesthetic injection in, 76, 78, 79f
    at distal insertion in elbow, 107-108
    etiology, 74
    examination, 65, 69f, 70, 73f
Biofeedback, 304
  in chronic persistent pain, 288-289
  in Raynaud's disease, 133-134
Bite plate, in temporomandibular joint dysfunction
    syndrome, 28, 29f
Bowleg, 235
Bowler's thumb, 124

Breast, proper brassiere to minimize neck pain, 44, 45f
Briquet's syndrome, 281
Bruxism, in temporomandibular joint dysfunction
    syndrome, 27
Bunion, 258-259
Bupivacaine, steroid injection with, 294. *See also*
    Anesthetics
Bursae
  development, 20
  fluid in, 20
  knee, 217, 218f, 229
Bursitis, 4
  at Achilles tendon, 248
  cervicothoracic, 42-43
    injection into, 43, 43f
  common sites, 4
  crystal deposition in, 21
  elbow
    at insertion of triceps, 107
    olecranon, 104, 106-107
  etiology and pathogenesis, 20-21
  heel pain due to, 249
  in hip pain, 212-214
  iliopectineal, 214
  iliopsoas, 214
  intermetatarsal, 254
  ischial, 200
  at knee, 229-231
    anserine, 230
    differential diagnosis, 230
    etiology, 230
    laboratory and radiographic evaluation, 230
    management, 230-231
    outcome, 231
    popliteal, 230. *See also* Baker's cyst
    prepatellar, 230
    septic, 231
  Milwaukee shoulder, 21
  olecranon, 104, 106-107
    aspiration and corticosteroid injection in, 106-107
    differential diagnosis, 106
    etiology, 104
    laboratory and radiographic evaluation, 104, 106
    management, 106-107
    outcome, 107
    septic, 104, 106
  prepatellar, 220, 221f
  septic, 21
  shoulder, 71-73
    loss of motion in, 65
    subacromial, 71-73
    subcoracoid, 72-73
  trochanteric, 213
    corticosteroid injection in, 298t

C2 nerve root irritation, 44
C5 nerve root irritation, 41-42
Calcaneocuboid joint sprain, 251
Calcaneus
  periostitis, 249
  spurs, 249
Calcifications
  of Achilles tendon, 248

in bursitis, 21
knee, 234, 234f
in quadriceps tendon, 225
with rotator cuff tear, 73
in shoulder
    etiology, 74
    radiographic findings, 72f, 75
of supraspinatus, 68, 72f
in tendon, 19
in wrist and hand, 115
Calcitonin, in osteoporosis, 155
Calcium, in osteoporosis therapy, 155
Calcium channel blockers, in Raynaud's disease, 132
Calf muscle rupture, 238
Camptodactyly, 112
Capsulitis, adhesive, 83-88. *See also* Shoulder, frozen
Carotid artery
    palpation causing pain referral, 31, 31f
    styloid process compressing, 32
Carotidynia, 31-32, 31f
Carpal tunnel syndrome
    corticosteroid injection in, 298t
    etiology and pathogenesis, 22-23
    forearm and arm symptoms in, 110
    pathologic findings, 23
    tarsal tunnel syndrome associated with, 261
    and thoracic outlet syndrome, 48-49
    at wrist, 128-131
        clinical features, 128
        diagnosis, 128-129, 128-129f
        etiology, 129-130
        exercises in, 131, 131f
        management, 130-131
        outcome, 131
        surgery in, 131
Causalgia, of upper extremity, 56-59. *See also* Reflex
        sympathetic dystrophy
Cerebral infarction, after chiropractic neck
        manipulation, 38-39
Cervical rib, and thoracic outlet syndrome, 48
Cervical sprain, 34
Cheiroarthropathy, diabetic, 112, 114-115
Chemonucleolysis, in disc herniation, 196
Chest
    corticosteroid injection in, 298t
    exercises for, 147, 147f, 148t
    expansion measurement, 145-146
    musculature effect on back support, 162
    thoracic outlet syndrome, 48-56
Chest pain, 141-156
    abdominal structures causing, 143
    chest wall structures causing, 143
        myofascial syndromes, 143-149
    danger signs, 141t
    decision chart for, 142t
    esophagus causing, 143
    history-taking on, 141-142
    intrathoracic, 141-143, 142t
    in mitral valve prolapse, 142-143
    pleural, 143
    psychogenic, 146-147
    spine disorders causing, 143
    superior structures causing, 141
    in thoracic outlet syndrome, 141
    in Tietze's syndrome, 149-150, 149f

Chest wall
    chest pain from, 143
    exercises in thoracic outlet syndrome, 55, 55f
    joint protection, 148t, 309-310t
    myofascial syndromes, 143-149
        costosternal syndromes, 144-145
        differential diagnosis, 146-147
        etiology, 146
        laboratory and radiographic evaluation, 146
        management, 147-149
        rib-tip syndrome, 145-146
        sternalis syndrome, 145
        tests and maneuvers for, 146
        trigger points, 144f
        xiphoidalgia, 145
Children, tarsal tunnel syndrome in, 261-262
Chiropractic
    in low back pain, 195-196
    neck manipulation causing cerebral infarction, 38-39
Chondrocalcinosis, in hypermobility syndrome, 118
Chymopapain, in disc herniation, 196
Clenched fist syndrome, 119, 121
Clubbing, 114
Coccygodynia, 199-200
Coccyx, joint protection, 311t
Cold exposure, and Raynaud's phenomenon, 131-132
Cold laser, 306
Compartment syndrome
    shin splints distinguished from, 237
    of wrist, 113
Compression syndrome. *See* Nerve entrapment
Contracture, Dupuytren's, 126-127, 127f
Conversion reaction, 275-276, 280-281
Corset, in low back pain, 186-187
Corticosteroids
    epidural injection in low back pain, 196
    injection, 293-299
        agents in current use, 297t
        anesthetic combined with, 294. *See also*
            Anesthetics
        benefit compared to anesthetic alone, 294
        in carpal tunnel syndrome, 130, 130f, 298t
        in chest wall pain, 147-148, 149f
        contraindications, 294-295
        in DeQuervain's tenosynovitis, 123, 124f
        in diabetic cheiroarthropathy, 115
        dose, 297t
        in elbow, 103, 103f, 106-107, 298t
        epidural, 196
        in fascia lata fasciitis, 212, 298t
        in fibrositis, 273
        in frozen shoulder, 86, 89f
        in gluteal muscles, 298t
        hazards, 295-297, 299
        indications, 294
        in infrapatellar fat pad, 228-229, 229f
        in knee, 298t
            in bursitis, 230, 231f
        in low back pain, 191, 193-194, 193f
        in olecranon bursitis, 106-107
        in plantar fascia, 251, 252f, 298t
        in shoulder, 76, 78, 78-79f, 82, 86, 89f, 298t
        in symphysis pubis, 198, 199f
        in tarsal tunnel syndrome, 261, 262f
        in temporomandibular joint, 30, 298t

Corticosteroids, injection (*Continued*)
  in tender point, 273
  in tendon, 295
  in tennis elbow, 103, 103f
  in trapezius, 298t
  in trigger finger, 126, 126f
  in trigger thumb, 124, 125f
  in trochanteric bursitis, 213, 213f, 298t
  in reflex sympathetic dystrophy, 58-59
Costochondral junction
  tender point in, 268t
  Tietze's syndrome, 149-150, 149f
Costochondritis
  chest pain in, 143
  scintigraphy in, 146
  terminology, 145
Costoclavicular maneuver, in thoracic outlet
    syndrome, 50, 52f
Costosternal syndrome, 144-145
Cyclobenzaprine, in low back pain, 190
Cyst
  elbow swelling, 107
  epidermoid, 136

Dawbarn's sign, 70
Dental care, in temporomandibular joint dysfunction
    syndrome, 28, 29f
DeQuervain's tenosynovitis, 21-22f, 121-123
Diabetes mellitus
  cheiroarthropathy in, 112, 114-115
  corticosteroid injection in, 295
  finger contractures in, 112, 114-115
  frozen shoulder in, 84
Diaphragm, irritation causing shoulder pain, 76
Diet, in osteoporosis, 155
Diflunisal, in low back pain, 191
Disability
  definition, 182
  evaluation in low back pain, 182-183
  psychological factors in, 10-12
  soft-tissue rheumatic disorders causing, 2-3
  work-related injury causing, 10
Disc herniation. *See* Intervertebral disc, herniation
DMSO
  in chronic pain, 287
  in rotator cuff disorders, 76
  in tennis elbow, 102-103
Drawer sign
  anterior, 221-222
  posterior, 222
Driving, lower back pain related to, 160, 161
Dupuytren's contracture, 126-127, 127f
  differential diagnosis, 127
  etiology, 126-127
  management, 127

Eagle's syndrome, 32
Elbow, 98-110
  bony landmarks, 98
  bursal and cystic swellings at, 107
  corticosteroid injection in, 298t
  danger signs for, 98t
  decision chart for, 100t
  examination, 98-99

  exercises for, 104t, 105-106f
  golfer's, 99
  history-taking for, 98
  joint protection, 99t, 309t
  muscle components, 98
  nerve entrapment syndromes, 108-110
    carpal tunnel syndrome, 110
    pronator syndrome, 109-110, 109f
    radial tunnel syndrome, 108-109, 109f
    ulnar nerve, 110
  olecranon bursitis, 104, 106-107
    aspiration and corticosteroid injection in, 106-107
    differential diagnosis, 106
    etiology, 104
    laboratory and radiographic evaluation, 104, 106
    management, 106-107
    outcome, 107
    septic, 104, 106
  tennis, 99, 101-104
    associated disorders, 99
    clinical features, 99, 101
    definition, 99
    differential diagnosis, 101
    etiology, 101
    management, 101-103
      DMSO, 102-103
      exercises, 102, 104t, 105f
      friction massage, 103
      steroid-anesthetic injection, 103, 103f
      tennis elbow band, 102, 102f
    pathology, 101
    prognosis, 103-104
Electromyography, in low back pain, 184
Endorphins, and pain perception, 282
Enthesis
  injury at, 20
  neck pain syndrome, 37
  tendinitis at, 19-20. *See also* Tendinitis
Entrapment neuropathy. *See* Nerve entrapment
Eosinophilic fasciitis, 276
Epidermoid cyst, 136
Epidural space, injection of corticosteroids into, 293-294
Episacroiliac lipoma, 171, 172f
  management, 194
Ergonomics, of lower back pain, 159-160
Erichsen's test, 208
Erythermalgia, in hands and feet, 134
Esophagus, chest pain of, 143
Estrogen
  deficiency related to osteoporosis, 152
  in osteoporosis therapy, 155
Exercises. *See also* Physical therapy
  abdomen strengthening, 188f
  active, 302
  active assisted, 302
  adverse effects, 303
  aerobic, 303
  for ankle, 258t
  back, 156f
  in carotidynia, 31-32, 32f, 33f
  in carpal tunnel syndrome, 131, 131f
  for chest, 147, 147f, 148t
  in chronic persistent pain, 288
  for conditioning and fitness, 303-304

contraindications, 304
DeLorme system, 302
for elbow, 104t, 105-106f
evaluation for, 302
in fibrositis, 274
finger extension, 119, 123f
in flatfoot, 257, 257f
for flexibility, 301
for foot, 258t
goals, 301, 302
hamstring strengthening, 226t
for hand and wrist, 122t
hip flexor and quadriceps stretch, 226t, 227f
and immune system, 301
jaw balancing, 40t
knee, 226t
knee-chest, 189f
in leg disorders, 258t
in myofascial pain, 9
in neck myofascial pain, 36f, 38, 40t
in night cramps, 240, 240f
passive, 302, 306-307
pectoral muscle stretching, 147f, 148t
pelvic tilt, 188f
postisometric, 302
during prolonged sitting, 303-304
quadriceps resistant, 225, 227f
quadriceps strengthening, 226t
resistive, 302
in Scheuermann's disease, 152
shoulder
    capsule stretch, 93f
    in frozen shoulder, 80-81t, 85-87, 88f
    passive stretching, 94f
    in rotator cuff disorders, 78-79, 80-81t, 82-83f
    scapula stretching, 90f
straight leg stretching, 190f
strengthening, 302
stretching, 301
in temporomandibular joint dysfunction syndrome, 28, 29f
in tennis elbow, 102, 104t, 105f
in thoracic outlet syndrome, 54-56, 54-55f
for toe, 258t
trapeze, 191f
trunk stretching, 190f
type appropriate for patient, 302-303
Extremities. See Lower extremity; Upper extremity

Fabere test, 207, 208, 211f
Face, pain, 30-34
Facet syndrome, 164-165
Fascia lata
    anatomy, 207
    fasciitis, 212, 213f
        corticosteroid injection in, 298t
Fasciitis
    eosinophilic, 276
    fascia lata, 212, 213f
    myofascial pain related to, 17
Felon, 136
Fibromyalgia, 267. See also Fibrositis
Fibrositis, 267-275
    aching, stiffness and fatigue in, 268-269

added onto systemic disorders, 270
chest pain in, 147
differential diagnosis, 272-273
etiology, 271-272
in hypermobility syndrome, 118
immunologic mechanisms, 271
laboratory tests in, 270, 272
of low back, 169-171
management, 273-274
    drugs, 273-274
    facilitating attitudinal and lifestyle changes, 274
    physical therapy, 274
    steroid-anesthetic injection, 273
osteoarthritis with, 272
outcome, 274-275
pathology of tender points, 271
perfectionistic personality in, 269-270
primary, 270
psychogenic rheumatism distinguished from, 272
radiographic evaluation, 272
reflex phenomena in, 271
rheumatoid arthritis distinguished from, 272-273
secondary, 270-271
sleep disorder in, 269, 272
tender points in, 16, 16t, 267, 268f, 268t, 269
terminology, 268
Finger(s)
    acute blue fingers in women, 134
    clubbing, 114
    contracture, in diabetes mellitus, 112
    examination, 112
    extension exercises, 119, 123f
    hypermobility syndrome, 115-119
    hypothenar hammar syndrome, 134
    in rheumatoid arthritis, 113-114
    thumb disorders, 121-124. See also Thumb
    trigger, 124-126
        etiology, 125
        management, 125-126, 126f
        steroid-anesthetic injection in, 126, 126f
Finkelstein sign, in DeQuervain's tenosynovitis, 121-122, 123f
Flatfoot
    differential diagnosis, 256-257
    etiology, 256
    examination, 245, 256, 256f
    flexible, 255-258
    management, 257
    outcome, 257-258
    radiographic evaluation, 256
    significance, 255-256
Flexibility, 301
Fluoride, in osteoporosis therapy, 155
Fluorimethane spray
    in chest wall pain, 148
    in low back pain, 190
    in scapula myofascial pain, 91
Foot, 243-265. See also Ankle
    danger signs, 244t
    decision chart for, 263t
    examination, 244-246, 246f
    exercises for, 258t
    flatfoot, 255-258
    heel pain, 249-250
    history-taking on, 243-244

Foot *(Continued)*
  importance of shoes, 243, 244f
  joint protection, 245t, 312-313t
  midfoot problems, 251-255
    calcaneocuboid joint sprain, 251
    first tarsometatarsal spur or fibroma, 251
    metatarsalgia, 252-254
    tendinitis of superficial extensor tendons, 251
  nerve entrapment in, 259-262, 264
    common peroneal nerve compression, 264
    Joplin's neuroma, 264
    Morton's neuroma, 264
    occupational disorders, 259-260
    plantar nerve, 264
    tarsal tunnel syndrome, 260-262, 264
  night cramps, 264-265
  plantar fasciitis, 250-251
  tarsal coalition, 247
  toe disorders, 258-259
Footdrop, 264
Forearm. *See* Elbow; Wrist
Fractures, stress, 238, 254-255, 255f
Friction massage, 307, 307f

Gait, in low back pain, 180
Ganglion
  in tuberculous tenosynovitis, 126
  wrist, 135f, 136
Gate control theory, 282-283
Genu recurvatum, 219
Genu valgum, 219, 235
Genu varum, 235
Glomus tumor, in hand, 136
Glossopharyngeal neuralgia, 33-34
Gluteal muscles
  corticosteroid injection in, 298t
  tender point in, 268t
  tendinitis, hip pain in, 207
  Trendelenburg test of, 208
  trigger point in, 170f, 171
Golfer's elbow, 99
Gracilis syndrome, 198-199
Groin pain. *See also* Hip pain
  differential diagnosis, 208
Growing pains, 239

Haglund's disease, 249
Hallux rigidus, 258-259
Hallux valgus, 258
Hammertoe, 259
Hand, 112-136. *See also* Fingers; Wrist
  acrocyanosis, 134
  calcific tendinitis, 115
  camptodactyly, 112
  corticosteroid injection in, 298t
  danger signs in, 114t
  decision chart for, 120t
  dorsal edema after trauma, 128
  Dupuytren's contracture, 126-127, 127f
  erythermalgia, 134
  examination, 112
  exercises for, 122t
  hypermobility syndrome, 115-119
    exercises for, 119, 122t

  joint protection, 121t
  prognosis, 119
  hypothenar hammar syndrome, 134
  infectious tenosynovitis, 126
  interosseous nerve syndrome, 131
  joint protection, 309t
  nerve entrapment disorders, 128-131
  neurovascular disorders, 131-134
  nodules, 134, 135f, 136
  palm disorders, 124-127
  psychophysiologic disorders, 119, 121
    clenched fist, 119, 121
    clenched hand, 119
    writer's cramp, 121
  in scapulocostal syndrome, 89
  systemic diseases involving, 113-115
  thumb disorders, 121-124
  trigger finger, 124-126
  trigger thumb, 123-124
Head and neck, 26-46. *See also* Neck
  anterior neck and face pain, 30-34
    Eagle's syndrome, 32
    myofascial, 32-33
    neuralgia, 33-34
    vascular, 31-32, 31f
  cervical syndrome, 34, 36-40
  danger signs, 26t
  decision chart for, 35t
  exercises for, 40t
  impingement of fifth cervical nerve root, 41-42
  joint protection, 39t, 308t
  muscle contraction headache, 43-44
  occipital neuralgia, 44, 46
  temporomandibular joint dysfunction syndrome, 26-30, 31t
Headache
  history-taking on, 44
  muscle contraction, 43-44
Heel pain, 249-250
  in apophysitis, 250
  black heel, 250
  in bursitis, 249
  in calcaneal periostitis, 249
  heel pad syndrome, 249-250
  piezogenic papules, 250
  pump bumps, 249
  rheumatoid nodules causing, 249
Hemochromatosis, nodules in, 136
Herniated intervertebral disc, 156
Hip. *See also* Hip pain
  examination
    in lower back pain, 180
    movements, 180
  occult fracture in elderly, 208
  snapping, 211-212
Hip pain, 207-216
  bursitis, 212-214
    iliopectineal and iliopsoas, 214
    trochanteric, 213
  danger list, 207t
  decision chart in, 210t
  differential diagnosis, 208, 211
  examination in, 207-208, 209f, 211f
  motion evaluation in, 207, 209f
  myofascial, 211-212

fascia lata fasciitis, 212, 213f
  snapping hip, 211-212
nerve entrapment causing, 214-216
  meralgia paresthetica, 214-215
  obturator nerve, 214
  sciatic pseudoradiculopathy, 215-216
  special maneuvers in, 208
History-taking
  in chest pain, 141-142
  for elbow region, 98
  in foot pain, 243-244
  in headache, 44
  in knee pain, 217-218
  in lower back pain, 173-174, 174f
  in pain, 4-5, 283
  pain drawing, 173, 174f
  PQRST questioning, 44
  in shoulder pain, 62-63, 63t
  in thoracic outlet syndrome, 50, 52
HLA-B27, in low back pain, 184
Hoffa's disease, 227
Hoffman's syndrome, fibrositis distinguished from, 273
Hoffman-Tinel test, 128, 128f
Homan's sign, in Baker's cyst, 233
Hooking maneuver, in rib-tip syndrome, 145, 145f
Hydroxyapatite deposition. *See* Calcifications
Hyoid syndrome, 32
Hyperabduction, in thoracic outlet syndrome, 50, 53f, 53-54
Hypermobility syndrome, 112
  back pain in, 118, 163
  chondrocalcinosis and osteoarthritis in, 118
  diagnostic features, 115, 115t
  etiology, 117, 118t
  fibrositis in, 118
  incidence, 117
  laboratory and radiographic features, 118-119
  management, 119
    exercises, 119, 122t
    joint protection, 121t
  outcome, 119
  in patella disorders, 228
  rib, 145
  in wrist and hand, 115-119
Hypochondriasis, 280
Hypothenar hammar syndrome, 134
Hypothyroidism, fibrositis distinguished from myopathy of, 273

Ice therapy
  in low back pain, 190
  in rotator cuff disorders, 76
  in shin splints, 238
Ilioinguinal pain syndrome, 200
Iliopectineal bursitis, 214
Iliopsoas bursitis, 214
Iliotibial band
  exercise for taut band, 212, 212f
  friction syndrome, 234
  Ober's test for contracture, 208, 211f
  slipping over greater tuberosity causing snap, 211-212
Iliotibial tract, 207
Ilium, osteitis condensans, 197-198

Immune system
  exercise effect on, 301
  and fibrositis, 271
  in frozen shoulder, 85
Impairment, in low back pain, 182-183
Impingement syndrome. *See also* Nerve entrapment
  after osteoporosis-related vertebral fracture, 155
  in shoulder, 66-68, 70f, 71, 71f
    etiology, 74
    management, 82-83
    with spur, 82-83
Infection
  knee septic bursitis, 231
  olecranon septic bursitis, 104, 106
  tenosynovitis in hand, 126
Infraspinatus muscle
  strengthening exercise 80t, 88f
  trigger point, 65, 68f, 90
Injection, 293-299. *See also* Corticosteroids, injection
  benefit of combining steroid with anesthetic, 294
  contraindications, 294-295
  frequency, 299
  hazards, 295-297, 299
  indications, 294
  pitfalls, 299
  technique, 297t, 298t, 299
  vasovagal reaction, 296
Injuries. *See* Trauma
Intervertebral disc
  herniation, 156
    chemonucleolysis with chymopapain in, 196
    diagnosis, 196
    examination in, 176, 178, 179f
    history-taking in, 173
    in runners, 195
    sciatica due to, 168
    surgery for, 196
  lifting influence on pressures at, 162
  position influence on pressures at, 162
Ischial bursitis, 200

Jaw
  balancing exercises, 40t
  exercises in temporomandibular joint dysfunction syndrome, 28, 29f
  temporomandibular joint dysfunction syndrome, 26-30, 31t
Joint protection, 307, 308-313t, 313
Joplin's neuroma, 264

Knee, 217-235. *See also* Knee pain
  arthroscopy, 222, 224
  Baker's cyst, 231, 232f, 233
  bowleg and knockknee, 235
  buckling, 217
  bursae of, 217, 218f, 229
  calcifications, 234, 234f
  congenital abnormalities, 219
  corticosteroid injection in, 298t
  danger signs for, 218t
  drawer test, 221-222
  examination, 218-222
    anterior drawer sign, 221-222

Knee, examination *(Continued)*
  Apley grinding maneuver, 222
  congenital abnormalities, 219
  McMurray sign, 222
  posterior drawer sign, 222
  prepatellar bursitis, 220, 221f
  stress testing, 220-221, 221f
  exercises, 226t
  internal derangements, 217
  joint protection, 219t, 311-312t
  jumper's, 227
  loose bodies, 222
  meniscus tear, arthroscopy in, 224
  movements, 217
  Osgood Schlatter disease, 238-239
  patella disturbances, 225-229. *See also* Patella
        disorders
  plicae, 224, 234-235
  popliteal tendinitis, 233
  prepatellar bursitis, 220, 221f
  quadriceps mechanism derangement, 224
    calcific tendinitis, 225
    disruption, 224
    disuse atrophy, 225
  stress testing, 220-221, 221f
Knee pain. *See also* Knee
  bursitis, 229-231
    anserine, 230
    differential diagnosis, 230
    etiology, 230
    laboratory and radiographic evaluation, 230
    management, 230-231
    outcome, 231
    popliteal, 230
    prepatellar, 230
    septic, 231
  cinema sign, 225
  decision chart in, 223t
  differential diagnosis, 220t
  etiology, 217-218, 220t
  history-taking in, 217-218
  in iliotibial band friction syndrome, 234
  infrapatellar fat pad hypertrophy, 227
  in infrapatellar tendinitis, 227
  overuse syndromes, 218
  patellofemoral pain syndrome, 225-227
  in Pellegrini Stieda syndrome, 233-234, 234f
  in runners, 234
  in traumatic prepatellar neuralgia, 227
Knee-chest exercises, in low back pain, 187, 189f
Knockknee, 219, 235
Knuckle pads, 127
Kyphosis, juvenile, 150-152

Laboratory tests
  in fibrositis, 270, 272
  in frozen shoulder, 85
  in low back pain, 184
  in olecranon bursitis, 104, 106
  in Raynaud's phenomenon, 132
  in rotator cuff disorders, 75
Lasegue's sign, 176, 179f
Laser therapy, 306
Lateral femoral cutaneous nerve entrapment, 214-215,
        214f

Leg, 237-242
  calf muscle rupture, 238
  exercises for, 258t
  growing pains, 239
  night cramps, 239-240
  night starts, 241
  postphlebitic syndrome, 240-241
  pseudorheumatoid nodules, 241-242
  psychogenic pain, 239
  reflex sympathetic dystrophy involving, 241
  restless, 241
  shin splints, 237-238
Leg length discrepancy, 208
Levator syndrome, 199-200
Lidocaine. *See also* Anesthetics
  steroid injection with, 293-299. *See also*
        Corticosteroids, injection
Ligaments, ankle sprains, 246-247
Lipoma, episacroiliac, 171, 172f, 194
Loose body, in knee, 222
Looser zones, 153, 154f
Lordosis
  low back pain related to, 163
  positions for reducing, 186
Low back loser, 172
Low back pain, 159-200. *See also* Back pain, lower
Lower extremity
  ankle and foot, 243-265. See also Ankle; Foot
  knee, 217-235. *See also* Knee
  leg, 237-242. *See also* Leg
  leg length discrepancy, 208
  overuse pain syndromes, 237-238
Lumbosacral strain, 164-165

Magnetic resonance imaging, in soft-tissue rheumatic
        disorders, 7
Malingering
  evaluation in low back pain, 180, 182
  patient characteristics, 11
Manipulation of spine, in low back pain, 195-196
March fracture, 254-255
Marfanoid syndrome, 118
McArdle's syndrome, fibrositis distinguished from, 273
McMurray sign, 222
Median nerve compression
  by pronator muscle, 109-110, 109f
  at wrist, 128-131
Meralgia paresthetica, 214-215
Metacarpals, trapezium-first metacarpal sprain, 113
Metacarpophalangeal collateral ligament stability test,
        112, 113f
Metatarsal(s)
  first tarsometatarsal spur or fibroma, 251
  stress fractures, 254-255, 255f
Metatarsal bar, 253, 253f
Metatarsalgia, 252-254
  etiology, 252-253
  management, 253-254
  shoe modifications for, 253, 260t
  of traumatic origin, 254
Midfoot, 251-255
Milkman's lines, 153, 154f
Milwaukee shoulder, 21, 73
Mitral valve prolapse, 142-143

Morton's neuroma, 264
Moseley test, 73
Motor vehicles, lower back pain related to driving, 160, 161
Movement
  active, 64
  active resistive, 64
  passive, 64
Muscle(s)
  aging effect on, 18-19
  of elbow, 98
  myofascial pain, 3-4. See also Myofascial pain
  pathologic studies in fibrositis, 271
Muscle contraction headache, 43-44
Muscle relaxants
  in chronic pain, 287
  in low back pain, 190-191
Musculocutaneous nerve compression, 109
Musculoskeletal disorders. See Soft-tissue rheumatic disorders
Myelography, in low back pain, 184
Myofascial pain, 3-4
  age factor in, 18-19
  biochemical factors in, 18
  in chest wall, 143-149
    costosternal syndromes, 144-145
    differential diagnosis, 146-147
    etiology, 146
    laboratory and radiographic evaluation, 146
    management, 147-149
    rib-tip syndrome, 145-146
    sternalis syndrome, 145
    tests and maneuvers for, 146
    trigger points, 144f, 146
    xiphoidalgia, 145
  diagnosis, 5-6
  etiology and pathogenesis, 16-19
  excluding systemic disease, 7-8
  exercises in, 302
  in face, 32-33
  in hip, 211-212
    fascia lata fasciitis, 212, 213f
    snapping hip, 211-212
  ischemia related to, 17
  lower back, 163, 169-171, 170f. See also Back pain, lower
    examination in, 176, 178f
    in sacrococcygeal joint, 199
    trigger points in, 170-171, 170f, 191, 193-194, 193f
  management, 7-10, 8f
    giving prognosis, 10
    pain relief, 9-10
    providing explanation to patient, 8-9
    recognizing and eliminating aggravating factors, 8, 9f
    self-help exercises, 9
  mobilization effect on, 18
  myopathy distinguished from, 18
  in neck, 34, 36-40
  in scapula, 89-92
  in shoulder, 65, 67f, 68f
  steroid-anesthetic injections in, 293
  in structural disorders, 18

in temporomandibular joint dysfunction syndrome, 27-28
  trauma role, 17-18
  trigger points in, 16-17, 16t, 284-285f
Myoglobin, leakage after muscle injury causing tender point, 17
Myopathy, myofascial pain distinguished from, 18
Myositis ossificans, in elbow tendinitis, 108

Naffziger's test, 180
Naproxen, in low back pain, 191
Neck. See also Head and neck
  cervical syndrome, 34, 36-40
    myofascial pain, 34, 36-40
    sprain, 34
    tension neck syndrome, 34
  cervicothoracic bursitis, 42-43
    injection into, 43, 43f
  chiropractic manipulation causing cerebral infarction, 38-39
  exercises for, 40t
  impingement of fifth cervical nerve root, 41-42
  isometric exercise in thoracic outlet syndrome, 54-55, 55f
  joint protection, 308t
  myofascial pain, 34, 36-40
    differential diagnosis, 37
    exercises in, 36f, 38, 40t
    management, 37-39, 40t
    outcome, 39-40
    radiographic findings, 36
  pain in
    aggravating factors, 39t
    cervical traction in, 39, 40, 41t
    differential diagnosis, 37
    enthesiopathies, 37
    myofascial, 34, 36-40
    pendulous breasts causing, 44, 45f
    preventive practices, 39t
    psychogenic, 37
  ponderous-purse disease, 1-2
  sprain, 34
  tension syndrome, 34
  torticollis, 40-41
Needles, in injection, 298t, 299
Nerve block, in reflex sympathetic dystrophy, 57, 58
Nerve conduction studies
  in carpal tunnel syndrome, 128
  in low back pain, 184
  in thoracic outlet syndrome, 51, 52
Nerve entrapment, 4
  abdominal cutaneous nerve, 200
  carpal tunnel syndrome, 22
  common sites, 22
  at elbow, 108-110
    carpal tunnel syndrome, 110
    pronator syndrome, 109-110, 109f
    radial tunnel syndrome, 108-109, 109f
    ulnar nerve entrapment, 110
  etiology and pathogenesis, 21-23
  in foot, 259-262, 264
    common peroneal nerve compression, 264
    Joplin's neuroma, 264
    Morton's neuroma, 264

Nerve entrapment, in foot *(Continued)*
    occupational disorders, 259-260
    plantar nerve, 264
    tarsal tunnel syndrome, 260-262, 264
  in hip pain, 214-216
    meralgia paresthetica, 214-215
    obturator nerve, 214
    sciatic pseudoradiculopathy, 215-216
  ilioinguinal pain syndrome, 200
  obturator nerve, 200
  in Pancoast's syndrome, 59
  in reflex sympathetic dystrophy, 56-59
  sciatica, 165, 168-169. *See also* Sciatica
  spinal stenosis, 169
  thoracic outlet syndrome, 48-56, 49f
  in wrist and hand, 128-131
    anterior interosseous nerve syndrome, 131
    carpal tunnel syndrome, 128-131
    ulner nerve, 131
Nerve roots
  irritation at fifth cervical nerve root, 41-42
  in low back pain, 180, 181t
Nervous system, in pain perception, 282-283
Neuralgia
  glossopharyngeal, 33-34
  in neck and face, 33-34
  occipital, 44, 46
  superior laryngeal, 34
  traumatic prepatellar, 227
Neuroma
  Joplin's, 264
  Morton's, 264
Neurovascular disorders, of wrist and hand, 131-134
Nifedipine, in Raynaud's disease, 132
Night cramps, 239-240, 264-265
Night starts, 241
Nodule
  at Achilles tendon, 249
  in hand, 134, 135f, 136
  pseudorheumatoid, 241-242
Nonsteroidal anti-inflammatory drugs
  in low back pain, 191
  in myofascial pain, 9-10

Ober's test, 208, 211f
Obturator nerve entrapment, 200, 214
Occipital neuralgia, 44, 46
Occupational disorders, 10
  carpal tunnel syndrome, 128-129
  foot nerve entrapment disorders, 259-260
  low back pain, 160-161
  neck pain, 37-38
  thoracic outlet syndrome, 54
  trigger finger, 125
Occupational therapy, 301, 307, 308-313t, 313
  back school, 313
  joint protection, 308-313t, 313
  work hardening, 195, 313
Olecranon bursitis, 104, 106-107. *See also* Elbow,
    olecranon bursitis
Omohyoid muscle, trigger point in, 33
Osgood Schlatter disease, 238-239
Osteitis condensans ilii, 197-198
Osteitis pubis, 198-199, 198f

Osteoarthritis
  with fibrositis, 272
  in hypermobility syndrome, 118
  in low back pain, 183
Osteomalacia, osteoporosis distinguished from, 152
Osteopenia, of thoracic spine, 152-155
Osteoporosis
  differential diagnosis, 154
  estrogen deficiency causing, 152
  etiology, 152-153
  management, 154-155
  radiographic findings, 153, 153f, 154f
  of thoracic spine, 152-155, 153f
  types, 152

Pain
  chronic persistent, 280-290
    classification, 280
    differential diagnosis, 283
    examination in, 283, 284-285f, 286
    history-taking in, 283
    laser therapy, 306
    management, 286-287
      acupuncture, 288
      behavior modification, 289
      biofeedback, 288-289
      drug therapy, 287-288
      exercise, 288
      facilitating communication, 286
      pain clinic, 289
      transcutaneous electrical nerve stimulation, 288
    personality characteristics in, 281-282
    psychogenic, 280-281
    transcutaneous nerve stimulation in, 305
  endorphins role in, 282
  gate control theory, 282-283
  history-taking for, 4-5
    drawing picture, 173, 174f
  myofascial, 3-4. *See also* Myofascial pain
  outcome measures of management, 12
  perception, 280, 282-283
  physical examination in, 5, 5f
  psychogenic, 280-281
  quantification, 286
  threshold for, 280
Pain amplification syndromes, 267
Pain centers, 196
  in chronic persistent pain, 289
Pain drawing, 173, 174f
Pain-prone disorder, 172, 281
Pancoast's syndrome, 59
Parathyroid hormone, in osteoporosis, 152
Patella, grasshopper eye, 226-227
Patella disorders, 225-229
  chondromalacia, 225
  etiology, 227-228
  Hoffa's disease, 227
  laboratory and radiographic findings, 228
  management, 228-229
  outcome, 229
  patellofemoral pain syndrome, 225-227
  surgery in, 229
  tendinitis, 227
  traumatic prepatellar neuralgia, 227
Patellofemoral pain syndrome, 225-227
  in adolescents, 229
Patrick's test, 207, 208, 211f

Pectoral muscle stretching, 147f, 148t
Pellegrini Stieda syndrome, 233-234, 234f
Pelvic tilt, in low back pain, 187, 188f
Pelvis, pain syndromes, 197-200. *See also* Hip pain
   coccygodynia, 199-200
   ischial bursitis, 200
   osteitis condensans ilii, 197-198
   osteitis pubis, 198-199, 198f
Pendulum exercises, in rotator cuff disorders, 79, 80t, 82f
Periostitis, calcaneal, 249
Perkin's test, 226
Peroneal nerve
   common, compression, 264
   deep, entrapment in anterior tarsal tunnel, 262, 264
Peroneal tendon dislocation, 247
Personality
   in chronic persistent pain, 281-282
   in fibrositis, 269-270
Pes planus. *See* Flatfoot
Phalen maneuver, 128, 129f
Physical examination
   of Baker's cyst, 231, 232f
   in bicipital tendinitis, 70, 73f
   chest expansion measurement, 145-146
   of elbow, 98-99
   of flatfoot, 256, 256f
   of foot and ankle, 244-246, 246f
   in hip pain, 207-208, 209f, 211f
   of knee, 218-222
   in low back pain, 174, 176-183
   in pain disorders, 5, 5f, 283, 284-285f
   in patellofemoral pain syndrome, 225-227
   of rotator cuff, 70-71
   of runners, 255
   of shoulder, 63-65, 64-69f
      in adhesive capsulitis, 84
      in rotator cuff disorders, 68, 70-71, 73f
   in supraspinatus tendinitis, 68, 70, 73f
   in tarsal tunnel syndrome, 260
   in temporomandibular joint dysfunction syndrome, 26, 27f
   for tender points, 268t
   in thoracic outlet syndrome, 49-50, 51-53f
   of wrist and hand, 112
Physical fitness
   adjuncts to exercise program, 304-306
   exercises for, 303-304
   passive exercises, 306-307
Physical therapy, 301-307. *See also* Exercises
   evaluation for exercise plan, 302
   in fibrositis, 274
   in frozen shoulder, 80-81t, 85-87, 88f
   goals, 301, 302
   in low back pain, 187-189
   in myofascial pain, 9
   in reflex sympathetic dystrophy, 58
   in scapula myofascial pain, 91
   in tennis elbow, 102-103, 104t, 105f
   in trigger finger, 125-126
   type of exercise, 302-303
Piezogenic papules, 250
Pillow, in neck myofascial pain, 39
Piriformis muscle, spasm causing sciatica, 168
Pisiform-triquetral joint sprain, 113

Plantar fascia
   corticosteroid injection in, 251, 252f, 298t
   examination, 246, 246f
Plantar fasciitis, 250-251
   corticosteroid-anesthetic injection in, 251, 252f, 298t
   etiology, 250
   examination, 250
   management, 251
   outcome, 251
   radiographic evaluation, 250-251
Plantar nerve entrapment, 264
Plastizote insole, 253-254, 254f
Pleural pain, 143
Plica syndrome, 234-235
Polymyalgia rheumatica, 276
Popliteal cyst, 231, 232f, 233
Popliteal tendinitis, 233
Posterior interosseous nerve compression, 109
Posterior joint syndrome, 164-165
Postphlebitic syndrome, 240-241
Posture
   and intervertebral disc pressures, 162
   in low back pain, 186
PQRST questioning, 44
Prepatellar bursitis, 220, 221f
Procaine, steroid injection with, 293-299. *See also* Corticosteroids, injection
Pronator muscles, 98
Pronator syndrome, 109-110, 109f
Prostaglandins, in myofascial pain, 18
Pseudofracture, in osteoporosis, 153, 154f
Pseudorheumatoid nodules, 241-242
Psychogenic pain disorder, 280-281
   alexithymia, 281
   Briquet's syndrome, 281
   conversion disorder, 280-281
   of hand, 119, 121
   hypochondriasis, 280
   lower back pain, 171-173
      tests for, 180, 182
   pain prone disorder, 281
   somatoform disorders, 280
Psychogenic rheumatism, 275-276
   clinical features, 275
   conversion reaction in, 275-276
   fibrositis distinguished from, 272
Psychological factors
   in chronic persistent pain, 281-282
   in disability, 10-12
   in lower back pain, 160
Pubis, osteitis, 198-199, 198f
Pump bumps, 249
Pyridoxine
   in carpal tunnel syndrome, 130-131
   deficiency, in wrist disorders, 129-130

Quadratus lumborum, trigger point in, 171
Quadriceps muscle
   calcific tendinitis, 225
   disruption, 224
   disuse atrophy, 225
   strengthening exercises, 226t
      in patella disorders, 228

Questionnaires, as outcome measure in soft-tissue rheumatic disorders, 12
Quinine, in night cramps, 240

Radial nerve, compression at lateral epicondyle, 108-109, 109f
Radial tunnel syndrome, 108-109, 109f
  clinical features, 108
  etiology, 108-109
Radiography
  in cervical syndrome, 36
  in fibrositis, 272
  in frozen shoulder, 85
  in low back pain, 183-184
  in osteoporosis, 153, 153f, 154f
  in Pancoast's syndrome, 59
  in patella disorders, 228
  in plantar fasciitis, 250-251
  in rotator cuff disorders, 75
  in Scheuermann's disease, 151, 151f
  of shoulder, 72f, 75
  in temporomandibular joint dysfunction syndrome, 28
Radionuclide imaging
  in low back pain, 184
  in reflex sympathetic dystrophy, 57
  in soft-tissue rheumatic disorders, 6-7
Raynaud's disease, 132-134
  diagnosis, 132
  treatment, 132-134
Raynaud's phenomenon, 131-134
  etiology, 131-132
Rectum, massage of lateral walls in coccygodynea, 199
Reflex sympathetic dystrophy, 56-59
  clinical features, 56
  differential diagnosis, 57
  etiology, 56-57
  laboratory and radiographic examination in, 57
  leg pain in, 241
  management, 57-58
  outcome, 58-59
  pathology, 57
  physical findings, 56
  stages, 56
  thoracic outlet syndrome with, 58
Rehabilitation, 301-313. See also Exercises; Occupational therapy; Physical therapy
Reserpine, in Raynaud's disease, 132
Restless leg syndrome, 241
Rheumatic disorders, soft-tissue. See Soft-tissue rheumatic disorders
Rheumatism, psychogenic. See Psychogenic rheumatism
Rheumatoid arthritis
  fibrositis distinguished from, 272-273
  hand in, 113-114
  nodules in, 134, 135f
  temporomandibular joint pain in, 30
Rheumatoid nodules, at Achilles tendon, 249
Rib
  cervical, and thoracic outlet syndrome, 48
  hypermobility, 145
  slipping, 145
Rib-tip syndrome, 145-146

Rotator cuff disorders, 65-68, 70-76, 78-83
  arthroscopy in, 71
  bursitis, 71-73
  cuff tear arthropathy, 75
  differential diagnosis, 75-76
  etiology, 74-75
  examination for, 70-71, 73f
  impingement syndrome, 66-68, 70f, 71, 71f
  laboratory and radiographic findings, 75
  management, 76-83
    corticosteroid-anesthetic injections, 76, 78, 78-79f, 82
    DMSO, 76
    exercises, 78-79, 80-81t, 82-83f
    ice, 76
  tears, 73-74
  tendinitis, 66, 68, 70-71, 72f, 73f
  types, 66
Running
  disc herniation due to, 195
  examination of lower extremity, 255
  foot injuries in, 255
  knee pain associated with, 234
  overuse leg pain syndromes in, 237
  shin splints due to, 237-238
  shoes for, 243, 244f
  stress fractures due to, 238

Sacroileitis, Erichsen's test for, 208
Scapula
  disorders at, 88-92
    fluorimethane spray in, 91
    physical therapy for, 91
    scapulocostal syndrome, 89, 90f
    snapping scapula, 88-89
  normal motion, 88
  snapping, 88-89
  stretching exercise, 90f
  trigger point at, 89, 90, 91f
  winging of, 92
Scapulocostal syndrome, 89, 90f
Scheuermann's disease, 150-152
  back pain in, 150
  differential diagnosis, 151-152
  etiology, 150-151
  exercises in, 152
  radiographic features, 151, 151f
  management, 152
Schober test, 176
Sciatic pseudoradiculopathy, 215-216
Sciatica, 165, 168-169. See also Back pain, lower
  back-pocket, 1-2
  clinical features, 165
  etiology, 159, 168-169
  examination, 176, 178, 179f, 180
  facet joints as source of pain in, 165, 168
  history-taking in, 173
  non-disc causes, 168t
Scleroderma, Raynaud's phenomenon in, 132
Semi-Fowler position, 180f, 186
Serratus anterior muscle, paralysis or paresis, 92
Shin splints, 237-238
  clinical features, 237
  compartment syndrome distinguished from, 237

differential diagnosis, 237-238
etiology, 237
management, 238
outcome, 238
Shoe(s)
  common modifications in foot disorders, 260t
  in flatfoot, 257
  and foot disorders, 243, 244f
  in metatarsalgia, 253-254, 254f, 260t
  plastizote insole, 253-254, 254f
  for running, 243, 244f
  in toe disorders, 258-259, 260t
Shoulder, 62-94
  abduction, 64, 64f
  abduction contracture, 94
  acromioclavicular joint pain, 93
  adhesive capsulitis, 83-88. See also Shoulder, frozen
  aggravating factors in pain, 62-63, 63t, 75
  arthrogram, 75
  bicipital tendinitis, 66, 68, 70-71, 72f, 73f
  bursitis, 71-73
    pathogenesis, 21
  calcification
    etiology, 74
    radiographic findings, 72f, 75
  capsule stretch exercises, 81t, 93f
  corticosteroid injection in, 298t
  danger signs for, 62t
  decision chart for problems in, 77t
  differential diagnosis of pain, 69f, 75-76
  droopy, 48
  etiology of soft tissue disturbances, 74-75
  examination, 63-65, 64-69f
    in adhesive capsulitis, 84
    in rotator cuff disorders, 68, 70-71, 73f
  exercises
    in frozen shoulder, 80-81t, 85-87, 86f, 88f
    in rotator cuff disorders, 78-79, 80-81t, 82-83f
    in thoracic outlet syndrome, 54, 54f
  extension, 64
  frozen, 83-88
    corticosteroid injection in, 86, 89f
    definition, 83-84
    diabetes mellitus related to, 84
    differential diagnosis, 85
    etiology, 84-85
    exercises for, 80-81t, 85-87, 86f, 88f
    immunologic disorder in, 85
    laboratory and radiographic studies in, 85
    management, 85-86
    manipulation under anesthesia, 87-88
    outcome, 86-88
    pathology, 84-85
    physical examination, 84
    after rotator cuff tear, 83
    symptoms, 84
  history-taking for, 62-63, 63t
  impingement sign, 67
  impingement syndrome, 66-68, 70f, 71, 71f
    management, 82-83
    with spur, 82-83
  joint protection, 308-309t
  Milwaukee, 21, 73
  motions of, 64, 64-66f
    limitation, 64-65

myofascial pain, trigger points in, 65, 67f, 68f
neurologic disorders causing pain, 69f
painful arc syndrome, 65
ponderous-purse disease, 1-2
radiography, 72f, 75
referred pain to, 69f, 76
rotation, 64, 65-66f
rotator cuff disorders, 65-68, 70-76, 78-83
  bursitis, 71-73
  impingement syndrome, 66-68, 70f, 71f
  outcome, 83
  tears, 73-74
  tendinitis, 66, 68, 70-71, 72f, 73f
  types, 66
scapular region disorders, 88-92
  myofascial pain, 89-92
  scapulocostal syndrome, 89, 90f
  snapping scapula, 88-89
soft tissue enlargement, 93-94
systemic disease involving, 62
winging of scapula, 92
Shoulder-hand syndrome, 56-59. See also Reflex
    sympathetic dystrophy
Sitting, proper position in low back pain, 186
Sleep disorder, in fibrositis, 269, 272
Soft tissue, injections into, 293-299. See also
    Corticosteroids, injection; Injection
Soft tissue incompetence, 163
Soft-tissue rheumatic disorders
  classification, 3t
  clinical features, 6, 6t
  diagnostic techniques in, 6-7
  etiology and pathogenesis, 16-23
  generalized, 267-276
    danger signs, 273t
    eosinophilic fasciitis, 276
    fibrositis syndrome, 267-275. See also Fibrositis
    polymyalgia rheumatica, 276
    psychogenic rheumatism, 275-276
  helpful hints in diagnosis and management, 6
  history-taking in, 4-5
  impact on society, 2-3
  myofascial pain, 3-4
  neurovascular entrapment, 4
  outcome measures, 12
  overview of diagnosis and treatment, 1-12
  physical examination in, 5, 5f
  structural disorders, 4
  tendinitis and bursitis, 4. See also Bursitis;
      Tendinitis
Somatoform disorders, 275
  pain in, 280
Spinal stenosis, 169
  with bilateral neurological impairment, 44, 46
  clinical features, 169
  history-taking in, 173-174
Spine. See also Back; Back pain; Intervertebral disc,
      herniation
  anatomy, 162
  C2 nerve root irritation, 44
  cervicothoracic bursitis, 42-43
    injection into, 43, 43f
  examination, 174, 176-183
  impingement of fifth cervical nerve root, 41-42
  intervertebral disc pressures related to position, 162

Spine (*Continued*)
  movements of, 176, 177f
  pathologic changes in, 162
  radiography in low back pain, 183-185
  Scheuermann's disease, 150-152
  thoracic, 150-156
    and chest pain, 143
    herniated intervertebral disc, 156
    kyphosis of Scheuermann's disease, 150-152
    osteoporosis and osteomalacia, 152-155
Spondyloarthritis, HLA-B27 in, 184
Sports, structural disorders in, 4
Spur, in low back pain, 183
Spurling maneuver, 41, 42f
  in thoracic outlet syndrome, 50
Stanozolol, in Raynaud's disease, 133
Stellate ganglion block, in reflex sympathetic
        dystrophy, 58
Sternalis syndrome, 145
Sternocleidomastoid, trigger point in, 32-33, 34, 36
Straight leg stretching, 190f
Straight-leg-raising test, 176, 178, 179f, 180
  reversed, 178, 180
Stress, hand disorders related to, 119, 121
Stress fractures, 238
Stroke, after chiropractic neck manipulation, 38-39
Structural disorders, 4
  myofascial pain in, 18
Subscapularis muscle, strengthening exercise 80t, 92f
Substance P, in pain perception, 282
Superior laryngeal neuralgia, 34
Supraspinatus muscle
  impingement syndrome, 66-68, 70f
  strengthening exercise 80t
  tender point in, 268t
  tendinitis, 68, 72f
    corticosteroid-anesthetic injection in, 76, 78, 78f
    examination 68, 70, 73f
  trigger point, 90
Surfer's nodules, 241
Surgery
  in carpal tunnel syndrome, 131
  in herniated intervertebral disc, 156
  in low back pain, 196
  in patella disorders, 229
  in plantar fasciitis, 251
  in thoracic outlet syndrome, 56
Swelling, evaluation, 5
Sympathectomy, in reflex sympathetic dystrophy, 58

Tarsal coalition, 247
Tarsal tunnel syndrome, 260-262, 264
  anatomical considerations, 260, 261f
  anterior, 262, 264
  in children, 261-262
  clinical features, 260
  corticosteroid-anesthetic injection in, 261, 262f, 298t
  diagnosis, 261
  etiology, 260-261
  examination, 260
Tarsometatarsal spur, 251
Temporal artery biopsy, in polymyalgia rheumatica,
        276
Temporomandibular joint dysfunction syndrome, 26-30
  bruxism in, 27

clinical presentation, 26
corticosteroid injection in, 298t
differential diagnosis, 28
etiology, 27-28
laboratory and radiographic evaluation, 28
management, 28, 29f, 30, 31t
outcome, 28, 30
physical examination in, 26, 27f
in rheumatoid arthritis, 30
Tender point(s)
  etiology and pathogenesis, 17, 271-272
  examination for, 268t
  in fibrositis, 267, 268f, 268t, 269
  injections in shoulder pain, 78
  in myofascial pain, 3-4
  pathologic findings in, 16, 17, 271
  trigger point distinguished from, 16, 16t
Tendinitis, 4
  of Achilles tendon, 248
  ankle, 247
  bicipital, 66, 68, 70-71, 73f
    corticosteroid-anesthetic injection in, 76, 78, 79f
    etiology, 74
    examination for, 65, 69f
  calcific, 19
  elbow
    distal insertion of biceps, 107-108
    at triceps insertion on olecranon, 107
  etiology and pathogenesis, 19-20
  of foot superficial extensor tendons, 251
  friction massage in, 307, 307f
  infrapatellar, 227
  overuse causing, 20
  pathology, 20, 21-23f
  popliteal, 233
  quadriceps, 225
  rotator cuff, 66, 68, 70-71, 72f, 73f
    corticosteroid injection in, 76, 78-79f
    exercises in, 78-79, 80-81t, 82-83f
  supraspinatus, 68, 72f
    corticosteroid-anesthetic injection in, 76, 78, 78f
  in systemic disorders, 19
  triceps, 89
  triggering in, 4, 19, 23f
  in wrist, 115
Tendon(s)
  Achilles. *See* Achilles tendon
  corticosteroid injection in, 295
  crystal deposition in, 19
  giant cell tumor of sheath, 134, 136
  impingement between bone or ligaments, 19
  pathogenesis of injury, 20
  peroneal dislocation, 247
  posterior tibial rupture, 238
Tendon sheath, 19
Tennis
  elbow disorder related to, 99, 101-104. *See also*
        Elbow, tennis
  shoulder pain related to, 63
Tennis elbow band, 102, 102f
Tenosynovitis
  DeQuervain's, 121-123
    corticosteroid-anesthetic injection in, 123, 124f
    diagnosis, 121-122, 123f
    management, 123

in fingers, rheumatic diseases causing, 114
of flexor carpi radialis tendon sheath, 124
infectious, in hand, 126
overuse, 20
of wrist, 112-113
TENS. *See* Transcutaneous electric nerve stimulation
Teres minor muscle, strengthening exercise, 80t, 88f
Thermography, in soft-tissue rheumatic disorders, 7
Thigh, 207-216. *See also* Hip pain
Thomas heel, in flatfoot, 257
Thompson test, 248
Thoracic outlet syndrome, 48-56
  carpal tunnel syndrome in, 48-49
  chest pain in, 141
  danger signs, 54t
  diagnostic workup, 52
  differential diagnosis, 52-53
  etiology, 48-49
  exercises in, 54-56, 54-55f
  history-taking in, 50, 52
  management, 53-56
  nerve conduction velocity in, 51, 52
  outcome, 56
  pathophysiology, 48, 49f
  physical examination in, 49-50, 51-53f
  reflex sympathetic dystrophy with, 58
  surgery in, 56
  vascular studies in, 51-52
Thorax. *See* Chest; Chest pain
Thrombophlebitis, Baker's cyst distinguished from, 233
Thumb, 121-124
  bowler's, 124
  DeQuervain's tenosynovitis, 121-123
  examination, 112
  trigger, 123-124
    steroid-local anesthetic injection in, 124, 125f
Tibial nerve, posterior, entrapment, 260-262
Tietze's syndrome, 149-150, 149f
Tinel test, in radial tunnel syndrome, 108
Toes, 258-259
  bunion, 258
  examination, 245-246
  exercises for, 258t
  hallux rigidus, 258-259
  hallux valgus, 258
  hammertoe, 259
Tomography, computed
  in low back pain, 184
  in soft-tissue rheumatic disorders, 7
Tonsil, trigger point in, 32
Torticollis, 41
Tourniquet test, 108
Traction
  cervical
    in impingement of fifth cervical nerve root, 42
    in neck pain, 39, 40, 41f
  pelvic, in low back pain, 186
Transcutaneous electric nerve stimulation (TENS), 305
  in chronic persistent pain, 288
  equipment for, 304-306f
  in low back pain, 195
  in reflex sympathetic dystrophy, 58
Trapeze exercise, 191f
Trapezium, first-metacarpal sprain, 113

Trapezius
  corticosteroid injection in, 298t
  tender point in, 268t
  trigger point in, 31, 32, 34, 36f, 90
    injection, 38, 38f
Trauma
  myofascial pain due to, 17-18
  psychology of, 10-12
  work-related, 10
Trendelenburg test, 208
Triceps tendinitis, 89
Trigger point(s), 284f
  in chest wall myofascial syndromes, 144f, 146
  corticosteroid-anesthetic injection in, 298t
    in reflex sympathetic dystrophy, 58
    in shoulder pain, 78
  in infraspinatus, 65, 68f
  in low back pain, 170-171, 170f, 176, 178f
    injection into, 191, 193-194, 193f
  in myofascial pain, 3-4
  in neck myofascial pain, 34, 36, 36f
  in omohyoid muscle, 33
  pathologic findings in, 16-17
  at scapula, 89, 90, 91f
  in scapulocostal syndrome, 89
  secondary, 3
  in shoulder pain, 65, 67f, 68f
  in sternalis syndrome, 144f, 145
  in sternocleidomastoid, 32-33, 34, 36
  tender point distinguished from, 16, 16t
  in thoracic outlet syndrome, 54
  in tonsillar crypt, 32
  in trapezius and posterior neck muscles, 31, 32, 34, 36f
    injection, 38, 38f
  zones of reference, 285f
Trigger thumb, 23f, 123-124
Triggering, in tendinitis, 4, 19, 23f
Triquetral joint-pisiform sprain, 113
Trochanteric bursitis, 213
  corticosteroid injection in, 298t
Trunk stretching, 190f
Tuberculosis, tenosynovitis of wrist and hand, 126

Ulna, laxity of distal portion, 113, 114f
Ulnar nerve entrapment
  at elbow, 110
  at wrist, 131
Ultrasonography, of rotator cuff, 75
Upper extremity. *See also* Elbow; Hand; Shoulder; Wrist
  intermittent obstruction of neurovascular bundle of, 48-56
  in Pancoast's syndrome, 59
  reflex sympathetic dystrophy, 56-59
  shoulder, 62-94. *See also* Shoulder

Vasovagal reaction, after injection, 296
Verapamil, in Raynaud's disease, 132
Vibration testing, in neck pain, 41
Vitamin D, in osteoporosis, 155

Wand exercises
  in frozen shoulder, 85, 88f
  in rotator cuff disorders, 79, 80t, 82f, 83f
Whiplash, 34
Winter's heel, 249
Work hardening, 195, 313
Work-related injury, 10
  psychological factors in, 10-12
Wrist, 112-136. *See also* Hand
  calcific tendinitis, 115
  carpal tunnel syndrome, 128-131
  compartment syndrome, 113
  danger signs in, 114t
  decision chart for, 120t
  examination, 112
  exercises for, 122t
  extensor strengthening, 119
  ganglion, 135f, 136
  hypermobility syndrome, 115-119
    distal ulna, 113, 114f
    exercises for, 119, 122t

prognosis, 119
joint protection, 121t, 309t
nerve entrapment disorders, 128-131
neurovascular disorders, 131-134
pisiform-triquetral joint sprain, 113
systemic diseases involving, 113-115
tenosynovitis, 112-113
trapezium-first metacarpal sprain, 113
Writer's cramp, 121
Wryneck, 40-41

Xiphoidalgia, 145
  epigastric tenderness of gastrointestinal disease
    distinguished from, 146

Yergason's sign, 70, 73f

Zygapophyseal joint, abnormalities in back pain, 162